"'If you would have a lovely garden, you should lead a lovely life,' an anonymous Shaker extolled. An herb garden—the herbal life—is a pathway to both. Going down that path together with a teacher inspired by decades of experience is what Juliet Blankespoor delivers in *The Healing Garden*. Practical, entertaining, and gorgeous, the book imbues love of plants, love of beauty, and love of life. In stunning detail, Juliet proffers homage to over 140 medicinal herbs (among them aromatic plants, fungi, trees, and wildflowers), their traditions, cultivation, and properties. Dozens of recipes prove that your food should be your medicine. Nearly 400 of Juliet's elegant photographs reflect the heart of each herb and provide visual detail along each step to enjoying herbs for life. *The Healing Garden* is a once-in-a-generation herbal for the 21st century."

—Steven Foster, herbalist, photographer, and co-author of *Peterson Field Guide to Herbs and Medicinal Plants*

"*The Healing Garden* contains all the encouragement and guidance I need as a new homesteader learning to grow my own herbs. The gorgeous photography and Juliet's personal plant stories makes me feel as if she is taking me under her wing and giving me a first-hand tour of her wondrous gardens. Juliet honors all lineage of plant tenders and calls us to experience the plants as our allies. The plant profiles and recipes in the book give me clear step-by-step inspiration for kitchen tinkering with herbal remedies and nourishing goodies. This book is something I will pass along to my children!"

—Mimi Hernandez, herbalist, RH(AHG), and Executive Director of the American Herbalists Guild

"A book with tremendous heart poured into every page. Juliet brings your hands into the soil from the start and makes herbalism accessible and pleasurable as she guides you from garden to kitchen to apothecary with her wisdom and passion for all things herbalism."

—Bevin Clare, herbalist, nutritionist, professor, Board Chair of the American Herbalists Guild, and author of *Spice Apothecary: Blending and Using Common Spices for Everyday Health*

"Juliet Blankespoor offers gardeners and authentic approach to growing relationships with plants, and cultivating a personal practice of herbalism that is dynamic and deeply rooted. With stunning photography and lyrical narrative, readers are transported to Juliet's own luscious garden to find inspiration and wisdom. As a teacher, this is the textbook I have dreamed of sharing with my students for decades. As a gardener, I can't wait to dig deeper into my backyard practice with new levels of confidence and inspiration."

—Emily Ruff, founder of the Florida School of Holistic Living and Director of Sage Mountain Botanical Sanctuary

"Juliet's approach to teaching herb cultivation as a gateway to crafting medicine embodies the importance of reciprocity with the plant world. *The Healing Garden* is a step-by-step guide on nourishing a personal relationship with medicinal plants that can be applied at any scale—from windowsill to farmstead. Juliet's tenderness and personal stories highlight how growing our own herbs and making our own medicine can heal ourselves, our communities, and the planet."

—Susan Leopold, PhD, Executive Director of United Plant Savers

"Even if you lack a green thumb (or land, for that matter), *The Healing Garden* will show you how to cultivate medicinal herbs and transform them into a powerful home apothecary. The recipes are as creative and enticing as the beauty of the book itself. The writing is as clear and concise as it is poetic. From seed to medicine to wellness, Juliet's masterpiece just might be the only herbal book you'll ever need."

—John Gallagher, co-founder of LearningHerbs and creator of HerbMentor

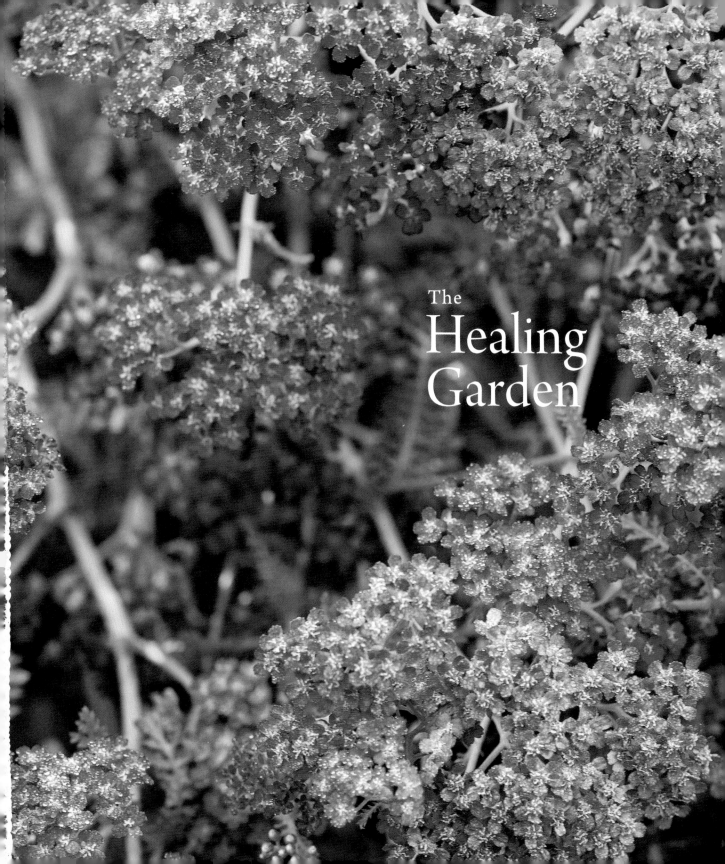

# The Healing Garden

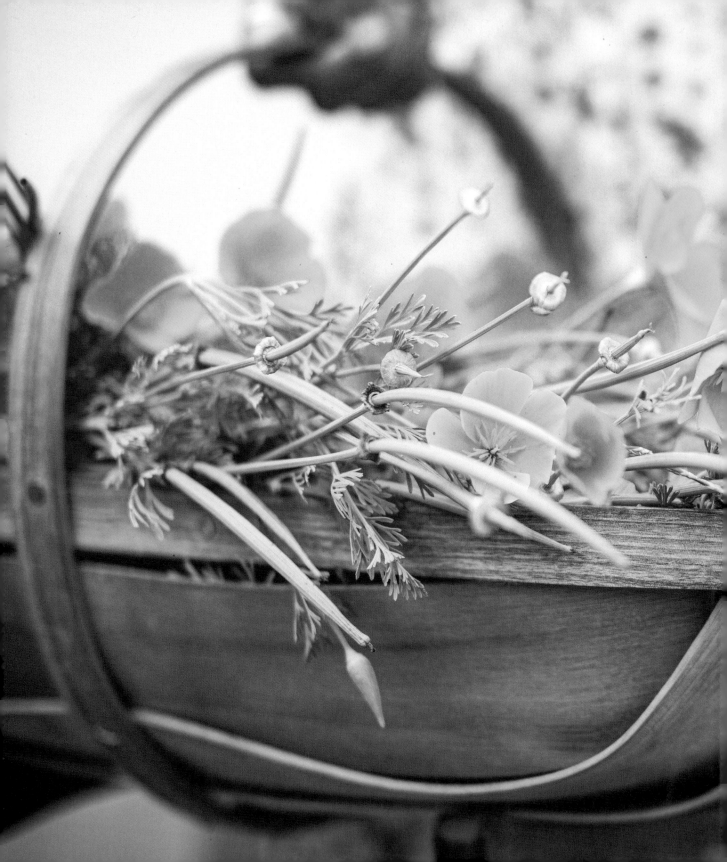

# The Healing Garden

## Cultivating & Handcrafting Herbal Remedies

Juliet Blankespoor

FOUNDER OF THE CHESTNUT SCHOOL OF HERBAL MEDICINE

HARVEST
*An Imprint of* WILLIAM MORROW

Boston  New York  2022

## The Healing Garden Gateway: Herb Gardening Mini-Course and Online Resources

*This book includes an online portal, or gateway, to free resources including video tutorials on growing herbs and making medicine, resources, printable seeding charts, and additional recipes. So many resources wouldn't fit in these pages or were better suited to the virtual sphere, so I created an online compendium for you. You'll also find regional profiles, written by the country's leading herb gardening experts, which explore the best herbs to grow in each climate or bioregion. You'll get lifetime access to the portal when you sign up for this free resource at the HealingGardenGateway.com.*

This book presents, among other things, the research and ideas of its author. It is not intended to be a substitute for consultation with a professional healthcare practitioner. Consult with your healthcare practitioner before starting any diet or other medical regimen, including herbal medicine. Make certain of your identification before harvesting or ingesting any plant. The publisher and the author disclaim responsibility for any adverse effects resulting directly or indirectly from information contained in this book.

THE HEALING GARDEN. Text and photography copyright © 2022 by Juliet Blankespoor.

All rights reserved. No part of this book may be used or reproduced in any manner whatsoever without written permission except in the case of brief quotations embodied in critical articles and reviews. For information, address HarperCollins Publishers, 195 Broadway, New York, NY 10007.

www.harpercollins.com

Book design by Jan Derevjanik

Library of Congress Cataloging-in-Publication Data has been applied for.
ISBN 978-0-358-31338-0 (hbk)
ISBN 978-0-358-27894-8 (ebook)

Printed in Italy

24 RTLO 10 9 8 7 6 5

## CREDITS

page 8: photograph by Asia Suler

page 65: From "Making Family" in *Earth Medicine* by Jamie Sams. Copyright © 1994 by Jamie Sams. Used by permission of HarperCollins Publishers.

page 72: photograph © Cathyrose Melloan/Alamy Stock Photo

page 119: "Silently a flower blooms" by Zenkei Shibayama from *Life Prayers* by Elizabeth Roberts and Elias Amidon. Copyright © 1996 by Elizabeth Roberts and Elias Amidon. Used by permission of HarperCollins Publishers.

page 129: "Spring Team Poem" by Keewaydinoquay Peschel. Used by permission.

page 193: From *Meditations with Hildegard of Bingen*, edited by Gabriele Uhlein. Published by Inner Traditions International and Bear & Company, © 1983. All rights reserved. http://www.Innertraditions.com. Reprinted with permission of publisher.

page 210: photograph © blickwinkel/Alamy Stock Photo; photograph © elakazal/Shutterstock

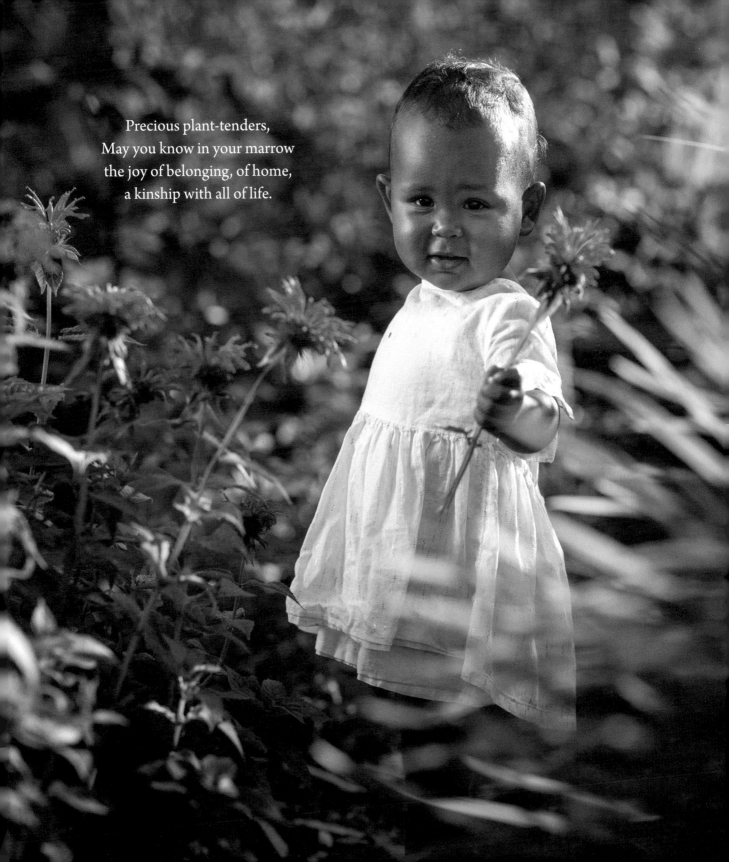

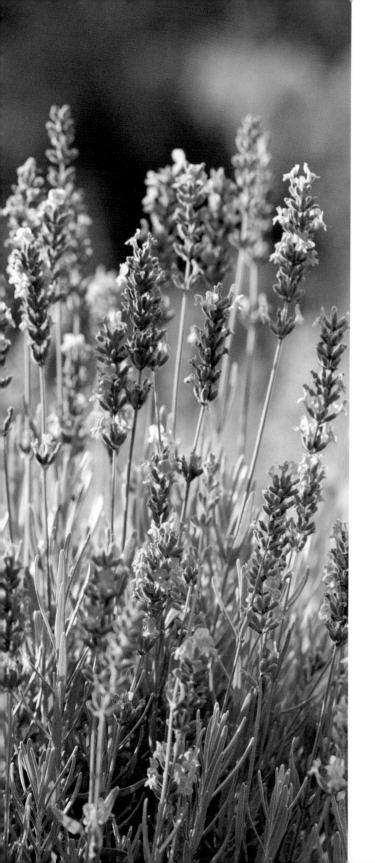

# Contents

INTRODUCTION 1

PART ONE
## Cultivating Medicine

CHAPTER ONE
**Planning Your Dream Herbal Landscape** 12

CHAPTER TWO
**The Nitty-Gritty on Soil** 44

CHAPTER THREE
**Holistic Solutions for Plant Diseases & Problematic Insects** 64

CHAPTER FOUR
**Growing Medicinal Herbs in Containers** 76

CHAPTER FIVE
**Plant Propagation** 84

PART TWO
# Making Medicine

CHAPTER SIX
Harvesting & Drying Herbs   118

CHAPTER SEVEN
Preparing Botanical Medicine & Healing Food   128

PART THREE
# Botanical Medicine

CHAPTER EIGHT
Foundations in Herbalism:
Herbal Action Terms, Energetics & Safety   192

CHAPTER NINE
Herbal Profiles & Recipes   202

Anise hyssop (*Agastache foeniculum*)   209
Ashwagandha (*Withania somnifera*)   213
Basil (*Ocimum basilicum*)   217
Bee balm (*Monarda* spp.)   223
Black cohosh (*Actaea racemosa*)   229
Calendula (*Calendula officinalis*)   235
Chickweed (*Stellaria media*)   247
Dandelion (*Taraxacum officinale*)   257
Echinacea (*Echinacea purpurea*)   267
Elderberry (*Sambucus canadensis*)   271

Elecampane (*Inula helenium*)   277
Goldenrod (*Solidago* spp.)   281
Goldenseal (*Hydrastis canadensis*)   287
Gotu kola (*Centella asiatica*)   293
Hibiscus (*Hibiscus sabdariffa*)   299
Lavender (*Lavandula angustifolia*)   311
Lemon balm (*Melissa officinalis*)   319
Meadowsweet (*Filipendula ulmaria*)   323
Milky oats (*Avena sativa*)   329
Mint (*Mentha* spp.)   335
Motherwort (*Leonurus cardiaca*)   341
Passionflower (*Passiflora incarnata*)   345
Prickly pear (*Opuntia* spp.)   351
Rose (*Rosa* spp.)   359
Skullcap (*Scutellaria lateriflora*)   367
Spilanthes (*Acmella oleracea*)   371
Stinging nettles (*Urtica dioica*)   377
Tulsi (*Ocimum tenuiflorum*)   387
Valerian (*Valeriana officinalis*)   393
Vervain (*Verbena* spp.)   397
Violet (*Viola sororia* and select species)   401
Yarrow (*Achillea millefolium*)   413

ACKNOWLEDGMENTS   418

REFERENCES   422

HERBAL RESOURCES   426

COMMON TO SCIENTIFIC NAME INDEX   428

INDEX   432

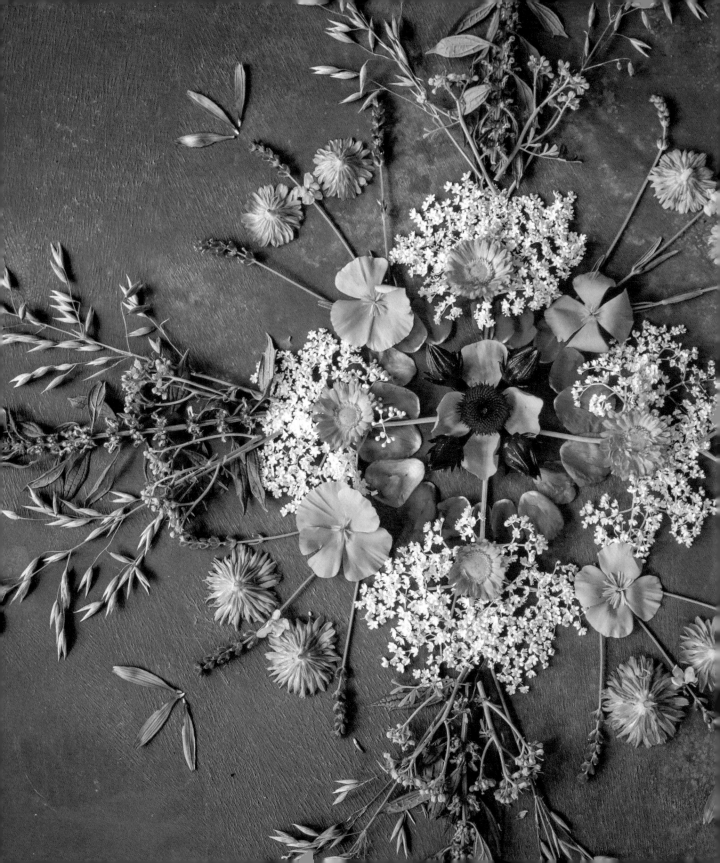

# Introduction

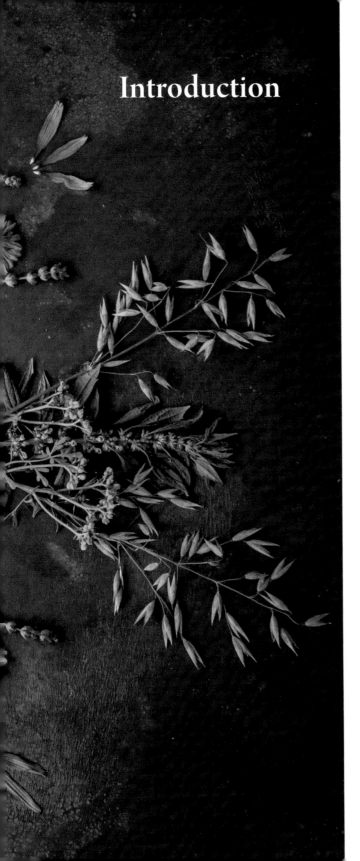

Gardening is medicine for our spirit, mind, and body. When we grow a garden that is in tune with the elements and the earth's ebbs and flows, we're cultivating more than meets the eye. We are, in essence, cultivating medicine. Medicine travels in many guises: it can take the form of connection—to our bodies, to the earth, to the healing plants. This rootedness is potent, a remedy for our times. Herb gardening is profoundly empowering: by nurturing a plant from seed to harvest and ultimately into a healing remedy, we're practicing ancient skills that all our ancestors once knew. Of course, we're also growing medicine in the literal sense. Herbs are the most ancient form of medicine and their usefulness persists into modern life. Medicine abounds, underfoot and towering above—healing plants range from lowly "weeds" to shrubs and trees. No matter where you live, there is an abundance of botanical medicine you can easily grow in your garden. Herbal medicine provides us with a natural and safe way to address everyday health challenges and minor upsets, along with plenty of tools for promoting vitality and overall wellness—it truly shines as preventative medicine.

Preparing homemade remedies from organic, homegrown herbs is one way we can tread more lightly on the earth. By that token, we're cultivating medicine for the earth as well as for ourselves. Our gardens beckon us outdoors and keep us moving, two vital foundations of happiness and wellness. Herbalism also provides a framework for gaining intimacy with our bodies and with wellness. When we grow and harvest our own medicine, the remedy is full spectrum—it contains the intangible and unquantifiable medicine of kinship.

*Being naturalized to place means to live as if this is the land that feeds you, as if these are the streams from which you drink, that build your body and fill your spirit.... To become naturalized is to live as if your children's future matters, to take care of the land as if our lives and the lives of all our relatives depend on it. Because they do.*

*~Robin Wall Kimmerer, Braiding Sweetgrass: Indigenous Wisdom, Scientific Knowledge and the Teachings of Plants*

# Cultivating a Relationship with Healing Plants

In our modern era, it's easy to feel profoundly disconnected not only from nature but also from our ancestors, sustenance, and medicine. The antidote to this cultural chasm is a *connection to place*. This connection is a web with pulsing threads fastening you to your neighbors, garden, medicine, ancestors, and heritage, which in turn resurrects a sense of belonging—a deep knowing that you have a rightful place in the world. Imagine yourself as a bright patch of cloth sewn into a vibrant quilt that stretches far into the past and deep into the future.

Befriending living plants keeps me close to my roots, literally and figuratively. When I want to know more about a plant, I bring it into the garden. From there, we slowly begin the dance of plant–human reciprocity, a friendship of sorts, born of companionable silence throughout the seasons. We become acquainted as I weed around the plant's roots, pick insects from its leaves, and share water with it during dry spells. This communion ultimately brings me to a deep-seated and intimate knowledge of the medicine itself.

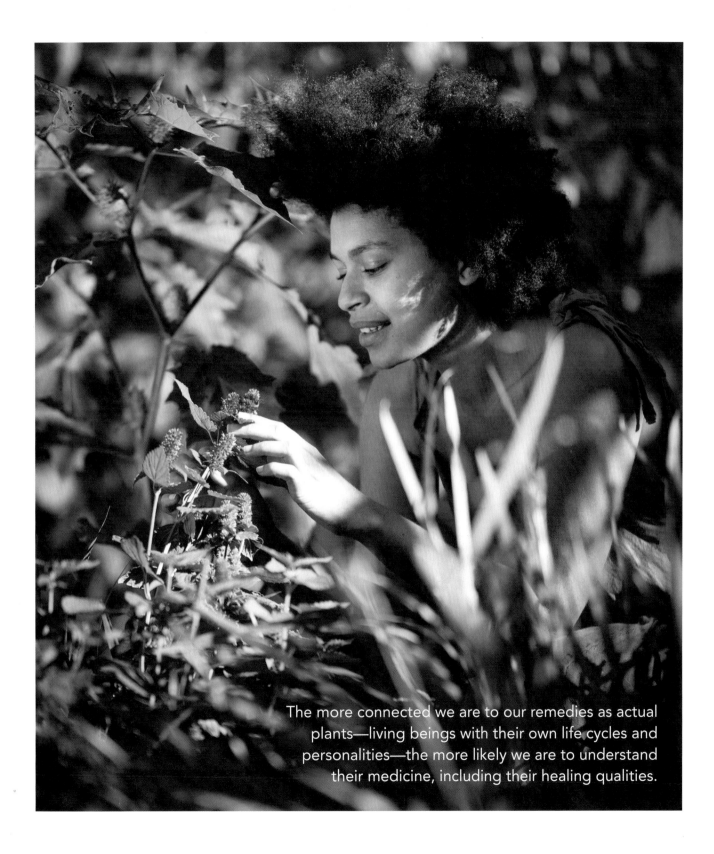

The more connected we are to our remedies as actual plants—living beings with their own life cycles and personalities—the more likely we are to understand their medicine, including their healing qualities.

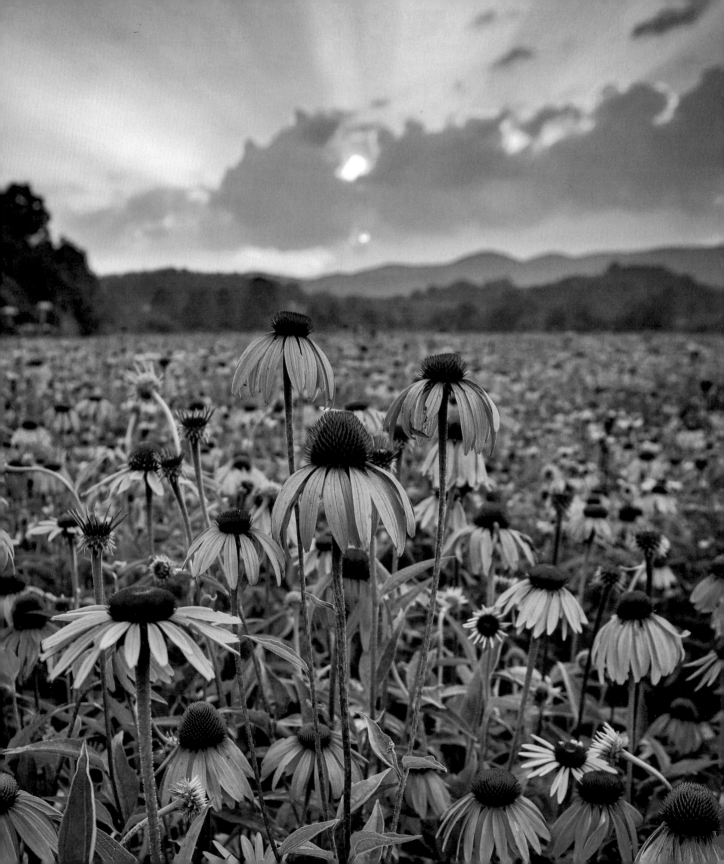

# Medicine for the Earth

An increasing number of people in industrialized nations are using medicinal herbs for their health and well-being. Nearly one-third of Americans use medicinal herbs, and the World Health Organization estimates that 80 percent of people worldwide continue to rely on herbs as their primary form of health care. According to a 2017 study published in the American Botanical Council's peer-reviewed journal *HerbalGram*, consumer spending on herbal dietary supplements in the United States has surpassed $8 billion annually. Most of that medicine is being grown overseas, often in countries with appalling labor and agricultural practices. Just as locally grown food is key to long-term sustainability, so is locally grown medicine. By organically growing your own herbs and preparing medicine at home, you're reducing fossil fuel use by cutting out transportation and packaging. As long as you're vigilant about plant identification and cleanliness in medicine making, homegrown medicine also ensures that you have the correct herb and that your medicine hasn't been adulterated or contaminated, issues that sometimes occur with commercially sourced herbs.

# My Dance with the Plants

My infatuation with herbal medicine started with college botany classes. Stamens, stigmas, and anthers were my first dates in what would become a lifelong love affair with plants. Today, I plan my vacations around botanical gardens, and I keep random pieces of colorful bark in my pocket in case I need an icebreaker in an awkward social situation. Three decades into this journey as a plant–human matchmaker, I've owned just about every type of herbal business you can imagine: an herbal nursery, a medicinal products business, a clinical practice, and now an online herbal school specializing in bioregional, hands-on herbalism.

But I wasn't always so inclined. As a child, I was an introverted bookworm who loved the solitude and magical freedom of the woods but had zero interest in plants. I was very close to my grandpa Joe (Joachim Naphtali Simon), an eccentric intellectual who was a vegetable gardener and a naturalist. On his own initiative, grandpa Joe labeled all the trees—with their common and scientific names—that grew on the path that led home from our school so all the kids could learn them. My Dutch dad—also an avid gardener—and my grandpa both tried to rope me into gardening, to no avail.

Field of purple coneflower (*Echinacea purpurea*) growing at Gaia Herbs' organic herb farm

Lucky for me, the seeds they planted sprouted when I left home and first learned about the environmental crisis, organic gardening, and plant medicine. I suddenly wanted to learn everything I could about plants. My conversion resulted in complete botanical bewitchment. I built my first garden—a monumental flop on all counts but one that nonetheless filled me with pride and joy. This burgeoning love of plants was my saving grace: my passion for herbs blossomed at a low point in my life, when I was consumed with self-doubt and felt lost. My kinship with plants fills me with connection, purpose, and belonging. I hope that I can share some of that beauty with you in the pages of this book.

Lest you think my journey was all about the plants, let me assure you it also included the *people* who taught me about the plants. For starters, my botany professor at the University of Florida, Dr. Terry Lucansky, encouraged me to pursue a career in science and showed me the magic of microscopic plant anatomy. Under his tutelage, I went on to earn my botany degree in the early 1990s. Meanwhile, I picked up the few herbal books I could find at the local bookstore (this was three decades ago—there was no internet and very few herbal teachers or authors) and started learning about growing and gathering herbs. I'd learn about a plant in a botany class and, recognizing the scientific name from one of my herbal books, I'd furiously ride my bike home to devour everything I could find about the herb in those tattered pages.

One day, in my native plant identification class, my professor introduced me to the herb bayberry. In my after-school research, I learned the root bark was the medicinal part of the plant. *Root bark*? I had no idea roots even had bark! So, I pulled out a shovel and dug up the plant's roots to see for myself. I experimented with decoctions of the bark whenever my friends got the sniffles or had a sore throat. In this fashion, I was able to learn how to make medicine and harvest plants (I had proper identification on my side from my university botany studies—*safety first, friends, always!*).

After years of self-study, I finally found a real, live herbalist: 7Song became my first plant medicine teacher. At the time, he ran an off-the-grid herbal school out of his tiny cabin in Ithaca, New York. I felt a natural affinity to his hands-on approach to herbal medicine, which focused on using local, abundant plants. (Plus, he has a wicked sense of humor and an encyclopedic plant brain.) I went on to study clinical herbalism with James Snow in California, and then, after a brief fling with seaweed on Orcas Island in Washington State, I sat at the feet of the late Michael Moore (the herbalist, not the filmmaker) in Bisbee, Arizona. Michael was a central player in the resurgence of herbalism among white healers in the 1970s and 1980s (many Black and Indigenous communities never stopped using herbs and thus didn't experience a "resurgence" because they had intact lineages and living knowledge). He passed on in 2009, but his legacy lives on in his irreverently hilarious and informative books on Western herbs.

Michael learned about the traditional uses of Southwestern plants from Indigenous and Latinx village healers, whose practice centers on local remedies. He also extensively studied the works of the Eclectics, an influential group of herbal physicians in North America who flourished in the late 19th and early 20th centuries. The Eclectic *materia medica* (study of each herb's therapeutic uses) is rooted in the knowledge of European herbalists—both studied and folkloric—and Indigenous and Black healers from North America. Much of the information

---

My former home and herb gardens, which also housed my herbal nursery, all on an acre and a half

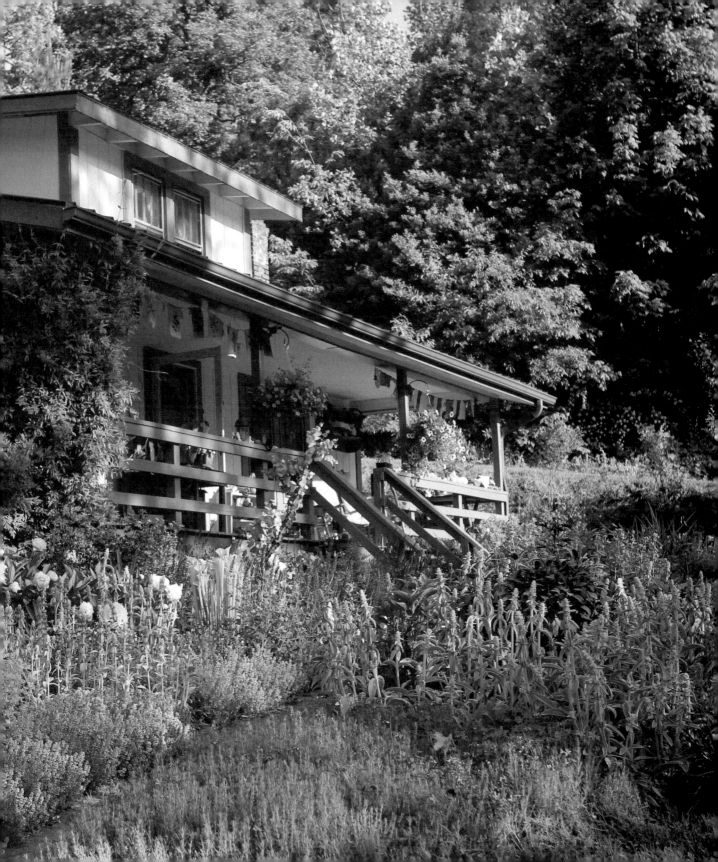

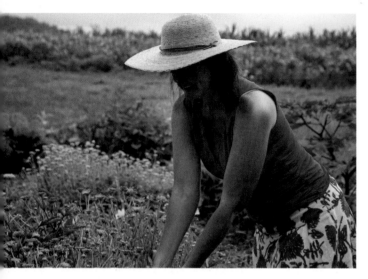

Me, picking calendula in my herb garden; photo by Asia Suler

contained in the earliest herbal books—primarily written by white men—has extensive roots in the traditional knowledge of Black, Indigenous, and white folk healers, often women.

This book is a convergence of my life as an herbalist: the knowledge I learned from my teachers and the experience I gained through my herbal endeavors is infused into these pages. I started my herbal journey as a medicine maker and owned an herbal products line, featuring homegrown and sustainably wildcrafted herbs, for close to a decade. My love for medicine making and healing food is woven into the pages of Chapter Seven, Preparing Botanical Medicine and Healing Food. My next project was the Chestnut Herb Nursery, an organic medicinal plant nursery. Every spring we grew tens of thousands of herb babies, which taught me about plant propagation and controlling plant diseases and problem insects. We painstakingly recorded all of our nursery statistics—successes and failures—which informed the technical propagation data I've included in Chapter Five, Plant Propagation. Finally, I founded the Chestnut School of Herbal Medicine in 2007 and spent a decade teaching all-outdoor herbal programs that focused on bioregional herbalism. Now the school is entirely online, with thousands of students from around the globe. Around the same time that I formed the school, I acquired my first camera and learned to use computers (I didn't want much to do with technology in those early years). I started writing and photographing for my blog *Castanea* and for herbal publications; these creative pursuits lit the fire for this book.

Shortly after Michael Moore died, I had a dream in which my apprentices and I took some of his old musty herbal books (Michael collected historical herbals), tore the faded pages free from the failing binding, and placed them into the fresh soil of a newly dug garden bed. My dream-self knew the pages would nourish the herbs we would plant in the garden, and then I would teach about those herbs to my students. And so the lineage lives on in your gardens and medicine cabinets.

> SAFETY NOTE: *Read over the Herbal Safety information in Chapter Eight and in the Precautions section of each herbal profile before you gather any herbs or ingest a new botanical. You need to be more than 100 percent positive of your identification before gathering an herb, even if you planted it, because there are deadly poisonous plants out there. To that end, read about plant identification and poisonous plants on page 199.*

# How This Book Will Grow You

This book is your gateway to a lush herbal garden and a pantry full of homegrown herbal remedies and concoctions. You'll learn how to grow herbs from seeds, cuttings, or root divisions and how to nurture plants through the seasons, right up to harvest. You'll learn how each botanical can be harvested and brought into the kitchen and medicine cabinet. With 75 pages devoted to medicine making and 82 herbal recipes, *The Healing Garden* is part "grow" and part "make." The recipes range from culinary to medicinal, including teas, tinctures, syrups, poultices, salts, pestos, and more. You'll find household first aid remedies for life's minor upsets—sunburns, bug bites, scrapes, rashes, cuts, and muscle aches. And you'll encounter recipes for botanical remedies to address common ailments like colds, sinus congestion, allergies, sore throat, coughs, insomnia, and more. There are tonic medicines—teas, vinegars, and broth—for fostering overall resilience and vitality. The culinary recipes include tasty infused vinegars and oils; herbal cocktails and mocktails; and herbal twists on familiar dishes and sauces, like lemon balm pesto and nettles pâté. Through growing these botanicals, I know you'll make lifelong herb friends and that your life will be richer, your health more vibrant, and your gardens more spectacular.

I wrote this book for aspiring and community herbalists who want to grow their own medicine in their garden or even on the porch or patio. It's equally helpful for the home vegetable gardener who wants to branch out to herbs and for homesteaders and permaculturists striving for greater self-sufficiency. Even skillful herbalists will find value in these pages, which are sown with seeding charts, propagation techniques, and sumptuous recipes. The gardening information and herbal profiles apply to most temperate gardens throughout North America, Europe, Japan, and the less tropical regions of Australia and New Zealand.

You'll come away with an intimate knowledge of more than 30 medicinal herbs, having learned exactly how to grow and harvest each one.

If you're new to gardening or don't feel like you have a "green thumb," take heart—you can learn to grow herbs! Gardening is a skill that anyone can pick up. Start small and visit your garden daily so your herbal charges are on your radar. You'll make mistakes, but these will only serve to make you a more skillful gardener. You'll be rewarded with the sweetest bounty: empowerment, plant friendships, a beautiful garden, greater health, and a cabinet full of potent medicine.

Elderflower (*Sambucus nigra* var. *canadensis*)

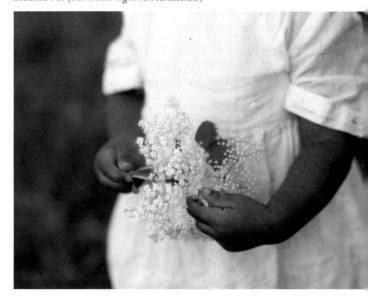

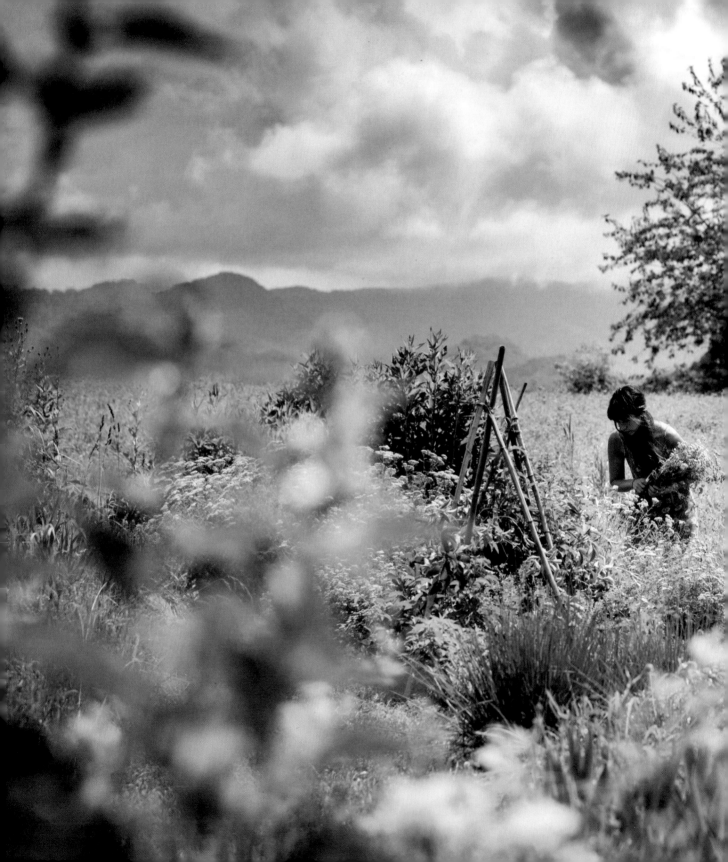

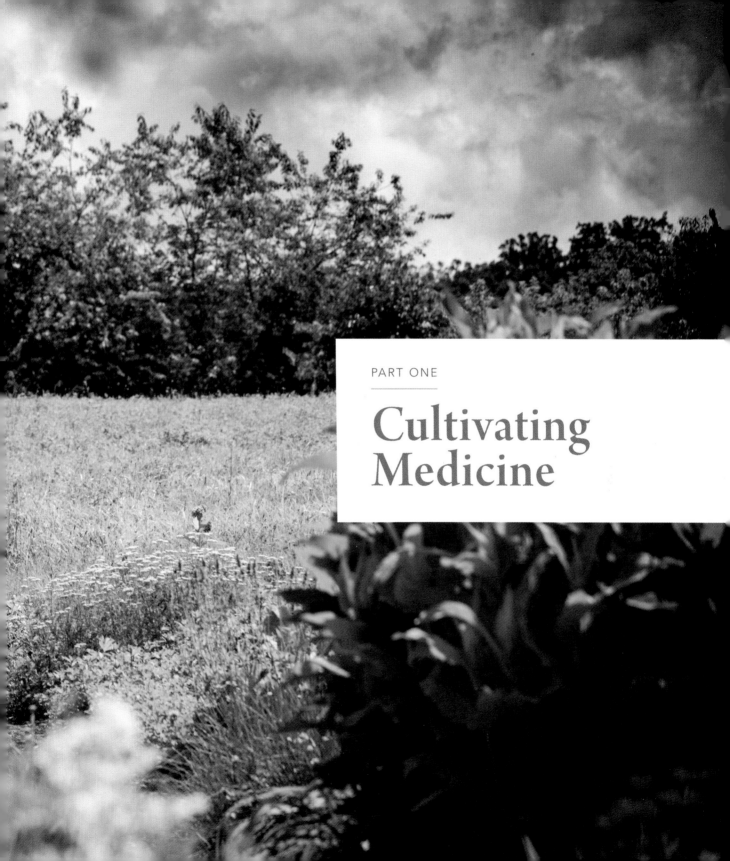

PART ONE

# Cultivating Medicine

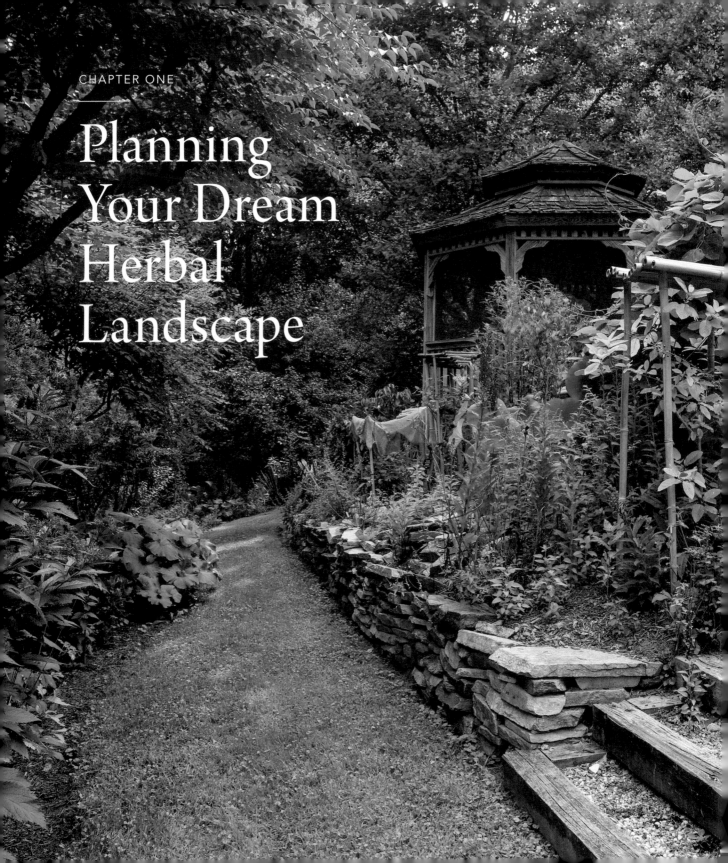

CHAPTER ONE

# Planning Your Dream Herbal Landscape

> The glory of gardening: hands in the dirt, head in the sun, heart with nature. To nurture a garden is to feed not just the body, but the soul.
> ~ Alfred Austin

# Organic Holistic Herb Gardening

My approach to holistic herb gardening mirrors my approach to holistic healing and herbalism. In holistic healing, we explore the *whole* individual—body, mind, temperament, home, work, diet, lifestyle, and community—and not just their disease or disorder. The holistic approach to remedying imbalances isn't limited to herbs; it also includes strategies aimed at improving diet, sleep, lifestyle, relationships, and community. Much as whole foods are more nourishing to the body than relying on supplements alone for nutrition, nourishing and building soil is more effective in supporting plant life than counting on fertilizer alone, even if it's organic.

You've heard the saying "An ounce of prevention is worth a pound of cure." Well, the same is true for plants. A healthy plant, one whose needs are met by the garden and gardener, is more

The medicinal herb gardens created by the late Dr. Jim Duke: the Green Farmacy Gardens in Fulton, Maryland resistant to disease and problematic insects and is more resilient to stressful conditions such as drought or extreme temperatures. Holistic herbalists look for the safest, most effective botanical remedies available. Similarly, holistic herb gardeners use environmentally sound solutions for garden problems. It is sadly ironic when medicinal herbs are grown with chemicals like herbicides, fungicides, and pesticides, which are linked to the increased incidence of cancer and the disruption of healthy hormone function. There's something inherently wrong with poisoning the planet and our bodies to grow a plant that is meant to heal.

Much of my approach to gardening is inspired by the idea of permaculture—a set of practices geared toward designing sustainable and regenerative agricultural and cultural systems. It's rooted in traditional Indigenous systems of agriculture and knowledge of natural ecosystems. Permaculture is a living, evolving set of ideas and principles that can be applied to many aspects of gardening, landscaping, building, and human relationships. It focuses on close observation of interconnectedness with an eye toward cocreating a vibrant and sustainable whole for all of life, elements, and planetary and societal health. To learn more, I recommend *Gaia's Garden: A Guide to Home-Scale Permaculture* by Toby Hemenway.

**1** BUILD THE SOIL INSTEAD OF FERTILIZING PLANTS. Nourishing the soil is a long-term strategy that honors your garden's place in the intricate web of life. Build your soil by adding copious amounts of organic matter, introducing and supporting healthy soil organisms, and growing cover crops. Foster ongoing soil fertility by mulching and reducing tillage, thus allowing soil microbes and beneficial garden animals to flourish. Building soil fertility may be more work initially, but it amounts to less work in the long run, as the plants are happier and healthier on a whole-foods diet of luscious dirt! We'll explore soil fertility in Chapter Two.

**2** GROW PLANTS THAT LOVE YOUR CLIMATE. Choose plants that are suited to your climate and you're more likely to meet with success and a greater harvest of medicinals. It's less work to grow herbs that don't need a lot of inputs like irrigation and soil amending. You'll find siting charts—recommended herbs by climate and landscape—on page 38. You'll also find extensive Regional Profiles in the Healing Garden Gateway (healinggardengateway.com), which cover the herbs best suited to the climate and soils for each bioregion.

**3** PREVENTION OVER TREATMENT. Nurture plant and animal diversity in your landscape for garden and planetary health. You'll invite a vibrant community of pollinators and beneficial insects through creating varied habitats, interplanting multiple species of herbs, and growing native flora. A balanced ecosystem encourages healthy plants by reducing disease and unchecked insect infestation. Chapter Three explores holistic solutions for plant diseases and problematic insects.

**4** YOU ARE WOVEN INTO THE RICH TAPESTRY OF LIFE. Consider how your actions affect the water, soil, air, and other organisms you share this planet with. Is your garden problem worth creating a legion of issues for generations to come? Choose the simplest remedies to reduce garden pests and forgo powerful insecticides—organic and non-natural alike—that harm all neighboring insects and not just the pest at hand. For example, instead of choosing quick measures like herbicides to control weeds, consider mulching, which keeps opportunistic plants at bay while nourishing and cooling the soil.

# Designing Your Herbal Landscape

You might envision a traditional herb garden as a small separate area of the landscape, filled with tidy, low-growing culinary herbs. And while that kind of garden certainly has its place, we can expand our scope by imagining a variety of herbs, tall and short, spreading and climbing, woven throughout the landscape, providing textural beauty, color, windbreak, shade, aromas, food, medicine, flavoring, and shelter for native wildlife. Here, we have a full-blown herbal landscape—with medicinals that serve plentiful functions for the gardeners and increase biodiversity—rather than an isolated herb garden. Before we discuss how you might plan for your herbal landscape, it's helpful to first define what an herb is. An herb is a useful plant that provides one or more benefits to humans: medicine, flavoring, dye, fragrance, or ceremonial material. Depending on the species, the parts used may include the flowers, fruit, bark, roots, leaves, or seeds. Some herbs are both medicinal and edible, whereas others are primarily

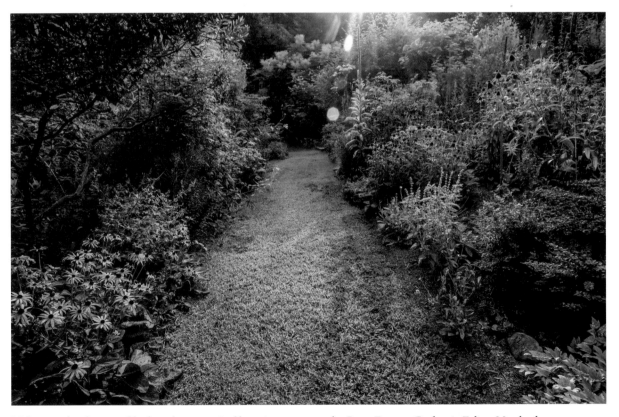

Wide-mowed pathways and herb gardens, organized by organ systems, at the Green Farmacy Gardens in Fulton, Maryland; note the medicinal trees and shrubs interplanted with perennial herbs

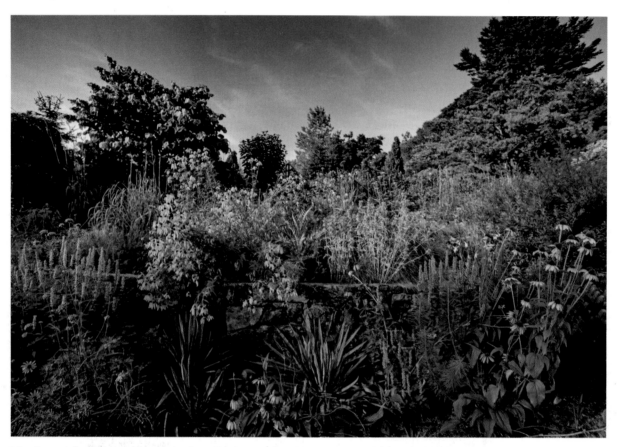

Mixed native plants, perennial ornamentals, and herbs at Longwood Gardens in Kennett Square, Pennsylvania

culinary (used to flavor food in small to modest amounts) with secondary medicinal uses, and some are solely medicinal. An herb plant can take many forms. In addition to the classic garden herbs, which are familiar perennials or annuals, some herbs are shrubs, vines, or groundcovers. An herb can be an evergreen tree, such as a pine, spruce, or juniper, or a deciduous tree, like ginkgo, slippery elm, or elderberry, which loses its leaves in the fall.

Many medicinals are exceptionally ornamental and can be planted in one's front walkway, alongside a patio, or under a shade tree, providing visual interest for you and your family and passersby. Instead of planting flowers, groundcovers, and shrubs purely for their pretty foliage or flowers, think about growing herbal flowers, groundcovers, and shrubs that are both attractive and useful. Depending on where you live, some herbs will be native to your bioregion and others will be introduced. Growing native wildflowers, shrubs, and trees is the best way you can support native populations of birds, butterflies, moths, mammals, and amphibians. Many of these native plants are also medicinal or edible!

Now that we've expanded our vision of an herbal landscape, let's think about how your existing outdoor space can become the canvas for your needs and desires. To do this, you'll need to observe your surroundings, ideally over several seasons. How much sun do you have throughout the year in the various areas of the landscape? Is there an area where prevailing winds enter your space? Take note of how water travels through the area, paying attention to drier or wetter spots. Take a visual tour to determine if there are areas you'd like to be more private, or views you'd rather not take in. Which existing features do you like and which would you rather improve upon or eliminate?

Now, let's explore your needs. Think hard about how much time and space you have to dedicate to your herbal plantings. Spend a moment envisioning what you would like to do with your herbs. Do you want to mostly grow culinary or edible herbs, or do you also want to make herbal teas, tinctures, or syrups? Perhaps you'd like to make natural body care products or grow aromatic plants. Now, think about how your garden can enrich your life. Do you want it to be a place of refuge, with quiet nooks and gurgling fountains? Do you need stylish outdoor spaces, such as a patio, porch, or deck, for entertaining? If you have children in your life, think about creating hidden nooks, places where their imagination can run free, or a small lawn for play. If you have a sunny yard, you might create shady spots, such as a large arbor or pergola covered with medicinal vines or a hedge of evergreen medicinal trees. If you live in a neighborhood and want more community, think about outdoor spaces in your front yard or stoop where you can interact with the people around you. Perhaps you'd like to grow plants that will encourage native pollinators and support wildlife. Then, think about how your garden will evolve with time and which needs are the most important and should be prioritized.

One of the biggest harvests we reap from the herb garden can't be dried for tea or prepared into a tincture: this invisible reward is a deeper connection with our medicine. The best way to become familiar with medicinal herbs is by growing them. Seeing an herb every day can inspire curiosity, which leads to learning medicinal attributes and traditional preparations. This intimate connection to our herbs is potent medicine in its own right.

If you're not sure which features you'd like to incorporate, I recommend strolling around a neighborhood you like and jotting down all the features in people's yards or landscape you enjoy. You can similarly cruise Pinterest or garden design books for inspiration. If you want to dive in further and mine gardening ideas, I recommend Rosalind Creasy's *Edible Landscaping*. But here is a brief introduction to the elements of garden design.

LIKELY SUSPECTS: WHICH HERBS TO PLANT. If you're a newbie herb gardener, consider planting some of the herbs from the Top 20 Garden Herbs, listed on page 18. Research which of these herbs might do well in your region by consulting the siting charts on page 38. Ask neighboring herbalists and plant lovers which herbs thrive for them. Finally, if you have limited time to devote to your garden, start with only a handful of plants and build your garden as time allows. If your gardening time is limited but you're blessed with lots of space, consider planting medicinal trees and shrubs, which require less input over time than smaller plants. Medicinal trees and shrubs include black walnut, wild cherry, ginkgo, elderberry, rose, cramp bark, black haw, bayberry, red bay, juniper, loquat, sassafras, slippery elm, black birch, chaste tree, spruce, pine, and mimosa (be sure it's not invasive in your landscape by checking invasive.org). Depending on where you live, many of these trees may be native and will support biodiversity in your landscape, help with insect control, and attract native wildlife. Planting perennial herbs instead of annuals is also a time-saver because perennials come back year after year.

## Top 20 Garden Herbs

I chose these plants based on ease of cultivation along with medicinal usefulness and versatility. That's to say, these are some of the easiest herbs to grow with a lot of medicinal uses!

Anise hyssop (*Agastache foeniculum*)

Bee balm or wild bergamot (*Monarda* spp.)

Black cohosh (*Actaea racemosa*)

Calendula (*Calendula officinalis*)

Echinacea (*Echinacea purpurea*)

Elderberry (*Sambucus canadensis*)

Elecampane (*Inula helenium*)

Gotu kola (*Centella asiatica*)

Lemon balm (*Melissa officinalis*)

Meadowsweet (*Filipendula ulmaria*)

Milky oats (*Avena sativa*)

Mint, garden varieties (*Mentha* spp.)

Motherwort (*Leonurus cardiaca*)

Prickly pear (*Opuntia* spp.)

Rose (*Rosa* spp.)

Spilanthes (*Acmella oleracea*)

Tulsi (*Ocimum tenuiflorum*)

Valerian (*Valeriana officinalis*)

Vervain, blue or European (*Verbena hastata* or *V. officinalis*)

Yarrow (*Achillea millefolium*)

HOW MANY OF EACH HERB DO I NEED? If you're a seasoned gardener, you already know that it's far too easy to plant a bazillion seeds in the springtime, when your garden beds are ripe with promise. *What's an extra calendula tucked in here, another sweet little valerian plant over there?* It can quickly add up to a lot of extra work to care for plants that you'll never harvest. Come summertime, when the bugs are buzzing and the sun is blazing overhead, you may be cursing your spring-self who thought it prudent to plant *all* those seedlings.

Think seriously about your needs, and limit yourself to the plan, especially when it comes to perennials, as your overzealousness can turn into overwork for many years to come. If you're growing medicine for your own needs, you don't need that many plants of each herb. For perennial herbs with medicinal roots, you can rotate the harvest from two to three plants in a regenerative fashion, which keeps the plants alive. For perennial herbs from which you harvest the aboveground parts (leaves, flowers, and stem), you'll typically need only one or two plants, especially if you can obtain two to three harvests from that herb during the growing season. There are exceptions—if you use a lot of a particular herb as a beverage tea, for example.

WHERE TO PLANT AND GARDEN BEDS. There are many styles of garden beds, with varying levels of ease and expense involved in their construction. If you have a small area, you might consider wooden raised garden beds, which can be constructed in the sunniest edges of the yard or lawn. You can purchase attractive garden bed kits made from rot-resistant, food-safe wood at garden supply centers or online. You might plant lemon balm, bee balm, mint, motherwort, edible flowers, and culinary herbs in your raised beds. Alternatively, you can build mulched perennial herb gardens around your front walkway or patio and plant ornamental herbs, which will both beautify your landscape and provide medicine for your family. Anise hyssop, lavender, rose, calendula, echinacea, California poppy, and wild bergamot are all showy herbs.

If you have shade trees in your yard, consider planting native woodland herbs underneath. Black cohosh and goldenseal are both fairly easy to grow and beautiful. Elevated raised garden beds can be placed in the perimeter of sunny decks and patios—these thigh-high gardens are an excellent option for those with limited mobility. Again, you can find kits online or at garden supply centers. A few potted herbs on a back deck, front stoop, or patio will also give a bit of medicine. You'll find helpful tips for growing herbs in raised garden beds and pots in Chapter Four, Growing Medicinal Herbs in Containers.

For larger gardens with heavy or average soil, raised, borderless beds (as typically seen in vegetable gardens), with small footpaths between, are a solid option. Garden beds can be created by hand with no special tool other than a shovel, and the design is conducive to weeding with a hoe. In areas with compacted soil or poor drainage, raised beds are highly recommended for increasing soil porosity. Aim for garden beds 3 to 4 feet wide, depending on your agility.

When choosing which plants to grow, you'll want to consider the needs of each herb with respect to sun requirement, growth pattern, ultimate size, and soil preference. See the siting charts starting on page 38 and the herbal profiles beginning on page 202 to help you plan. It's helpful to group plants with similar soil and solar needs. For example, I have areas in my garden that I've amended with sand to increase drainage where I plant the herbs that prefer well-drained soil, like lavender, white sage, and prickly pear. Similarly, I group wetland herbs, like meadowsweet, blue vervain, and marshmallow, in the lowest spot in my garden that retains the most moisture. Medicinals that prefer shade can be planted close to one another for ease of care.

If you're new to gardening, consider trying a mix of different types of garden styles, and see which suits you. For example, try a wooden raised garden bed next to a patio or a sunny fence; grow a few potted herbs; prepare a modest shaded garden bed under a deciduous tree and a mulched herb garden bed in a sunny area alongside your front walkway or in another prominent area. After a year, you can see if you have plenty of plants to keep you happy or if you'd prefer to grow more and which plants and configurations are working best for you.

Plant the herbs that need more attention near your home or in an area where you pass by daily. For example, calendula flowers need to be picked every few days to ensure continuing floral production. A bonus is seeing the flowers as you come and go and enjoying the pollinators. Another plant that requires regular attention is tulsi, or holy basil. The flowering stalks need to be periodically cut, which helps the plants put more energy into leaf production and grow larger. I plant culinary herbs right out my front and back doors so I can quickly grab an aromatic handful when I have a pot simmering on the stovetop.

THEME GARDENS. Specialty gardens provide an intriguing way to group herb plantings. You might create mini-gardens around similar usage, land of origin, or botanical relationship. For example, you could plant mullein, elecampane, lobelia, and licorice in a garden of respiratory herbs. This type of planting is especially useful in an educational setting. With a land-of-origin theme, you might interplant lavender, rosemary, sage, and thyme to create a Mediterranean herb garden. For those of you with an alchemical bent, consider concocting a moon garden with herbs that flaunt nocturnal blooms or arresting silvery foliage.

## Plant Communities: The Art of Interplanting

**GROW WITH CULTIVATED WILD ABANDON.** Traditional cottage gardens are my favorite type of garden with their informal appearance, painted by a rich palette of assorted herbs with varying heights and textures. Such gardens are reminiscent of a verdant meadow at the forest's edge, dotted with golden wildflowers. When I visit formal gardens planted with repetitive brushstrokes of botanical monotony, I find them stifling and uninspiring, but it's more than an issue of style. When plants grow with only their kind, they are easy targets for pathogens and problem insects. Conversely, when plants are interspersed with other species, it makes it more challenging for diseases and insects to spread.

To create your own cottage garden, plant herbs of varying heights: groundcovers in between knee-high perennial herbs, punctuated by a few deciduous shrubs. Plant taller herbs toward the back of the border and shorter plants like thyme, chives, spilanthes, and gotu kola next to walkways. Loose repetition and a color strategy tie it all together and keep it from feeling haphazard. For example, spread a few anise hyssop plants throughout a small area but not side by side. You might also group purple-flowered lavender and purple bee balm for splashes of purple throughout the landscape. I find silver

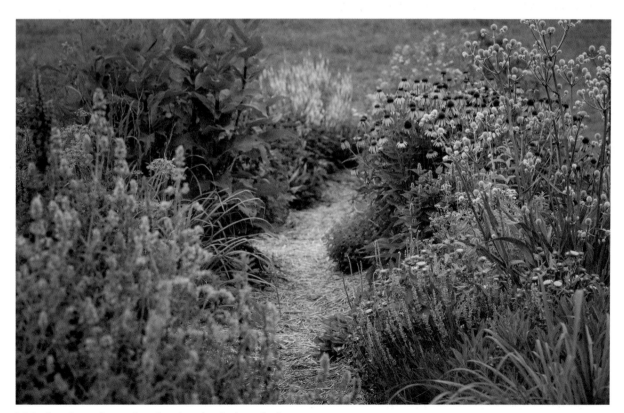

My herb garden with interplanted medicinal and culinary herbs

foliage especially attractive next to purple flowers, so I might add some white sage, lavender, and silver thyme in between the other herbs. This is just one idea—let your climate, soil, and plant preferences inspire you.

POLYCULTURES AND OPPORTUNISTIC PLANT ALLIES (EDIBLE AND MEDICINAL WEEDS). In traditional agriculture, gardens are patches of cohabitating food crops with useful edible and medicinal weeds filling the gaps in between. The "weeds" are allowed to grow and are loosely tended, as they are an essential component of the garden's productivity. You've likely heard how many Native American peoples have long planted the three plant sisters: corn, beans, and squash. The beans help the "family" by fixing nitrogen and feeding the hungry corn, and in return, the corn gives the beans a surface to climb up. The squash grows in between, acting as a living mulch, holding in the moisture, and providing habitat to beneficial animals (which prey on the insects that eat the plants). In the southwestern United States, native peoples know a "fourth sister"—the Rocky Mountain bee plant (*Cleome serrulata*), which is a "weedy" native wildflower with edible shoots. Its flowers also attract pollinators, which serve to increase bean and squash production by increasing pollination and fruit set. The three sisters method of planting is the best-known example of a *polyculture*—a fancy word for *manygrowing*, or growing a diverse array of many crops together. A polyculture is the opposite of a monoculture.

An example of an herbal polyculture that has worked well in my garden is passionflower, lemon balm, and gotu kola. The passionflower climbs up a trellis made out of a bamboo tripod, which creates a leafy cone of shade and moisture, which the gotu kola prefers. The gotu kola spreads, acting as a living mulch, holding in moisture and suppressing weeds. I place the lemon balm plants around the perimeter of the tripod. Both passionflower and lemon balm attract bees and other pollinators into the garden, helping to increase the fruit set of nearby vegetables.

Another example involves four-foot-tall roselle hibiscus in the center surrounded by shin-high tulsi and sprawling spilanthes underneath as a living medicinal groundcover. A woodland polyculture might include goldenseal, black cohosh, and ginseng. You'll see other examples throughout the book and read about them in the herb profiles. With a little observation and imagination, you can design your own mini herbal plant communities as suited to your climate.

## Garden Materials and Hardscaping

PATHWAYS. There are many types of garden pathways, including mowed greenery, mulch, wood chips, gravel, stones, recycled concrete "stones," and bricks. Each option has its pros and cons, which we'll touch on a bit here. Primary paths should be a minimum of 3 feet wide to accommodate a cart or wheelbarrow for materials distribution. For secondary footpaths, 18 inches in width should suffice. If your garden will be used for educational or social purposes or visited or maintained by people in wheelchairs, wider paths are in order.

Probably the simplest option is to sow a low-growing, nitrogen-generating cover crop, such as white clover, as a green pathway. Periodically mow the clover path, and apply the clippings as mulch or add them to your compost pile. Wood mulch makes for a pleasing pathway; it has to be reapplied every year but requires little maintenance other than that. Utility companies or city dumps often give away fresh wood chippings from sawed-off tree limbs.

Gravel or rock pathways require less maintenance than the choices above, especially if they are built right, with a ground cloth to suppress weeds, and the path is lined with a border. Keep gravel pathways separate from mowed areas—when rocks find their way into lawns, they can pose a hazard when mowing. Gravel and ornamental rock can be pricey, but the paths will last for many years. A strikingly sustainable option is "urbanite," large chunks of repurposed, used concrete. Flatter segments of urbanite can be used like flagstone pavers.

PLANNING FOR COMPOSTING AND OTHER AMENDMENTS. Place your composting area out of the way from entertaining and relaxation zones but close enough to your home that it won't be neglected. This same area might be used to store extra amendments and mulch. You might want to create a visual enclosure (compost piles aren't always pretty) by planting a hedge or building a privacy fence. If you have a larger garden, planning a central location where vehicles can deliver amendments, such as mulch, compost, manure, and soil, can make for a smoother flow throughout the garden.

MULCH. I am a big proponent of mulching (spreading a natural material on top of the soil), which I credit to my formative suburban years. My father indoctrinated me into the "cult of mulch" every spring by corralling me into his gardens to spread bark mulch while extolling its many virtues—weed suppression, moisture retention, and soil building as it degrades. Mulch also keeps the soil cooler in the summer and prevents dirt, along with potential plant diseases, from splashing up onto crops. Basically, mulch turns into soil goodness *and* holds in existing soil goodness. I generally apply mulch in the fall after the plants have begun to die back and then reapply a fresh layer, a few inches deep, in the spring.

Despite the miraculous merits of mulch, it has several drawbacks. Mulch can harbor slugs and snails, so you may choose to avoid mulching plants that are especially alluring to slugs, such as elecampane, spilanthes, and anise hyssop. Damp mulch touching the base of plants can cause rot and disease, so give plants a few inches of breathing space from the mulch. This is especially true when applying mulch to trees and shrubs.

There are plenty of options when it comes to mulch: grass clippings, hay, straw, bark, raked leaves, and pulled weeds. Keep fresh grass clippings from touching tender young plants by either giving a wide berth around plant stems or drying the clippings in the sun a bit before adding them to the garden beds. Hay often harbors weed and grass seeds, so be prepared to deal with periodic flushes of germinating seeds. The second cutting of hay usually has fewer seeds. You may be able to find moldy hay available for free or for super cheap. Straw is typically more expensive than hay, and depending on where you live, it may be imported some distance. Straw is often free of weed seeds, but it can contain grain seeds.

Wood bark mulch is a superb option for perennials, as it's long-lasting and quite effective at weed suppression. It's fairly economical when purchased by the yard (loose and not bagged). Bagged leaves are available for free by raking your own leaves or trolling neighborhood curbs in the fall. Try to collect bags from people who don't spray. You'll want to either compost the leaves over the winter or break them up before applying them to the garden because leaves can stack up and form an impenetrable barrier, preventing rain from reaching the soil.

---

Wide paths made of crushed rock accommodate for wheelchairs and large groups at the Robison Herb Garden at Cornell Botanic Gardens

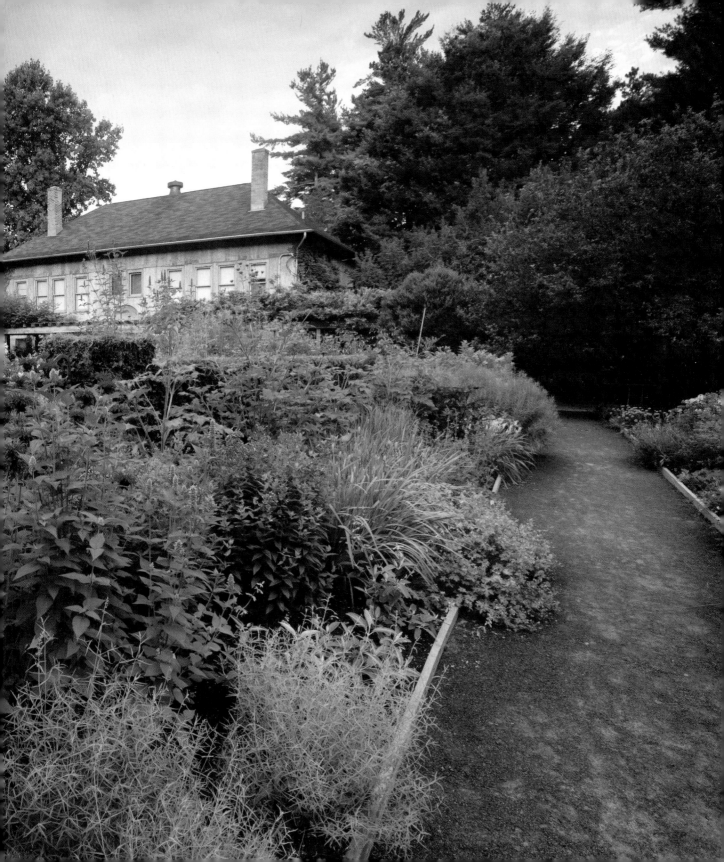

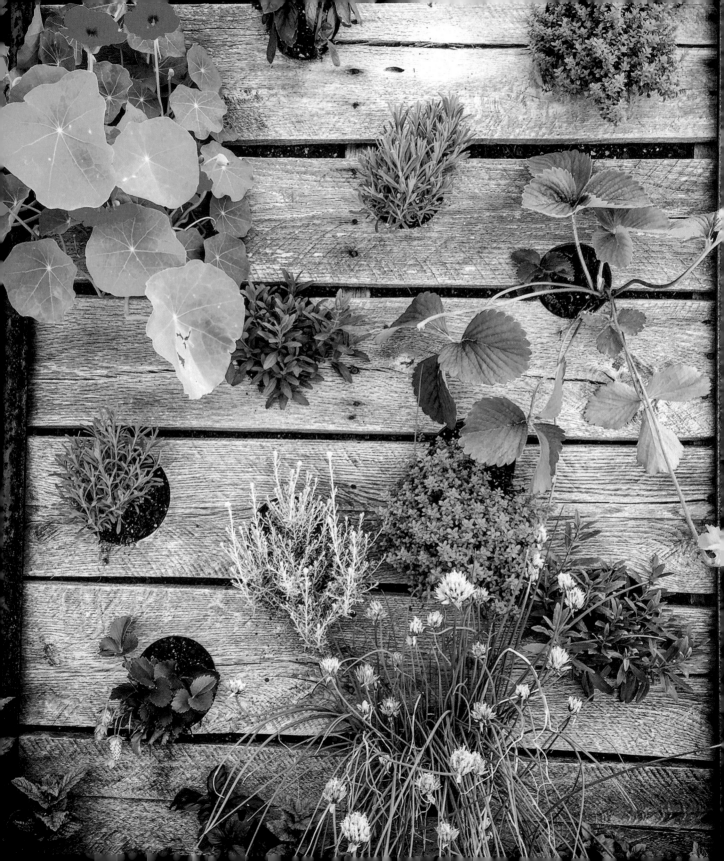

# Getting the Most Out of Small Gardens

Not everyone wants or has the space for a huge garden. If you have limited outdoor space, here are some tips to get the most out of your plantings.

**1 THE SKY'S THE LIMIT: GO VERTICAL.** Train vining herbs such as passionflower, hops, raspberry, jiaogulan, and climbing roses up onto a trellis, arbor, or pergola. Hops can grow to gigantic proportions, so you'll need to tame it by cutting it back, or simply let the vine have its way with a large fence or wall of a building. Many of these vining herbs also spread by runners and can quickly take over a garden. Planting in containers or using a rhizome barrier can help to limit their spreading. (Be especially careful with jiaogulan, as it can be seriously invasive in a woodland setting.)

**2 COME AGAIN? REPEAT HARVESTING.** Certain herbs can be harvested multiple times throughout the year in a "cut-and-come-again" style (similar to microgreens cultivation). Give the plants a "haircut" early enough in the season, and they grow right back. I harvest the following herbs in this fashion, two to three times during the growing season: gotu kola, tulsi, spilanthes, thyme, California poppy, passionflower, comfrey, basil, rosemary, chickweed, violet, lemongrass, garden sage, boneset, bee balm, meadowsweet, anise hyssop, white sage, and lemon balm. Growing these cut-and-come-again herbs can effectively double or triple your yield for every square foot of precious dirt.

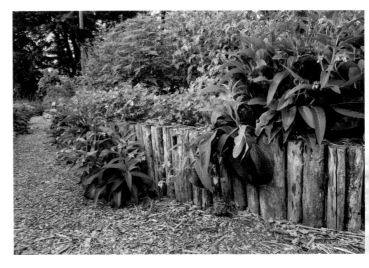

Urban terraced garden beds with rot-resistant wood retaining walls and wood chip mulch pathways in V Kapoor's garden in Asheville, North Carolina

**3 THINK INSIDE THE BOX.** A time-tested solution for growing in a limited space is container gardening. Larger ceramic pots, retired bathtubs, and wooden barrels can hold a surprising number of herbs, especially if you plant trailing herbs at the perimeter and taller plants at the rear. See Chapter Four to learn more about container gardening.

Vertical herb garden at the North Carolina Arboretum in Asheville, North Carolina

# Reining in Exuberant Garden Companions

Various species of medicinal plants will spread by seed throughout the garden if you don't mulch and you leave their seed heads intact. These plants produce plentiful seeds—typically spread by wind (or sometimes critters)—which germinate the following growing season. When unplanted seedlings germinate throughout the garden, the plants are said to *self-sow*. Herbs can also spread locally by runners and dominate a small patch of ground. Before planting milk thistle, mugwort, horehound, mimosa, or shiso, I recommend researching whether those plants are already present in your area and are invasive. If they are, find a nearby place to harvest them, and don't exacerbate the problem by planting more.

HERBS THAT "SOW THEIR WILD OATS." Depending on your climate, the following herbs may self-sow: lemon balm, valerian, feverfew, spilanthes, echinacea (all species), calendula, shiso, elecampane, motherwort, California poppy, borage, tulsi (holy basil), catnip, horehound, lobelia, angelica, and nasturtium. Many medicinals that have earned "weed" status spread quite prolifically: chickweed, violet, mugwort, mullein, burdock, milk thistle, yellow dock, stinging nettles, and dandelion are a few examples. To control their spread, cut back the developing seed heads after the plants flower (the seed heads develop from flowers after pollination and fertilization) and mulch heavily.

SOME HERBS GET AROUND. Herbs that spread by runners (horizontal underground stems or roots) or clump vigorously include mints, bee balm, wild bergamot, hops, stinging nettles, yarrow, comfrey, jiaogulan, passionflower, gotu kola, and certain species of goldenrod. Plant them out of the way, where they can do their thing, or place barriers in the soil to control their runners—a half-buried rhizome barrier (available from garden supply companies and bamboo sellers) will keep them in their place quite nicely. Another option is to place these roaming herbs in a container before they develop any wild ideas.

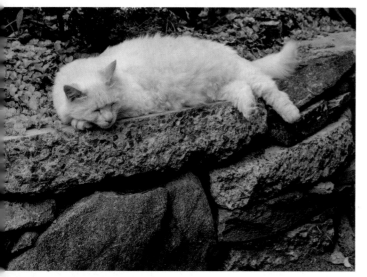

Retaining wall made from urbanite, or repurposed demolished concrete; V Kapoor's garden

Mulched perennial herb beds, mowed pathways, and boulder-lined terraces at Herb Mountain Farm in Weaverville, North Carolina

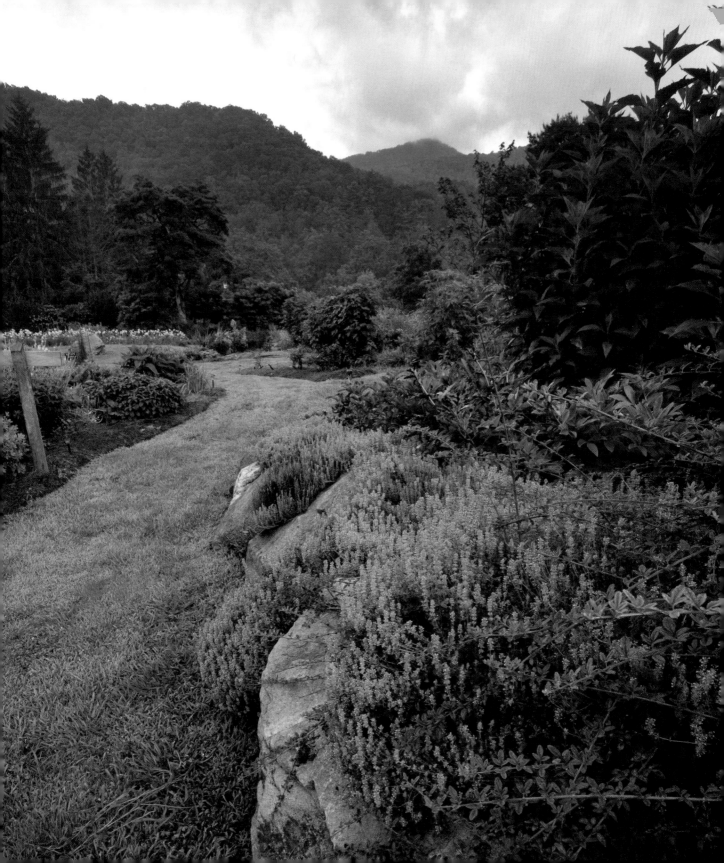

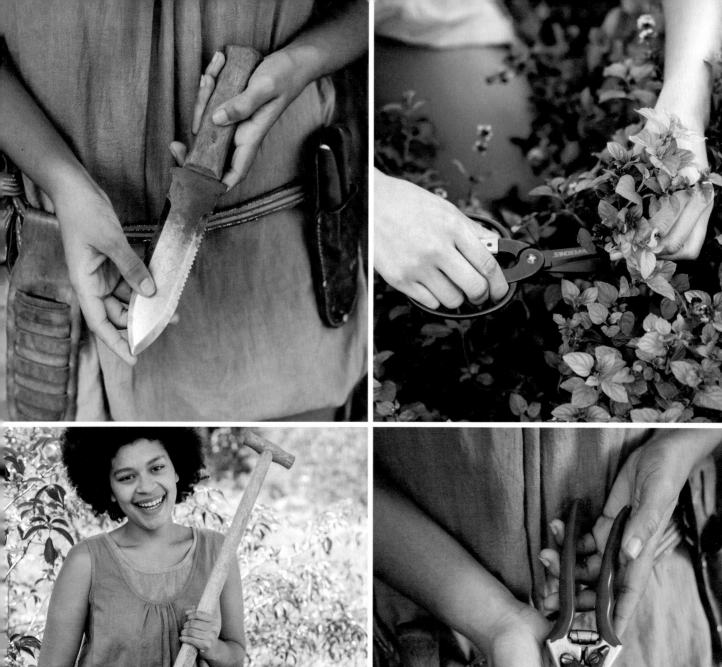

# Essential Gardening Tools

Having the right tools for the job makes all the difference and can save you precious time by increasing your efficiency with garden chores. Investing in high-quality tools will also save you money over time because you'll need to spend less on repairs or replacements. I still have the same pruners and weeding knife I purchased 25 years ago!

HIGH-QUALITY PRUNERS OR GARDEN SHEARS. You'll use your pruners for many garden chores and to harvest and process plants in medicine making. I recommend Felco brand pruners, as they are built to last. They can be sharpened, and the blade and spring can be replaced. A holster is indispensable for safety and for keeping pruners in handy reach. High-end pruners come in a variety of models—look for a pair that fits your hand. The pruner handles, when fully opened, should not exceed the width of your extended grasp. You may want to go to the store and try out different models to see which feels the best.

HORI-HORI OR WEEDING KNIFE. I keep this heavy-duty and compact tool at my side, along with my pruners, whenever I am gardening. Also called a Japanese garden knife, this sturdy garden implement is a match for clayey soils (unlike a trowel, it won't bend or break when digging in heavy soils). It's also helpful for dividing roots and can even pry rocks out of the ground. Look for models with a "lip" at the base of the blade—this safety feature guards your hand from the sharp blade. A holster will help you keep track of your garden knife and protect you from the blade.

*Clockwise from top left:* Hori-hori; garden shears; pruners; digging fork

DIGGING FORK. This is one of my most-used garden and harvesting tools. Digging forks have square, sturdy tines, unlike the manure fork or hayfork, which has flat, bendable tines. Don't confuse the two when digging, or you'll ruin the hayfork! Use the digging fork to turn over garden beds, harvest roots, and loosen and aerate soil.

SHOVELS. Flat-ended shovels are helpful for spreading materials and for root division, and shovels with a pointed blade are helpful for digging in compacted soil.

BUCKETS OR GARDEN TUBS. You can use repurposed food-grade buckets; 3- and 5-gallon sizes are handy. Newer on the scene are pliable bucket-tubs or garden trugs with handles. Both are useful for weeding, harvesting, and spreading amendments.

WHEELBARROW OR GARDEN CART. Helpful for carting amendments, mulch, and weeds throughout the garden.

BASKETS, ALWAYS BASKETS. I like to keep a variety of baskets on hand for harvesting and drying herbs. It's helpful to have some with handles and some that are flat and wide for drying flowers, bark, and fruit.

HEAVY-DUTY GARDEN GLOVES. These are especially needed when harvesting stinging nettles and prickly plants like raspberry.

# Woodland Herb Cultivation

Many of our cherished medicinals—herbs like ginseng, goldenseal, black cohosh, and wild yam—are rare woodland understory plants. Cultivating them, along with protecting their habitat, is essential to their future, which is why I've included a section on growing these threatened herbs. As roads, development, lawns, and agriculture replace wildlands, we're losing vast populations of native flora, including woodland herbs. Growing these plants reduces the demand for overharvested wild herbs. Many forest understory herbs are easy to grow; if sited properly, they can fend for themselves after the first year or two of life and require few or no inputs. If you have a shade tree in your yard, you can cultivate woodland herbs underneath. Many are highly ornamental and will beautify your landscape—black cohosh, bloodroot, trillium, wild geranium, lady's slipper, false unicorn root, and wild ginger are especially attractive. If you're serious about growing woodland herbs, consult *Growing and Marketing Ginseng, Goldenseal, and Other Woodland Medicinals,* by Jeanine Davis and W. Scott Persons. And you'll also want to join the United Plant Savers, a nonprofit organization dedicated to the preservation of threatened and endangered medicinal plants.

The first step in growing forest medicinals is to look at the type of forest you have, including the soil pH. The existing trees can tell you a lot about the soil pH and, thus, which herbs will thrive in the understory. Neutral to alkaline soils are primo for ginseng, goldenseal, wild geranium, black cohosh, blue cohosh, and wild yam. In central and eastern North America, look for tulip poplar, sugar maple, yellow buckeyes, white ash, basswood, and wild cherry as good indicators of an ideal habitat for these herbs. Outside this region, look for oak, maple, birch, linden, ash, hickory, and beech. Trees and shrubs that indicate acidic soils include pine, hemlocks, rhododendron, Douglas fir, and mountain laurel. Habitat under these plants is more suitable to acid-soil medicinals such as partridgeberry, pipsissewa, and pink lady's slipper. See the Woodland Medicinal Herbs, Shrubs, and Trees chart on page 39 for an idea of what you might grow where. Also consult the Shade and Shade-Tolerant Herbs chart on page 40 for botanicals that will thrive at the wood's edges.

If you live in a hilly or mountainous region, you'll want to take slope orientation into account. North-facing and east-facing slopes are cooler and moister—ideal habitat for many woodland herbs that prefer rich, moist soil. South-facing slopes tend to be drier and hotter. That said, creeks and springs create extra moisture, so take multiple factors into account when picking your ideal site. The presence of thriving woodland herbs and indicator trees should be the most influential factors in deciding where to plant.

Even if you don't have ideal mature woodlands to plant in, you can still grow forest medicinals. Before planting, loosen the soil, amend it with copious organic matter, including pine bark fines and composted leaves, and then mulch heavily, and water during dry periods. By following these strategies, I was able to grow ginseng, goldenseal, trillium, and black cohosh in my backyard, where I have an acidic young forest with damaged soil from years of overgrazing. See the picture on the following page of these herbs growing in less than ideal habitat. You can even grow certain woodland herbs in containers. I've seen goldenseal, blue cohosh, black cohosh, and

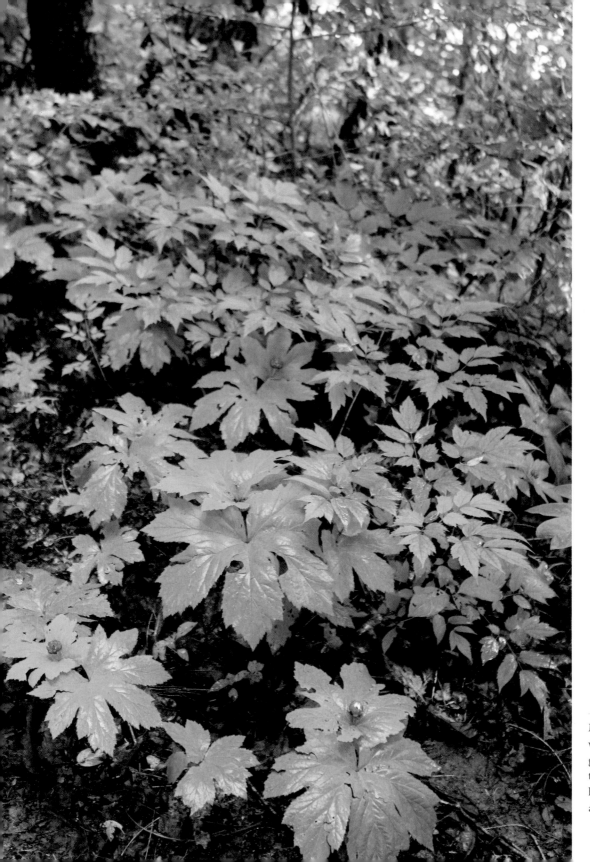

My backyard woodland herb garden, in a less than ideal soil, with happy goldenseal and black cohosh wild geranium thriving in pots and raised container beds sited in the shade.

Planting woodland herbs is a bit different from planting in a field or garden. For starters, there are tree roots, and sometimes big rocks, to avoid. Work around these obstacles and loosen the soil with a garden mattock or digging fork. Composted leaves make an extraordinary soil amendment for woodland herbs. Mulch heavily to hold in the moisture and increase organic matter. If you plant several individuals of each species, they'll begin to spread through seed.

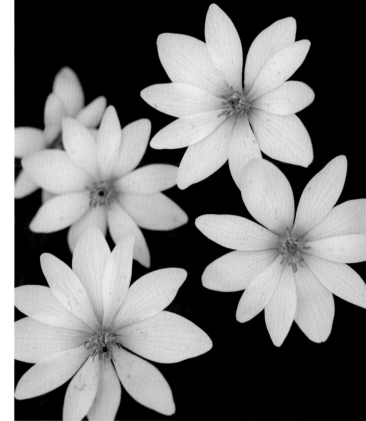

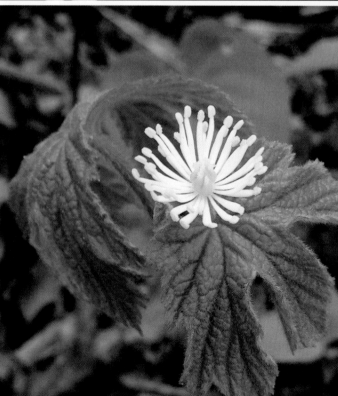

***From left to right:*** Bloodroot (*Sanguinaria canadensis*); blue cohosh (*Caulophyllum thalictroides*); pink lady's slipper (*Cypripedium acaule*); goldenseal (*Hydrastis canadensis*); fringe tree (*Chionanthus virginicus*); yellow trillium (*Trillium luteum*)

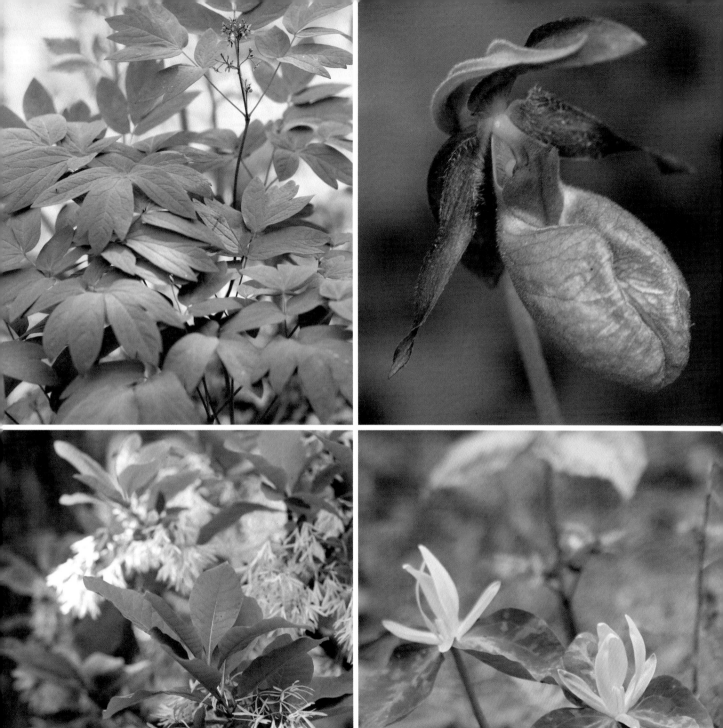

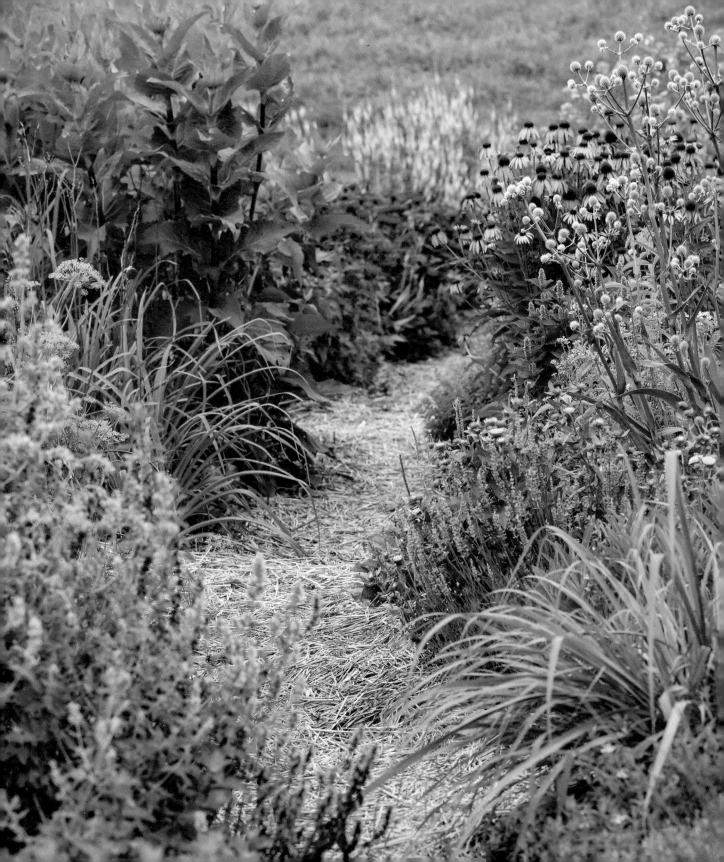

# Step-by-Step Guide to Creating a New Garden Bed with Tilling

Tilling refers to digging up and turning over the soil. I have used this double tilling method many times to create new garden beds from lawn or field. If you're blessed with fertile, loamy soil, you may not need to till. But for compacted soils that are relatively infertile, tilling at the outset of a garden's formation will yield dramatic results for decades to come. Tilling is an easy way to incorporate large amounts of organic matter into the soil and increases soil porosity.

The fall or early spring is an ideal time for tillage because grass and other existing plants are less likely to sprout up from roots. If you can prepare your garden in the fall, consider planting a fall cover crop—a planting designed to protect the soil from erosion and build soil fertility—after tilling to suppress weeds and improve the soil. This is the best way to ensure you've eradicated the grass, especially if you have a particularly invasive or tenacious grass species. Come springtime, you can till or dig the crop into the soil to build its fertility and structure. Contact your local agricultural extension agent to find out which fall cover crops are best for your area, and read more about cover crops in Chapter Two. Planting a bean-family cover crop will help build nitrogen levels and contribute organic matter to the soil. You can rent tillers from local equipment rental facilities, borrow a neighbor's, or hire a local farmer or landscaper to come out and till for you. If you have a small garden and tilling isn't practical, use a pointed shovel to break up the soil and incorporate amendments.

*My herb garden, one year after its creation using the double tilling method*

## Double Tilling to Create a New Garden Bed

**STEP 1:** Prepare for your garden's creation by testing your soil's pH and nutrient levels and deciding which amendments you'd like to add. (See page 49 for more on soil amendments.) In general, I like to add as much organic matter as possible to new garden beds along with a smattering of organic fertilizer. In the past, when I've added only organic matter without fertilizer, plants have been stunted during the garden's first year. It takes a while to build soil fertility, and fertilizer can help nurture plants in a new garden bed until the soil matures.

In general, sandy soil benefits from the incorporation of leaf mulch, pine bark fines, and aged manure and compost. Clay is also a useful addition and helps with water and mineral retention. Many of these amendments are available by the truckload from mulch yards, farms, and nursery supply outfits and can be delivered to your site. If you aren't familiar with the wonders of pine bark fines, prepare to become a convert! They are a by-product of the pulp and logging industries, consisting of the ground-up bark of pine trees. Also sold as "soil conditioner," this extraordinary brown fluff assists with drainage and water retention, has a near-neutral pH, and slowly degrades into the lushest of organic matter over time.

Compacted or clayey soils benefit from materials that assist with drainage, such as coarse sand or pine bark fines, in addition to aged manure and compost. You'll often hear that you should never add sand to clayey soils because it can create a near-concrete hardness, but in my experience, if you add enough organic matter with the sand, it shouldn't be a problem. Coarse sand is especially helpful if you want to grow plants that thrive in well-drained soils, such as Mediterranean herbs. Let the results of your soil test dictate which organic fertilizers and amendments to use.

STEP 2: Till your garden area with a walk-behind rotary tiller (a rototiller, for example) or a tractor. If you're working with a shovel, you can similarly turn over soil and break it up into smaller pieces. If you have large clumps of soil or plants left behind, break them up with a hoe or shovel. Using a hard rake, gather any sod and compost it. Let the ground sit for two to three weeks.

STEP 3: Add the organic matter and amendments you chose in the first step, and till a second time to mix them in and further break up the soil. Wearing safety goggles, spread powders or lightweight fertilizers on a relatively still day. After the initial tilling, the exposed roots and unearthed seeds will have sent out a flush of greenery. This second tilling will knock back the emerging weeds and grass. If your soil is still relatively compacted, run the tiller through a third time.

STEP 4: After the equipment has run through the beds a few times, you'll want to come in with hand tools to finish the job. Use a hard rake to gather any remaining sod and compost it. Rotary tilling breaks up a shallow layer of the soil, leaving the deeper layers untouched. Use a shovel or a hoe to break up any large clumps and lightly loosen the lower layers of soil, or double-dig the garden beds by removing the upper 8 inches of topsoil and placing it aside. Then, break up the subsoil layer, loosening the soil to about 8 inches deep. Replace the topsoil and break that up, too.

STEP 5: Prepare and flatten the garden beds 3 to 4 feet wide. Flattening and shaping garden beds is best achieved with a flat, hard metal rake (often called a bow rake). Stake out the ground using strings as guides to help keep the beds straight and of equal width if you're going for uniform beds.

STEP 6: Mulch the prepared beds if you're planting seedlings right away. If you're planting seeds or a cover crop, there's no need to mulch. Mulching soon after disturbing the soil keeps sprouting weeds to a minimum. If you originally had tenacious grass in the garden area, mulching will keep any remaining roots from emerging. After mulching, you can plant your seedlings right into the mulch. Behold the pictures of my most recent garden, created with this very method.

ONGOING MAINTENANCE: After this initial tilling and garden bed creation, you may not need to till in subsequent years, especially if you generously add mulch, frequently plant cover crops, and side-dress (add amendments and soil conditioners around the base of established plants) with compost and manure. The primary advantage to not tilling is that you maintain the integrity of the soil strata with their finely tuned communities of beneficial soil microbes and earthworms. Tilling compromises the structure of the soil and disrupts soil microbe communities. That said, the benefits of initial tilling in garden creation outweigh the cons.

---

(A) Spreading composted manure on the beds after the initial tilling; (B) spreading organic fertilizer before the second tilling; (C) the second tilling incorporates the organic matter and amendments; (D) heavy mulching after tilling prevents weed seeds and grass from sprouting; (E) freshly planted herbs in the newly created garden beds; (F) the garden, six months after its creation

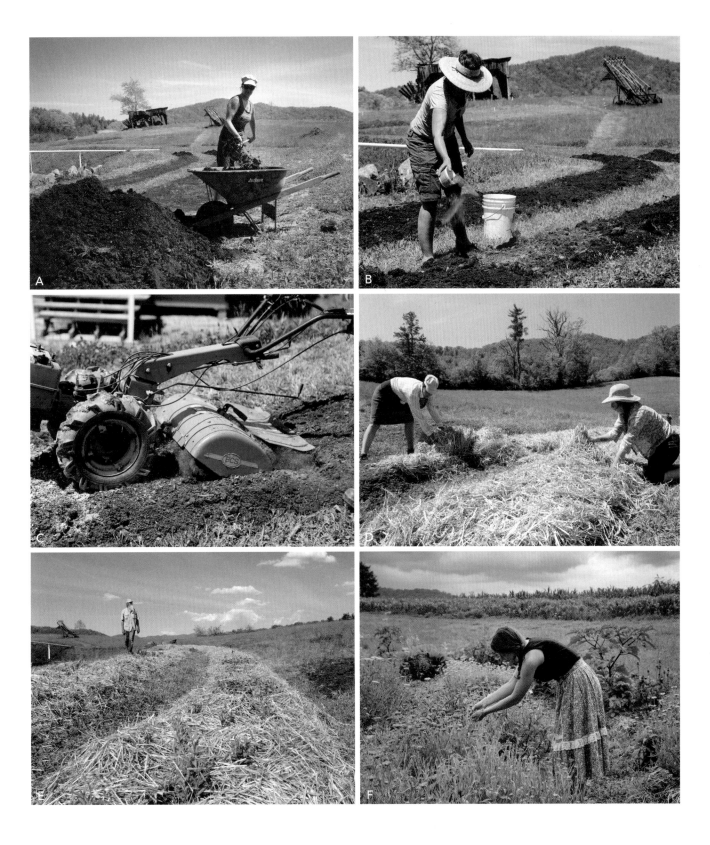

# Siting Charts: Herbal Habitats

Use these charts to give you an idea of the best herbs to grow in your climate and throughout your landscape. You'll also find extensive Regional Profiles in the Healing Garden Gateway (HealingGardenGateway.com), the online portal that accompanies this book. The Regional Profiles cover the best herbs to grow in various bioregions, suited to particular climates and soil types.

KEY

**M** = *Prefers moist soils and/or habitat (many of these species can be grown in rich soil and heavily mulched if moist soils aren't present in the landscape)*

**W** = *Prefers very moist soils (that are periodically submerged or near the edge of the water)*

**S** = *Grows in submerged soils (under the water)*

**P** = *Porous, wet soils; plants that grow well in sandy, moist soils*

## Wetland and Water-Loving Herbs

| COMMON NAME | SCIENTIFIC NAME | OTHER |
|---|---|---|
| Bayberry | *Morella cerifera* | M–W, P |
| Bee balm | *Monarda didyma* | M |
| Blue flag | *Iris versicolor* | W |
| Blue vervain | *Verbena hastata* | M |
| Boneset | *Eupatorium perfoliatum* | M |
| Brahmi | *Bacopa monnieri* | M–W |
| Calamus/Sweet flag | *Acorus americanus* | M–W |
| Cranberry | *Vaccinium oxycoccos, V. macrocarpon* | M–W |
| Culver's root | *Veronicastrum virginicum* | M |
| Elderberry | *Sambucus nigra, S. nigra var. canadensis* | M–W |
| Gotu kola | *Centella asiatica* | M, P |
| Horsetail | *Equisetum* spp. | M–W |

| COMMON NAME | SCIENTIFIC NAME | OTHER |
|---|---|---|
| Marshmallow | *Althaea officinalis* | M |
| Meadowsweet | *Filipendula ulmaria* | M |
| Skullcap | *Scutellaria lateriflora* | M |
| Stinging nettles | *Urtica dioica* | M |
| Sweetfern | *Comptonia peregrina* | M, P |
| Valerian | *Valeriana officinalis* | M |
| Violet, select species | *Viola* spp. (research individual species) | M |
| Wasabi | *Wasabia japonica* | M–W |
| Water lily | *Nymphaea odorata* | S |
| Watercress | *Nasturtium officinale* | M–W–S |
| Willow | *Salix* spp. | M–W |
| Witch hazel | *Hamamelis virginiana* | M |

## Shade-Loving and Partial-Shade Herbs

KEY

**W** = *Woodland herb*
**FS** = *Full sun*
**Sh** = *Shade*
**PSh** = *Partial shade*
**A** = *Grows in acidic soil*

*Note: Gardeners in hot or dry climates can experiment with planting full-sun plants in partial shade to moderate the heat and sunshine. Conversely, partial-shade plants can grow in full sun when planted in colder climates. Many plants that prefer full sun will tolerate partial shade but will produce fewer flowers and grow more slowly.*

## Woodland Medicinal Herbs, Shrubs, and Trees

| COMMON NAME | SCIENTIFIC NAME | OTHER |
|---|---|---|
| Basswood/Linden/Lime tree | *Tilia* spp. | W–PSh |
| Black cohosh | *Actaea racemosa* | W–PSh |
| Bloodroot | *Sanguinaria canadensis* | W |
| Blue cohosh | *Caulophyllum thalictroides* | W |
| False unicorn root | *Chamaelirium luteum* | W |
| Fringe tree | *Chionanthus virginicus* | W–PSh |
| Ginseng | *Panax* spp. | W |
| Goldenseal | *Hydrastis canadensis* | W |
| Oregon grape | *Mahonia aquifolium* | W–PSh, A |
| Partridgeberry | *Mitchella repens* | W, A |
| Pedicularis, eastern | *Pedicularis canadensis* | W |
| Pink lady's slipper | *Cypripedium acaule* | W, A |
| Pipsissewa | *Chimaphila umbellata; C. maculata* | W, A |
| Sassafras | *Sassafras albidum* | W–PSh |
| Slippery elm | *Ulmus rubra* | W–PSh |
| Solomon's seal | *Polygonatum biflorum* | W–PSh |
| Spikenard | *Aralia racemosa* | W–PSh |
| Trillium | *Trillium* spp. | W |
| Wild geranium | *Geranium maculatum* | W–PSh |
| Wild yam | *Dioscorea villosa* | W |
| Wintergreen | *Gaultheria procumbens* | W–PSh, A |
| Witch hazel | *Hamamelis virginiana* | W–PSh |

## Shade and Shade-Tolerant Herbs

| COMMON NAME | SCIENTIFIC NAME | OTHER |
|---|---|---|
| Aloe | *Aloe vera* | PSh–Sh (indoors: north- or east-facing in a window) |
| Angelica | *Angelica* spp. (depends on species) | FS–PSh |
| Anise hyssop | *Agastache foeniculum* | FS–PSh |
| Bee balm | *Monarda* spp. | FS–PSh |
| Blue vervain | *Verbena hastata* | FS–PSh |
| Boneset | *Eupatorium perfoliatum* | FS–PSh |
| Calamus/ Sweet flag | *Acorus americanus* | FS–PSh (FS if near water) |
| Cleavers | *Galium aparine* | FS–PSh |
| Comfrey | *Symphytum officinale* | FS–PSh |
| Elderberry | *Sambucus nigra, S. nigra var. canadensis* | PSh–FS (FS if near water) |
| Elecampane | *Inula helenium* | FS–PSh |
| Eleuthero/ Siberian ginseng | *Eleutherococcus senticosus* | PSh |
| Ginger | *Zingiber officinale* | PSh |
| Gotu kola | *Centella asiatica* | FS–PSh (will tolerate FS in moist soils and cold climates) |
| Jiaogulan | *Gynostemma pentaphyllum* | PSh |
| Lady's mantle | *Alchemilla vulgaris* | FS–PSh (give some shade in warm or dry climates) |
| Lemon balm | *Melissa officinalis* | FS–PSh |

| COMMON NAME | SCIENTIFIC NAME | OTHER |
|---|---|---|
| Marshmallow | *Althaea officinalis* | FS–PSh |
| Meadowsweet | *Filipendula ulmaria* | FS–PSh |
| Oregon grape | *Mahonia aquifolium* | FS–PSh to Sh |
| Peppermint | *Mentha x piperita* | FS–PSh |
| Poor man's ginseng | *Codonopsis pilosula* | PSh |
| Schisandra | *Schisandra chinensis* | FS–PSh (more shade, closer to equator) |
| Self-heal | *Prunella vulgaris* | PSh |
| Skullcap | *Scutellaria lateriflora* | FS–PSh |
| Spearmint | *Mentha x spicata* | FS–PSh |
| Spikenard | *Aralia racemosa* | W- PSh (wet soils) |
| Stinging nettles | *Urtica dioica* | FS–PSh |
| Sweet woodruff | *Galium odoratum* | PSh–Sh |
| Tea | *Camellia sinensis* | FS–PSh (depending on climate and variety) |
| Turmeric | *Curcuma longa* | PSh–Sh |
| Uva-ursi | *Arctostaphylos uva-ursi* | FS–PSh, A |
| Valerian | *Valeriana officinalis* | FS–PSh |
| Violet | *Viola* spp. (depends on species) | FS–Sh |
| Wild bergamot | *Monarda fistulosa* | FS–PSh |
| Wild geranium | *Geranium maculatum* | W–PSh |
| Wild indigo | *Baptisia tinctoria* | PSh, A |
| Wintergreen | *Gaultheria procumbens* | PSh, A |

# Arid Climate Herbs

| COMMON NAME | SCIENTIFIC NAME |
|---|---|
| Aloe | *Aloe vera* |
| Arizona cypress | *Cupressus arizonica* |
| Ashwagandha | *Withania somnifera* |
| Bay laurel | *Laurus nobilis* |
| Black sage | *Salvia mellifera* |
| California poppy | *Eschscholzia californica* |
| Catmint | *Nepeta x faassenii* |
| Cayenne | *Capsicum annuum* |
| Curry plant | *Helichrysum italicum* |
| Desert willow | *Chilopsis linearis* |
| Epazote* | *Dysphania ambrosioides* |
| Ephedra/*Ma huang* | *Ephedra sinica* |
| Fennel | *Foeniculum vulgare* |
| Hops | *Humulus lupulus* |
| Horehound | *Marrubium vulgare* |
| Horsemint | *Monarda punctata* |
| Hyssop | *Hyssopus officinalis* |
| Juniper | *Juniperus communis* (and other species) |
| Lavender | *Lavandula angustifolia*, and other species |
| Lemon | *Citrus x limon* |
| Lemon balm | *Melissa officinalis* |
| Lemon verbena | *Aloysia citriodora* |
| Lemongrass | *Cymbopogon citratus* |
| Mexican tarragon | *Tagetes lucida* |
| Mimosa* | *Albizia julibrissin* |
| Mugwort, Western* | *Artemisia douglasiana* |

| COMMON NAME | SCIENTIFIC NAME |
|---|---|
| Mulberry, white* | *Morus alba* |
| Mullein, common* | *Verbascum thapsus* |
| Ocotillo | *Fouquieria splendens* |
| Olive | *Olea europaea* |
| Oregano | *Origanum vulgare* |
| Oregon grape root/ Algerita | Select *Mahonia* spp. |
| Passionflower | *Passiflora incarnata* |
| Pineapple sage | *Salvia elegans* |
| Prickly ash | *Zanthoxylum clava-herculis, Z. americanum* |
| Prickly pear | *Opuntia* spp. |
| Red root/New Jersey tea/California lilac | *Ceanothus* spp. |
| Rosemary | *Salvia rosmarinus* |
| Sage, garden | *Salvia officinalis* |
| St. John's wort* | *Hypericum perforatum* |
| Thyme | *Thymus* spp. |
| Uva-ursi/Bearberry | *Arctostaphylos uva-ursi* |
| Vitex/Chaste tree | *Vitex agnus-castus* |
| White sage | *Salvia apiana* |
| Wild bergamot | *Monarda fistulosa* |
| Wild indigo | *Baptisia tinctoria* |
| Wormwood | *Artemisia absinthium* |
| Yarrow | *Achillea millefolium* |
| Yaupon holly | *Ilex vomitoria* |

* May become invasive; research its potential to spread before planting

## Subtropical and Tropical Herbs (Moist and Humid Climates)

| COMMON NAME | SCIENTIFIC NAME | COMMON NAME | SCIENTIFIC NAME |
| --- | --- | --- | --- |
| Ashwagandha | *Withania somnifera* | Kava kava | *Piper methysticum* |
| Basil | *Ocimum basilicum* | Lemon | *Citrus x limon* |
| Brahmi | *Bacopa monnieri* | Lemongrass | *Cymbopogon citratus* |
| Calendula | *Calendula officinalis* | Mimosa* | *Albizia julibrissin* |
| Cardamom | *Elettaria cardamomum* | Passionflower | *Passiflora incarnata* |
| Cayenne | *Capsicum annuum* | Prickly ash | *Zanthoxylum clava-herculis* |
| Chickweed | *Stellaria media* | Prickly pear | *Opuntia* spp. |
| Cinnamon | *Cinnamomum verum* | Red bay | *Persea borbonia* |
| Curry leaf | *Murraya koenigii* | Rue | *Ruta graveolens* |
| Elephant garlic | *Allium ampeloprasum* | Saw palmetto | *Serenoa repens* |
| Epazote* | *Dysphania ambrosioides* | Spilanthes | *Acmella oleracea* |
| Eucalyptus* | *Eucalyptus* spp. | Stevia | *Stevia rebaudiana* |
| Fringe tree | *Chionanthus virginicus* | Tulsi | *Ocimum tenuiflorum* |
| Garlic chives | *Allium tuberosum* | Turmeric | *Curcuma longa* |
| Ginger | *Zingiber officinale* | Yaupon holly | *Ilex vomitoria* |
| Gotu kola | *Centella asiatica* | | |
| Hibiscus (Roselle) | *Hibiscus sabdariffa* | | |
| Hibiscus, cranberry | *Hibiscus acetosella* | | |
| Jamaican dogwood | *Piscidia piscipula* | | |

Research each species for its cold-hardiness. Some species are slightly frost-hardy and others are highly sensitive to frost.

* May become invasive; research its potential to spread before planting

Urban permaculture oasis with herbs, vegetables, and fruit trees, at V Kapoor's garden in Asheville, North Carolina

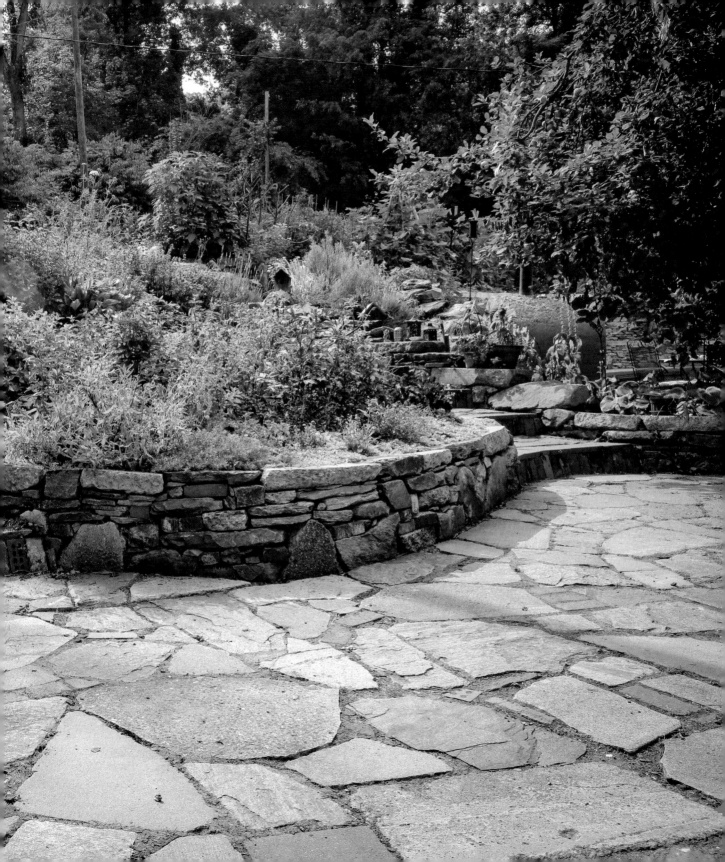

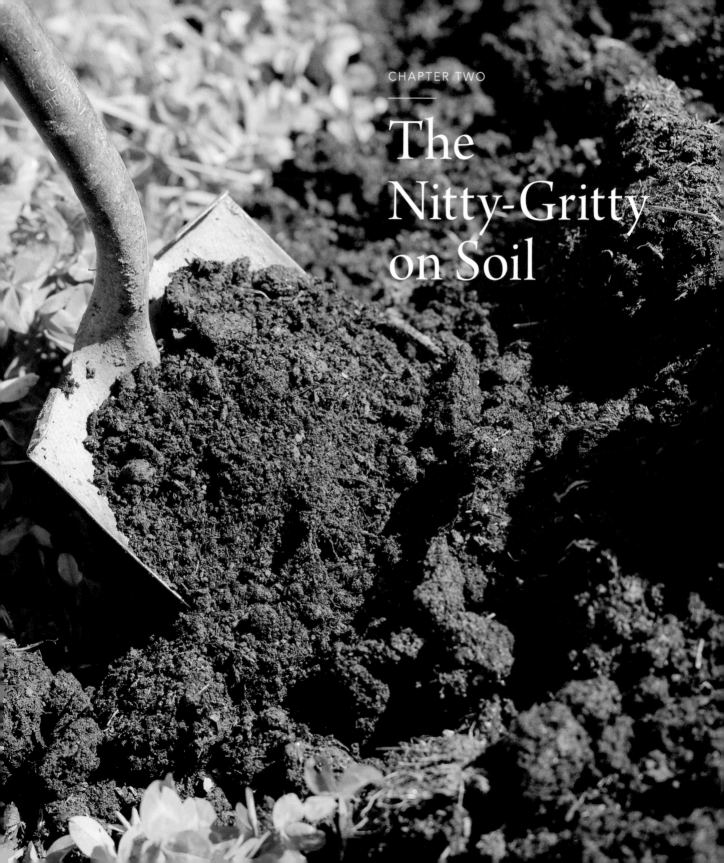

CHAPTER TWO

# The Nitty-Gritty on Soil

> The soil is the great connector of lives, the source and destination of all. It is the healer and restorer and resurrector, by which disease passes into health, age into youth, death into life. Without proper care for it we can have no community, because without proper care for it we can have no life.
> ~ Wendell Berry, *The Unsettling of America: Culture and Agriculture*

# Soil Is the Heart & Health of the Garden

The heart of our gardens lives and beats underground. Nourishing the soil—by improving its texture, fertility, and subterranean ecosystem—is the cornerstone of organic cultivation. The vitality of our garden's plants is wholly rooted in the soil's underground metropolis of bacteria, fungi, worms, and all manner of creepy-crawlies. These organisms are the humble but mighty alchemists of soil, adding nutrients in the ever-flowing cycles of renewal: decay to rebirth. In this chapter, we'll first pull out our proverbial microscopes to examine soil up close and then look at how we can optimize its structure and nutrient levels and, in turn, nurture the beneficial organisms that call it home.

Soil is composed of air, water, organic matter, living organisms (bacteria, fungi, earthworms, and insects), and mineral

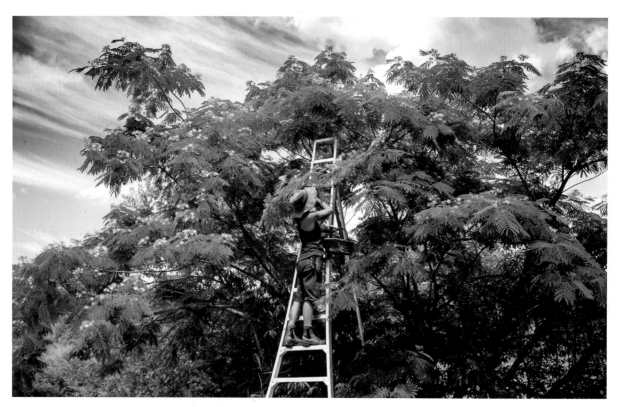

Mimosa is a nitrogen-fixing medicinal tree that can enrich the entire garden.

particles. The three types of mineral particles in descending order of size are sand, silt, and clay. Compact, or heavy, soil is dominated by clay particles, whose tiny size allows them to fit together snugly. This compact configuration means there's less space for air and plant roots. On the other hand, sandy soils are overly porous because sand particles are so large—there's abundant air between the grains of sand, which means these soils drain quickly, which can leach nutrients. Straddling between sandy and clayey soils are loamy soils—the gold standard of soil texture—primarily composed of equal parts sand and silt, with lesser amounts of clay. Too much water, and we have waterlogged ground. Not enough organic matter, and the soil's masses of microbes go hungry and move to greener pastures—the soil loses its heart and cannot nourish healthy plants.

Fertile soil is lush with organic matter, nutrients, and soil flora, fungi, and fauna. It is dark, loose, and crumbly; it holds moisture yet drains water in a slow and steady procession. This desirable texture is also called optimal soil *tilth*. Microscopic plant root hairs easily penetrate the soil's crevices, freely taking in water, oxygen, and nutrients. In short, soils with good tilth are well balanced and poised to nurture plant life. Before you grow covetous, take heart: the majority of gardeners do not start out with this kind of soil! We diligently work toward this dirt-nirvana wheelbarrow by wheelbarrow. But if there *were* a golden ticket to this luxurious dream garden soil, you would certainly purchase it with organic matter.

## Organic Matter

If soil is the heart of your garden, organic matter is its lifeblood. This brown, fluffy stuff helps with soil texture, pH balance, and the retention of moisture and nutrients. Organic matter decreases erosion and feeds the hungry subterranean masses. It's the best antidote for soil issues. Organic matter breaks up heavy soils, helping to increase the soil's porosity and texture; conversely, it helps make sandy soils more fertile and less porous.

WHAT EXACTLY IS ORGANIC MATTER? Organic matter is a mixture of decaying plant and animal matter, the microscopic life-forms eating the decaying matter, and the end product of their decomposition: humus. The crown jewel of organic matter, humus is potent and persistent, helping to maintain an ideal soil structure for the long term.

HOW DO YOU ADD ORGANIC MATTER TO THE SOIL? You can mix amendments such as compost, aged manure, leaf mold, and pine bark fines directly into your garden beds when tilling or preparing beds for the growing season. Adding thick layers of mulch around your plantings every season is another way to increase the organic matter content of the soil. Growing cover crops (discussed below) and applying them as mulch—or incorporating them into the earth—is another method.

I recommend acquiring a book that covers organic gardening in detail—the general information on soil building, composting, and plant nutrients are wholly applicable to the herb garden. (See the Recommended Reading at HealingGardenGateway.com for my favorite books.) Because you can find this material in other works, I've set my focus in this chapter on topics that you won't find in most gardening books: homemade herbal fertilizers, herbal nitrogen fixers, and dynamic accumulators that can help you improve your garden soil.

# Building Soil Fertility

Before you can build your soil, you need to know what you're working with. A soil test is a good starting point. Available from your local agricultural extension office or online, these test your soil pH and nutrient levels and will help you decide which amendments or fertilizers you want to add to your garden. I also recommend asking neighboring organic gardeners and farmers, master gardeners, and the local extension office for local recommendations.

Just be aware that there are regional differences in soil—there's no magic formula! When I was gardening in Florida, I added clay, along with copious organic matter, to the super-sandy soil, and now, in North Carolina, I add sand, along with copious organic matter, to help break up our super-clayey soil. I know I've already waxed poetic over it, but do you notice the theme here? When in doubt, add organic matter. If you're just starting your garden, organic fertilizers can provide the necessary nutrients to your plants while you're building up the soil. As your soil's fertility and texture gradually improve, you'll no longer need to rely on fertilizers.

## Plant Nutrients

In addition to oxygen, carbon dioxide, and water, plants have nutritional needs that the soil provides. Plants need the primary nutrients—nitrogen (N), phosphorus (P), and potassium (K)—in large quantities for their growth processes and overall health. You've probably seen these three nutrients listed on fertilizer labels as the NPK levels. These essential nutrients tend to get depleted from the soil every year, which is why we continually add fertilizers and amendments to our soil. Other nutrients used by plants include calcium (Ca), magnesium (Mg), and sulfur (S), and the trace elements, or micronutrients, which include boron (B), copper (Cu), iron (Fe), chlorine (Cl), manganese (Mn), molybdenum (Mo), zinc (Zn), cobalt (Co), and nickel (Ni). You can learn more about plant nutrients, including organic sources, and symptoms of deficiencies in books covering organic vegetable gardening or from your local agricultural college or university. By following the organic gardening practices outlined in this book and building soil fertility through incorporating copious organic matter into the soil, fertilizing, and mulching, you'll likely provide most of the plant nutrients your plants need. Nonetheless, you'll want to start with a soil test to determine which amendments will be the most important for your garden.

Good organic sources of nitrogen include leguminous cover crops (like red clover, alfalfa, vetch, fenugreek, and field peas), blood meal, feather meal, fish meal, poultry manure, liquid fish emulsion, and alfalfa and soybean meals. If your soil is low in phosphorus, the best natural remedy is adding plenty of organic matter; other sources of the nutrient include rock phosphate and bone meal. Organic sources of potassium include composted animal manures (and organic matter in general), kelp meal or liquid kelp, wood ash, and liquid fish emulsion. Organic matter, azomite (naturally mined volcanic mineral), kelp powder, and liquid kelp all provide trace elements to plants.

## Soil pH

Soil pH is a measure of the soil's acidity or alkalinity on a scale of 0 to 14, with 7 being neutral. Acid soils have a pH lower than 7, and the pH of alkaline soils is higher than 7. Most herbs and vegetables grow optimally in soils that have a pH of 6 to 7 but will tolerate slight differences on either end of that range. Some plants have a preference for acidic soils and others for alkaline soils. Gardeners need to pay attention to soil pH levels because they significantly affect a plant's ability to absorb nutrients from the soil. Organic matter is the best buffer of soil pH on either end of the scale. You can remedy acidic soils by adding powdered lime (calcium carbonate), which is available from garden supply stores; follow the application rate on the label. Recheck your soil pH periodically; you may need to reapply lime over time as it leaches from the soil. The best option for remedying alkaline soils is adding plentiful organic matter to your soil and then retesting after six months to see if the pH is less alkaline. You can also add elemental sulfur to bring down the pH (it will take a few months before the pH is altered), but for soils that are high in calcium carbonate, or free lime, it can be difficult to lower the pH with sulfur. Instead, you'll want to focus on adding plenty of organic matter and growing plants that are tolerant of alkaline soils.

# Soil Amendments & Fertilizers

Many gardeners use the terms "amendment" and "fertilizer" interchangeably, but it's helpful to conceptualize their difference. A fertilizer supplies nutrients directly to the plant, whereas amendments build the texture of the soil, feed the soil's organisms, and may provide limited nutrients. Examples of amendments include composted plant matter, aged manure, leaf mold, green manures, and pine bark fines. Examples of fertilizers include animal-based products like bonemeal, blood meal, fish emulsion, and composted chicken manure; plant-based products like alfalfa meal, cottonseed meal, kelp, and seaweed; and rock-based products like greensand, rock phosphate, and langbeinite. A growing number of high-quality organic fertilizers are available. You can check whether a product is suitable for organic gardening by looking for the Organic Materials Research Institute (OMRI) seal on the package or by visiting omri.org. Try to pick products sourced from renewable ingredients and manufactured close to home. Here are some additional considerations when choosing a fertilizer or amendment.

WHERE WAS THE AMENDMENT PRODUCED? How far did it have to travel to reach you? Look for locally sourced, renewable materials, which include worm castings, compost, aged manure, or pine bark fines. Amendments that can be sourced on site (you make them!) include worm castings, compost, green manures from cover crops, leaf mold, and manure if you have chickens, horses, or cattle.

HOW MUCH DOES THE AMENDMENT COST? CAN YOU BUY IT IN BULK (NOT BAGGED)? There are many ways to add organic matter to your soil, many of which are free or affordable. Purchasing bulk amendments such as compost, pine bark fines, or composted manure by the truckload is substantially cheaper by volume than purchasing bagged materials, and it forgoes the plastic. Collect bagged leaves in the fall from the neighborhood. Compost vegetable scraps from your kitchen and nearby restaurants. Manure is often free if you dig it from stalls; compost it before you add it to the soil.

WAS THE AMENDMENT COMMERCIALLY MINED? Most of the powdered rock amendments, such as greensand and lime, are mined with heavy equipment in big pit mines.

FOR ANIMAL PRODUCTS SUCH AS BONEMEAL, BLOOD MEAL, AND MANURE, HOW WAS THE ANIMALS' QUALITY OF LIFE? Most of the products available commercially are not sourced from humane operations. Inquire with the manufacturer or visit the farm yourself if applicable.

## Applying Fertilizers

There are several ways you can add fertilizer to your soil or garden plants. If you're creating a new garden or fluffing up an older bed, mix the fertilizer with your organic matter into the soil. To determine how much to add, follow the directions for the product or specific amendment you're applying.

SIDE-DRESSING. For established plants, apply fertilizer as a side-dressing directly to the base of a plant. The soil of perennial herb beds can become

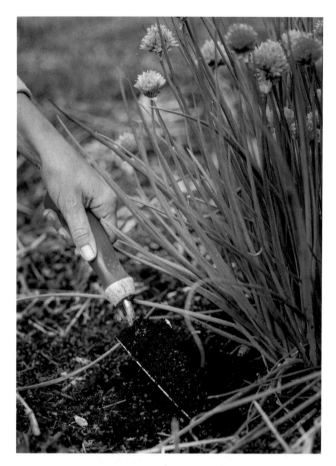

Side-dressing gussies up perennial herbs.

depleted—you'll often notice a decline in vigor after a few years of planting. I gussy up these fading starlets by preparing a homemade blend—think of it as a "green juice" for plants. To make your own Perennial Gussy Blend, mix 2 parts compost with 1 part worm castings and ½ part organic fertilizer. To apply, scrape back any mulch, apply a ring of the Gussy Blend an inch deep and a few inches wide around the plant, taking care not to let it touch the stem, scuffle it in, and reapply the mulch. For shrubs or trees, apply the blend to the drip line (the area under the outer circumference of the branches), where the feeder roots that take up nutrients reside.

FOLIAR FEEDING. Applying liquid fertilizer directly to plant leaves is a straightforward method of delivering nutrients almost instantaneously, making it a clever way to remedy nutrient deficiencies and promote seedling growth. Many types of liquid fertilizers can be used as foliar feeds, including fish emulsion, seaweed, commercial foliar feeding blends, and homemade herbal teas or ferments (see Herbal Fertilizers below). Applying nutrients to plant leaves may seem counterintuitive since plants take up nutrients through their roots, but they can also absorb nutrients through their epidermis (leaf "skin") and through the teeny-weeny holes (stomata) on their leaves, which also allow for gas exchange. (The air that you're breathing this very second contains oxygen that at one time traveled through these minuscule foliar portals.) If you're a foliar feeding newbie, try a premade blend containing fish emulsion and seaweed, and follow the manufacturer's recommendations for dilution rates.

A regular spray bottle won't deliver a fine enough spray for the leaves to absorb. You'll need a pressurized pump sprayer, which creates a fine mist of spray, perfect for evenly coating leaves. Sprayers are sold at farm and garden supply stores or online and come in a variety of sizes. For the home garden, a 1-gallon size is quite sufficient; larger sizes are better for bigger operations.

Despite its merits, foliar feeding has drawbacks. High-nitrogen applications can "burn" foliage. To avoid this, spray in the morning on a cloudy day when there is little chance of rain. (Sunshine increases the risk of burning the leaves, and rain will

---

*Clockwise from top left:* Chicken manure fertilizer; pine bark fines help with soil porosity and water retention; fully degraded compost is black gold for the soil; worm castings contain beneficial soil microbes and help with soil aeration and water retention.

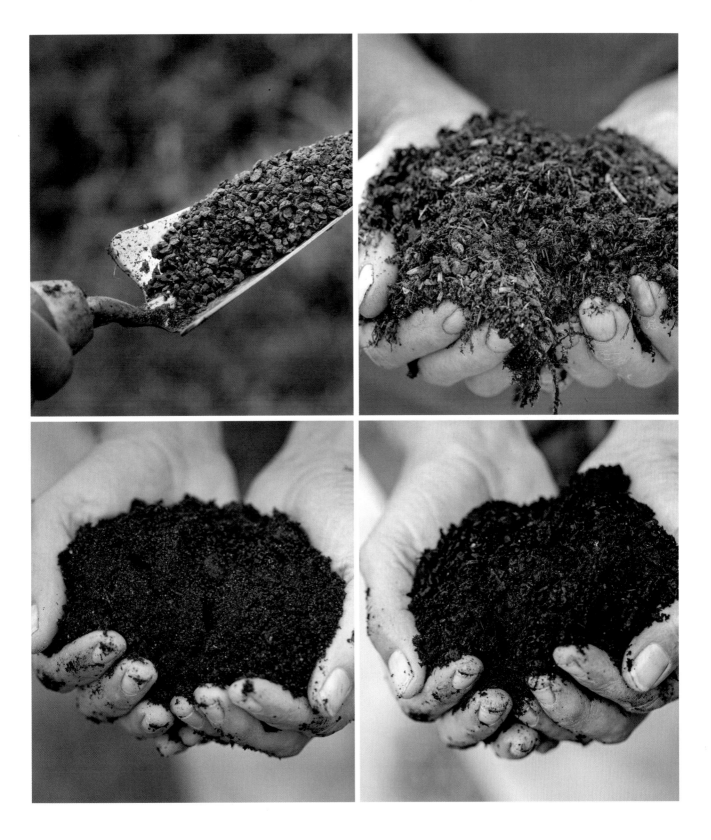

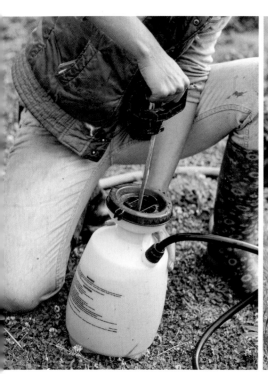
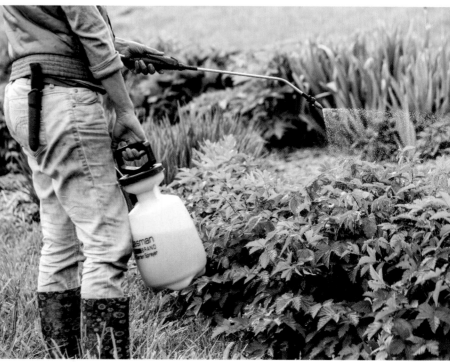

wash away the goodness.) Apply the spray evenly to the point of dripping; it's okay if the fertilizer drips down to the roots. Spot-test each species before spraying, and wait two to three days to see whether the plants respond negatively to the spray, as reactions vary among species. These sprays are quite stinky; avoid contact with clothing or skin if possible. Depending on your soil fertility, you may want to spray when plants are young or rapidly growing, or you may want to spray your plants every few weeks. When I had my herbal nursery, we sprayed our seedlings with a highly diluted fish and seaweed emulsion every three days. If you're going to spray that frequently, dilute your fertilizer beyond the recommended rate—it should be *highly* dilute. Just remember that foliar feeding doesn't feed the soil as other methods of amending and fertilizing do.

### Herbal Fertilizers

Herbs that are exceptionally high in minerals can be used to fertilize the rest of the garden. It's quite the party trick to grow your own fertilizer! Herbs and weeds that are considered nutritious for humans—that are high in minerals—likely also contain a variety of plant nutrients. Nettles, chickweed, and horsetail are commonly used, as are plain old weeds. The foliage of nettles is rich in nitrogen and even higher in potassium. Horsetail is high in silica and is a traditional fungicide against powdery mildew and damping-off in seedlings. Nettles, chickweed, and horsetail regrow quickly and can all be cut repeatedly throughout the growing season. There are several ways to use herbal fertilizers in your garden. The easiest method is to add an herb's foliage directly to your compost pile. Finally, you can make a tea and apply it as a foliar feed or liquid fertilizer. To prepare

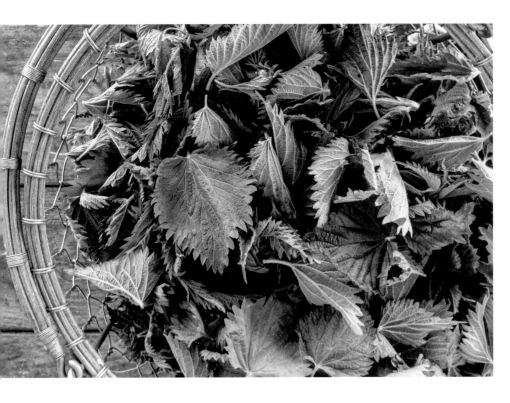

*Left to right:* Pumping air into a pressurized spray bottle in preparation for foliar feeding; foliar feeding meadowsweet plants with a homemade herbal fertilizer; stinging nettles (*Urtica dioica*)

an herbal fertilization tea, soak the leaves in a bucket of cold water for a few days, strain through an old pillowcase, and spray, following the directions above.

Alternatively, if you let the leaves sit longer, fermentation will take place. Fermenting the plant material increases the potency of the fertilizer and also introduces beneficial bacteria. Fermented herbal fertilizers are stink city—smelling distinctly like the morning breath of an ogre who's never met a toothbrush—so be sure to place them out of olfactory range while they ferment and when storing. Depending on the recipe you use, you'll need to dilute these homemade fertilizers before foliar feeding or fertilizing with them.

To make a fermented botanical fertilizer, take a food-grade 5-gallon bucket, a barrel, or a trashcan and fill it halfway with plant material (leaves and stems). You can use a blend of herbs and weeds or let one rock-star plant shine. Weigh down the plant material with bricks. Fill the container full with water and cover with a loose cloth tied around the edges to keep out critters and insects. Then loosely cover with a tarp to keep out the rain and reduce odors. Let sit for three to six weeks in the shade, and then strain through an old T-shirt or pillowcase. To use as a foliar spray, dilute the fermented tea with 15 times as much water (1 part fertilizer to 15 parts water). Make sure the color of your spray is no darker than weak iced black tea. Be sure to spot-test a few leaves before you spray a wide area. To add the fertilizer to the soil, dilute the fermented tea with five times as much water (1 part fertilizer to 5 parts water); avoid allowing it to touch the foliage of garden plants. (Note: Comfrey is a common ingredient in botanical fertilizers. See the discussion on page 201 regarding the possible transfer of harmful compounds into the fertilizer.)

# Cover Crops, Nitrogen Fixers, & Dynamic Accumulators

When we understand the soil in our gardens as a colorful tapestry woven from countless life-forms, we can blossom into dexterous gardeners. By growing plants imbued with exceptional qualities—cover crops, nitrogen-fixing plants, and dynamic accumulators—in addition to everyday garden herbs and vegetables, we can grow our own organic matter, enrich the soil, and nourish the other plants in our garden.

## Cover Crops and Green Manures

Cover crops—a foundational feature of organic cultivation—contribute to the vitality and fertility of a garden or farm. Traditionally, these are crops that are grown solely for their benefit to the soil rather than food or medicine, although we'll be discussing some that you can use for medicine as a secondary function. The benefits of these plants include weed suppression, production of biomass, nitrogen fixation, soil retention, and loosening of heavy soil. When we till them into the soil, they are termed "green manures," and some people use the terms interchangeably. Planting cover crops increases the sustainability of a farm or garden, as they can take the place of resources that are typically found off-site, such as manure, soil conditioner, and amendments, lowering the amount of outside material you have to bring in. And if you grow medicinal cover crops, you'll be taking full advantage of these plants' merits!

There are several strategies for fitting cover crops into your garden. You can plant them in winter or very early spring, when food or medicine crops are not yet in the ground. Or you can incorporate them into a rotational system, with beds allocated for food or medicine production one year and planted with a cover crop in alternate years. Additionally, they can be interplanted with a vegetable or herb crop, such as red clover grown in between rows of corn or undersown in an orchard.

## Nitrogen-Fixing Plants

Some plants have a superpower: they're able to convert atmospheric nitrogen into a biologically active form of this plant nutrient and make it available for their own growth processes. Our planet is basically swimming in nitrogen (nitrogen gas comprises 78 percent of the air we breathe), yet it is the most common limiting factor for plant growth. Despite nitrogen's abundance in the air, it isn't readily available for plants to use as a nutrient. (Chemically speaking, the two nitrogen atoms in nitrogen gas are quite satisfied with their relationship and are not easily distracted from each other.) Needless to say, nitrogen fixation is quite the magic trick, and like most good works, it is brought about by the efforts of many. Plants cannot convert, or "fix," nitrogen on their own. They need the help of microscopic bacteria, who are the actual alchemists, transforming the nitrogen in the air ($N_2$) into ammonium ($NH_4$), an especially useful compound for plants. Nitrogen-fixing plants set up housekeeping with

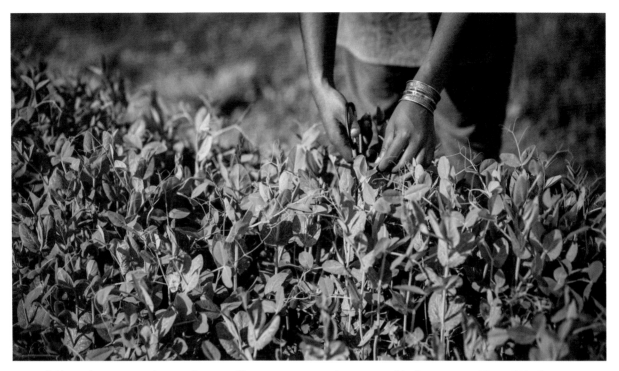

Winter field peas (*Pisum sativum*) are my favorite cold-season cover crop. They grow quickly, fix nitrogen, and have edible shoots that can be eaten raw or cooked.

these soil minions, offering them shelter and nutrients produced through photosynthesis in return for the valuable nitrogen produced and shared by these cohabitating bacteria.

The pea, or legume, family (Fabaceae) is known for its nitrogen-fixation capabilities. Close to 90 percent of Fabaceae members form "associations," or symbiotic relations, with soil bacteria called *rhizobia*. These associations are found in specialized nodules on the plant's roots—visible to the naked eye, they resemble little pearls strung along the length of the roots. If you cut open a nodule, you're essentially opening a "Whoville" composed of millions of beneficial bacteria, and you might even hear them cursing your curiosity if you listen closely. Common nitrogen-fixing medicinal cover crops include red clover and alfalfa. Some lesser-known nitrogen-fixing medicinal herbs include fenugreek, licorice, astragalus, mimosa, and wild indigo—these are described below.

INOCULATING NITROGEN-FIXING PLANTS. To encourage nitrogen fixation, at the time of planting you'll want to add nitrogen-fixing bacteria, in the form of inoculant, to the soil around the roots or seeds of nitrogen-fixing plants. Inoculant is typically sold in powder form at farm and garden supply stores. The bacteria found in the inoculant quickly multiply and begin forming root nodules, helping the plants they're associated with to grow. You can add the inoculant powder directly to the furrow at time of planting or moisten the seeds in a plastic

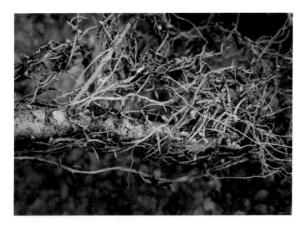

Rhizobia (the nipple-looking structures on this root) are "Whovilles" of nitrogen fixation.

bag, add the powder, and shake until the seeds are evenly coated. Follow the directions on the label for application rates. It's essential to match the type of inoculant with your specific plant. It's easy enough to match bean family cover crops and food crops with their correct inoculant, but you need to pay more attention with herbs. Choose the clover inoculant for red clover and Dutch white clover; alfalfa takes the same inoculant as clover. Use a cowpea inoculant for wild indigo and a milkvetch inoculant for astragalus. Prairie Moon Nursery (prairiemoon.com) sells specific inoculants for the following genera: *Astragalus*, *Baptisia*, and *Glycyrrhiza*.

SHARING THE BOUNTY OF NITROGEN WITH THE GARDEN. These garden superstars can serve as "fertilizer" for other plants. Nitrogen-fixing shrubs, trees, and perennials can be planted throughout the garden. If the plants are deciduous, their leaf droppings enrich the soil. Another way to share the nitrogenous bounty of shrubs and trees is to cut their woody portions back periodically. When you prune a woody shrub or tree, there is a proportional die-off of the root system. The dead portion of the roots decomposes, releasing nitrogen into the soil. This periodic release of nitrogen is appropriate for red root, mimosa, sweetfern, and bayberry. Consider planting smaller deciduous perennials, such as astragalus and licorice, in between rows of other perennial medicinals and letting the dropped leaves enrich the soil. Annual nitrogen fixers, such as fenugreek and alfalfa, can be incorporated into the ground or left as a mulch. Finally, nitrogen-rich cover crops can be mowed and left in place as mulch or added to compost piles.

## Nitrogen-Fixing Medicinal Herbs

FENUGREEK (*Trigonella foenum-graecum*) is a famous spice plant native to the Middle East. It's grown as an annual cover crop to help break up clayey soils and fix nitrogen. Sow the seeds from spring to late summer directly in prepared garden beds that receive full sun. You can eat the greens as sprouts or microgreens, and the tender young shoots are tasty as a cooking green. The seeds are a versatile medicinal, used in the treatment of respiratory conditions, digestive upset, reproductive hormonal imbalance, heart conditions, and diabetes. Fenugreek seed is one of the best breast milk promoters you'll find. The seed is hypoglycemic (lowers blood sugar), so diabetics must be careful to monitor blood sugar closely and consult with a medical practitioner. Do not use high doses of the seed in pregnancy (culinary use is fine).

---

*Upper image:* Harvesting mimosa (*Albizia julibrissin*) flowers
*Bottom left to right:* Fenugreek (*Trigonella foenum-graecum*); red clover (*Trifolium pratense*); wild indigo (*Baptisia tinctoria*)

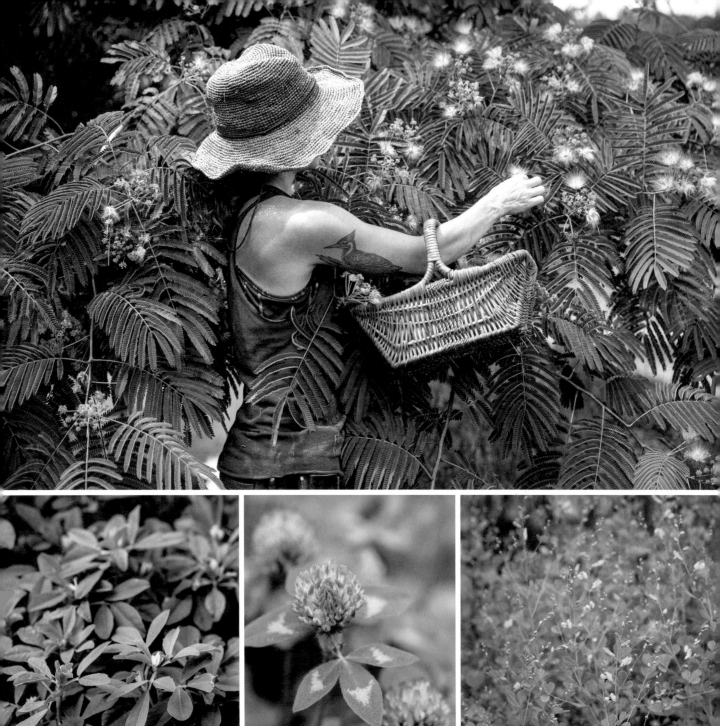
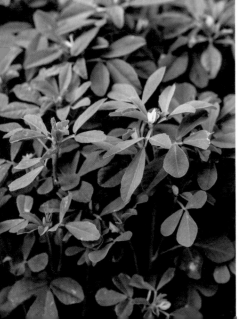
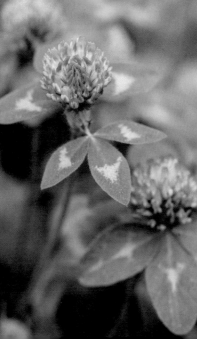
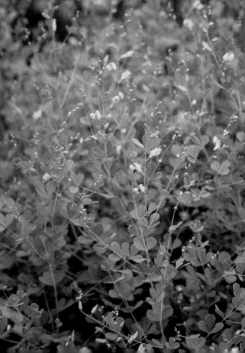

LICORICE (*Glycyrrhiza glabra*) has a rich tradition as a medicinal herb in India, China, and Europe. Common licorice is native to the Mediterranean and Russia and is an herbaceous perennial that spreads by stolons. It can be grown in zones 8–10. It does well in arid, full-sun conditions, with acidic to alkaline soils. The sweet-tasting root possesses a legion of medicinal actions, including demulcent, anti-inflammatory, carminative, phytoestrogen, expectorant, and alterative (see page 196 for definitions). It's a premier remedy for those who run dry, especially in the sinuses and lungs. Licorice is one of my favorite internal anti-inflammatory medicines for treating poison ivy or poison oak. Be aware that licorice has a fair number of medicinal contraindications. Those with congestive heart failure, high blood pressure, liver disorders, heart disorders with edema, and water retention, or edema, should avoid it. Do not use either licorice species during pregnancy.

CHINESE LICORICE (*G. uralensis*) is a cold-hardy herbaceous perennial native to China and Siberia. It prefers full sun and well-drained soil and will grow in zones 3–10. According to medicinal herb cultivation guru Richo Cech, it thrives on neglect. When happy, it can spread assertively and may require a root barrier to keep it from taking over. Chinese licorice is more cold-hardy than common licorice. Another species of Chinese licorice (*G. yunnanensis*) is hardy to zone 6; it is sometimes substituted for other licorice species in Chinese medicine.

ALFALFA (*Medicago sativa*) is a purple-flowered perennial native to the Middle East. It's grown as a cover crop and fodder plant throughout the world. As a forage plant, it's a premier choice for dairy cows to increase milk production. Alfalfa helps break up heavy soils, and the flowers are a good nectar source for many species of bees and butterflies. The leaves are employed medicinally as an all-purpose nutritive tonic. It is a traditional remedy for anemia, weakness, and fatigue. Alfalfa is typically planted as a perennial cover crop in the early spring in full sun.

ASTRAGALUS (*Astragalus propinquus*) is a prized tonic medicinal native to China. Also called *huang-qi*, the root is an immune supporter and respiratory herb. Astragalus root has a pleasant, sweet, "beany" flavor and can be used to make soup stock all throughout the winter. (See the Herbal Immunity Broth Concentrate on page 174.) Astragalus is an herbaceous perennial preferring well-drained, loose soil without a lot of fertility. Plant it in full sun to partial shade in zones 4–9. Astragalus is a long-term garden proposition, as the root is typically harvested in the fall of its third to fifth years.

MIMOSA (*Albizia julibrissin*) is a small, charismatic tree with pink powderpuff blooms. Native to Asia, its bark and flowers are revered in Chinese medicine as a remedy for disorders of the spirit—grief, loss, anxiety, insomnia, depression, and irritability. The bark and flowers are also used topically and internally as an anti-inflammatory. Mimosa can be quite invasive, especially in the southeastern United States and parts of the southwestern United States. Research this issue thoroughly at the Center for Invasive Species and Ecosystem Health (invasive.org) before planting. Plant the tree in full sun to partial shade; it tolerates a wide variety of soil types, from sandy to clayey. Mimosa grows in zones 6–9 and is quite forgiving of drought and summer heat.

RED CLOVER (*Trifolium pratense*) is one of the most commonly grown cover crops, as it produces ample biomass, fixes nitrogen, suppresses weeds, and breaks up heavy clay soil. The flower heads of red clover are used medicinally as a blood cleanser,

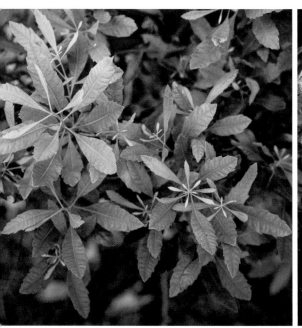 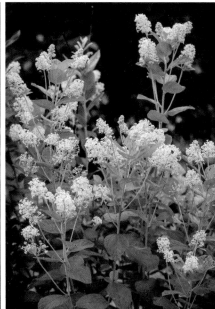 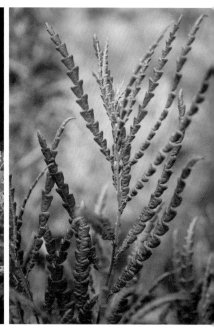

*Left to right:* Bayberry (*Morella cerifera*); red root (*Ceanothus americanus*); sweetfern (*Comptonia peregrina*)

cough remedy, and fertility and nutritive tonic. It is a short-lived perennial and is winter-hardy to zone 4. In the United States, red clover is grown as a winter annual in the Southeast and Pacific Northwest (zones 7 and warmer).

WILD INDIGO (*Baptisia tinctoria*) is a drought-tolerant herbaceous perennial, native to eastern and central North America, that grows in zones 3–9. It is adorned with blue-green leaves and little yellow, pea-like flowers. Its root is a potent antimicrobial and immune stimulant; it has been used to fight infections for centuries. Wild indigo is quite happy in soils that other plants scoff at—it does well in dry, rocky, and sandy soils. It's suited for harsh urban conditions (think median or hell strip) as well as rock outcroppings. Plant in full sun to part shade.

## The Non-Legume Nitrogen Fixers: Actinorhizal Plants

There is a lesser-known group of plants—called actinorhizal plants—that use a different mode of nitrogen fixation from legumes. Instead of root nodules, actinorhizal plants form symbiotic relationships with *actinomycetes* in the genus *Frankia*. Examples of medicinal actinorhizal plants include bayberry, sweet gale, sweetfern, and red root. The oleaster family (Elaeagnaceae) also fixes nitrogen in this fashion. The oleaster family includes notable edible members sea buckthorn, autumn olive, and gumi, and is thus popular in permaculture settings for its versatility in fixing nitrogen and producing highly nutritious fruit. At the time of this writing, there is no commercially available source of inoculant for the *Frankia* bacteria. When I plant actinorhizal plants, I add a bit of soil to use as an inoculant, dug from neighboring plants of the same species if possible.

## Actinorhizal Nitrogen-Fixing Medicinal Herbs

BAYBERRY, WAX MYRTLE, AND SWEET GALE (*Morella cerifera* and other *Morella* species; formerly *Myrica* spp.) are a group of aromatic shrubs that grow in sandy to damp but well-drained soil. Southern bayberry is one of the first medicinals I learned to identify, with its distinctive golden-dotted leaves and copious clusters of white, waxy fruit. The *Morella* genus is well known for its medicinal root bark, which is an unusual combination of astringent and warming aromatic spiciness. The tea and tincture of bayberry are used internally to alleviate sinus congestion, sore gums, periodontal disease, gastrointestinal inflammation, sore throat, and diarrhea. In the hot and humid climate of the southeastern United States, wax myrtle is popular as a low-maintenance ornamental evergreen hedge in parking lots, in woody landscapes, and along roadsides. I recommend researching the *Morella* species native to your area to find the right species for your climate, keeping in mind they vary in medicinal strength and traditional usage. (Note: Most botanists now place these shrubs in the *Morella* genus instead of *Myrica*; *Myrica gale* is an exception and remains in the old genus.)

SWEETFERN (*Comptonia peregrina*) is a low-growing aromatic medicinal shrub with softly toothed, feathery leaves. Rub your hand along its resinous foliage, and you'll be rewarded with its golden, sweet, and spicy aroma. Sweetfern is in the same plant family (Myricaceae) as bayberry and sweet gale and is highly useful as a companion plant in medicinal polycultures. It is drought and salt tolerant, a pioneer of disturbed land and infertile soils. Sweetfern leaves are used ceremonially by the Chippewa, and the smoke is a Potawatomi remedy for warding away biting insects. The astringent and warming tea made from the leaves is a remedy for diarrhea, intestinal cramps, and respiratory congestion. Perhaps the most popular use of sweetfern is as a wash to treat poison ivy. Plant sweetfern in full sun to light shade in dry to moist, well-drained sandy or rocky soil. It prefers slightly acidic to neutral soil in zones 2–7.

## Dynamic Accumulators

Plants that are dynamic accumulators mine nutrients such as nitrogen, potassium, phosphorus, and calcium from the soil, concentrating them in their leaves and then releasing the nutrients when the plants die or shed leaves. Many dynamic accumulators have deep taproots and act to break up the soil in addition to enriching it. Some accumulators are colonizers of disturbed soil and are especially adept at optimizing their own nutrition in poor soils, even without deep roots.

### Examples of Herbal Dynamic Accumulators

Alfalfa (*Medicago sativa*)

Chickweed (*Stellaria media*)

Comfrey (*Symphytum officinale*)

Dandelion (*Taraxacum officinale*)

German chamomile (*Matricaria recutita*)

Horsetail (*Equisetum* spp.)

Licorice (*Glycyrrhiza glabra*)

Linden (*Tilia* spp.)

Red clover (*Trifolium pratense*)

Stinging nettles (*Urtica dioica*)

Yarrow (*Achillea millefolium*)

Yellow dock and Sorrel (*Rumex* spp.)

# Composting

The compost pile fully embodies renewal: death and decay are transformed into a vital substance that can then nourish new life. In its purest essence, compost is degraded waste from the garden, yard, kitchen, or farm animals. Compost is aptly called "black gold" by gardeners because it improves the texture of soil and adds to soil fertility with essential nutrients and beneficial microorganisms. When added to sandy soils, it helps with moisture and nutrient retention, and when added to heavy soils, it "lightens" the earth by improving garden tilth. It's easy to make (the microbes and worms make it for you), requiring little upkeep and attention.

The first step is picking a composting system. There are plenty of choices, but, as a universal principle, it's helpful to have two rotating piles going at once: the first pile is where you're actively adding ingredients, and the second pile is "resting," in a state of decomposition. When the second pile is done composting, you'll add the finished compost to the garden, and that section will then become the active pile (where you add ingredients), while the other pile decomposes.

COMPOSTING SETUPS. You'll want to place your compost piles outdoors away from walkways or recreational areas, but not so far that they will be neglected. Compost needs air and moisture, so it's helpful if your setup allows for rainfall and airflow into the ingredients. An important consideration when choosing a setup is the unwanted critters you might attract, which might include dogs, opossums, raccoons, and rats or other rodents. If you live in an urban area with high rodent pressure, consider plastic tumbler bins, which are easy to turn

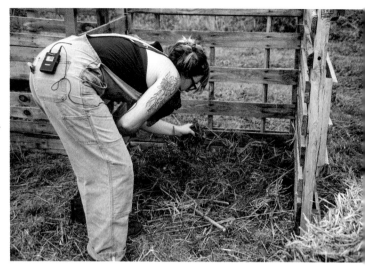

Layering browns and greens in a compost system made from repurposed pallets

and deter whiskered neighbors. Perhaps the most straightforward system is a wire circle, 3 feet in diameter, constructed of chicken wire or hardware cloth supported by stakes and fastened with wire. You can place two wire circles side by side. Pallets are available for cheap or free and can be used to construct three- or four-sided enclosures, fastened with chicken wire. Just be sure the pallets aren't constructed from pressure-treated wood (look for the green sheen, characteristic of pressure-treated lumber), which can leach toxins into your pile.

COMPOSTING 101. Heat, air, and moisture are necessary for happy, hardworking microbes and a productive compost heap. The more active the bacteria and fungi are, the speedier the decomposition process. You can introduce microbes to your pile by periodically adding a small amount of garden soil. Fermented herbal fertilizer (described on page 53) will also do the trick. Aerate the pile by turning it over monthly with a shovel or digging fork and

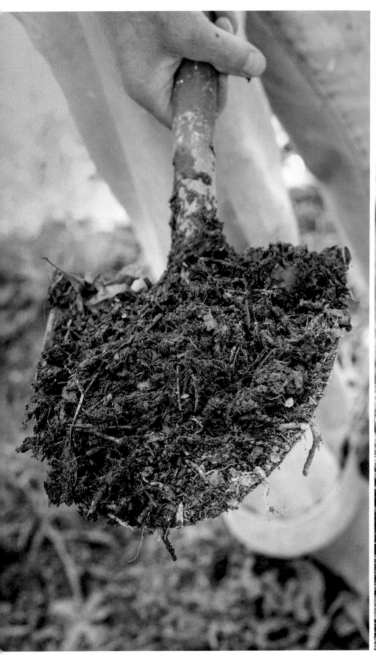

Composted leaf mold

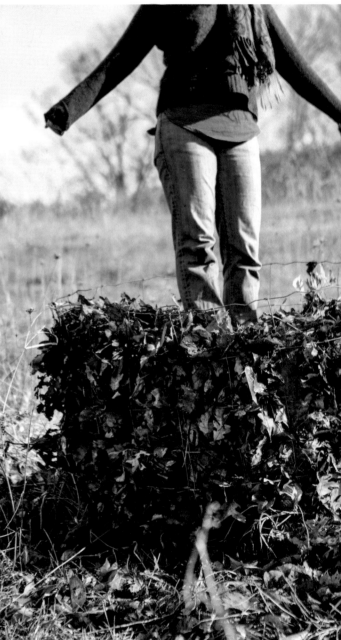

Leaf pile to be composted into leaf mold

layering in small sticks from time to time to allow for proper oxygenation. In the warmer months, when the microbes are active, water the heap during dry periods. If you live in an arid climate, cover the pile with a tarp to keep in moisture, and water every week or two. Conversely, too much moisture dampens the mood at the bacterial shindig; keep the compost heap covered during extreme downpours.

COMPOSTING INGREDIENTS. To feed your composting microbes, you'll want to dish up a blend of nitrogen-rich (green) and carbon-rich (brown) ingredients. Striking the right balance of nitrogen and carbon speeds along the decomposition process. "Green" ingredients include vegetable and fruit scraps, grass clippings, and weeds. Nitrogen-rich manure is considered a "green" ingredient (which can certainly be confusing because it's brown in color). Oftentimes, manure from farming stalls (delivered by the truckload) will contain bedding material (mulch or straw) and will thus be a mix of greens and browns. Bagged manure is often already composted. "Brown" ingredients include straw, hay, fall leaves, wood chips, and small twigs. To get the party started, layer ingredients in your compost in a 2:1 ratio, with 2 parts green ingredients for each 1 part brown ingredients. It's helpful to keep a pile of leaves, hay, or straw next to the compost area. That way, when you add some kitchen scraps, you can easily layer "brown" ingredients on top. Remember to periodically add soil or fermented herbal fertilizer, and keep the pile fresh by turning it over with a digging fork every month. No-no's of the pile include meat and dairy scraps, pet and human feces, invasive weeds that have gone to seed, and diseased garden plants.

ADDING COMPOST TO THE GARDEN. Depending on your expertise and level of attention, your compost will be ready in six months to one year. When it looks like rich, dark soil—without odors or visible vegetable scraps—you'll know it's ready for the garden. You can then add the compost to the garden by digging it into the soil, applying it as a side-dressing, or using it as a nutrient-rich mulch (it won't suppress weeds unless you cover it with a coarse mulch, like bark mulch).

## Leaf Mold

Made solely of decomposed leaves, this fertile soil amendment helps improve the tilth and water-absorbing qualities of soils and feeds the teeming underground menagerie of microbes and earthworms and builds the crown jewel of organic matter: humus. Leaf mold is one of the best amendments for growing woodland medicinal herbs.

Compost fall leaves in any of the compost setups listed above—it will take one to two years for the leaves to fully degrade into leaf mold. Speed the process along by mowing over the leaves several times with a lawnmower before composting them to shred them into smaller, easier-to-degrade pieces (it's fine if you get some grass clippings mixed in). While you don't need to add any "greens" to fallen leaves, if you add a bit of a high-nitrogen material, such as composted chicken manure or fish meal, it will speed up the decomposition process. When leaf mold is ready to use, it is dark and crumbly. If it's only partially decomposed, you can use it as a slow-release nutritive mulch. Be sure to keep the pile moist during the growing season.

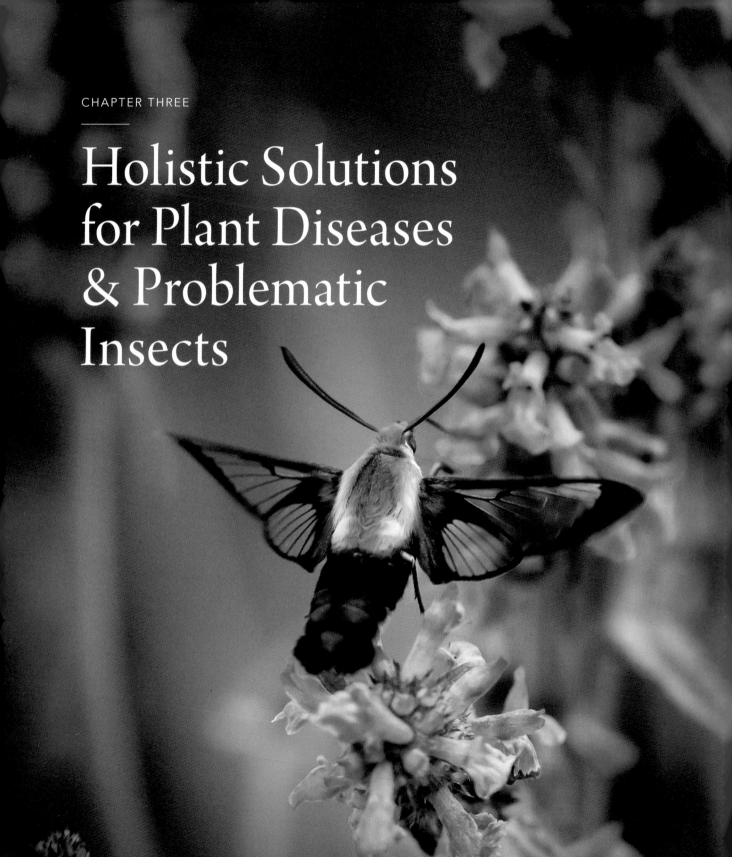

CHAPTER THREE

# Holistic Solutions for Plant Diseases & Problematic Insects

> Teach me every language of
> the creatures that sing to me,
> That I may count the cadence of
> Infinite lessons in harmony.
>
> ~ Jamie Sams, *Making Family*

I am a laid-back gardener. I don't get riled up when I see a few disfigured leaves, and honestly, I rarely take any action against problem insects that show up in my garden. Now, this approach is a luxury of *not* bringing herbs to the marketplace—farmers, by necessity, need to be more assertive with pest and disease issues because crop failure can be economically devastating. Similarly, when I operated my commercial nursery, I had to be more vigilant about slugs, aphids, flea beetles, and the like because people don't want to buy munched-up plant starts. But now that I grow solely for my own kitchen and apothecary, I've consciously adopted a laissez-faire approach toward garden problems.

    I focus on growing the healthiest plants possible, knowing that they'll be more likely to resist pests and diseases, rather than putting my attention toward garden problems, although, realistically, these need to be addressed from time to time in any garden, no matter how experienced the gardener. Gardens rich with different plant species and a variety of habitats for beneficial insects are going to be more resilient than a field containing only one crop. While I do sometimes use organic pest sprays, my primary strategies reside in the realm of preventive medicine. My mainstays of disease and pest management include fostering plant diversity, building soil fertility, and encouraging beneficial insects to move in and take care of garden rascals for me. That's not to say that I ignore the health and happiness of my plants—I simply don't react to "sniffles and sneezes," and instead encourage plant "immunity" through sound organic gardening practices.

I try to take the long view when considering how my actions will affect other organisms that I share this beautiful planet with. Therefore, I don't turn to chemical pesticides or fungicides, even if they might provide an immediate fix to the problem at hand. These chemical "solutions" will eventually cause newer and bigger problems: harm to life-forms and elements that my plants (and my human family and neighbors) count on. We're going to explore the topic of pest and disease management from this holistic and long-term perspective. We'll begin with preventive garden practices, like encouraging biodiversity, then home in on creating welcoming habitats for beneficial garden insects, and finally, we'll explore sustainable ways to address common garden problems.

## Preventive Garden Practices Minimize Disease and Pest Problems

**1** BUILD HEALTHY SOIL. This is the single most important thing you can do to prevent problems in your garden. Nourished plants are resilient plants. Add organic matter to your soil, grow cover crops, and encourage soil biodiversity (bacteria, worms, mycorrhizae, and more) through the addition of worm castings, compost, leaf mold, mulch, and inoculants. Be sure that your soil doesn't have nutrient deficiencies or pH imbalances—both of which can compromise plant "immunity." See Chapter Two for information on building soil fertility.

**2** MULCH IS MIRACULOUS. I've already waxed poetic over mulch's virtuous nature, but it bears repeating, as mulch truly encourages overall garden vitality. Mulch helps keep the soil moist and cool in sweltering summer heat, which makes life easier for plant roots and beneficial soil microorganisms. Mulch can also help prevent soil-borne pathogenic microbes from splashing up on plant leaves and provide habitat for beneficial ground beetles and spiders.

**3** DON'T FIGHT THE CURRENT. This is one of my primary garden strategies: accepting "what is" and having the grace to adapt to reality. One of the easiest ways to practice "garden Zen" is to choose plants that do well in your climate. Ask nearby herb growers and nurseries which plants thrive in your area. If you have an especially problematic insect in your region, some plants will be susceptible, while others aren't affected at all. Sometimes, going with the current means changing the time when you harvest an herb. One example of this approach involves red bee balm. Typically, bee balm is harvested when

---

*Clockwise from top left:* A legion of freshly hatched praying mantises, garden predator-ettes; anise hyssop is literally abuzz and aflutter with pollinators all day long; praying mantis on a wild bergamot (*Monarda fistulosa*); toads help balance insect populations in the garden and moonlight as diversions for young gardeners; soldier beetles, beneficial garden insects, enjoying a special moment on yarrow (*Achillea millefolium*); flower fly, or syrphid fly, on a calendula (*Calendula officinalis*)

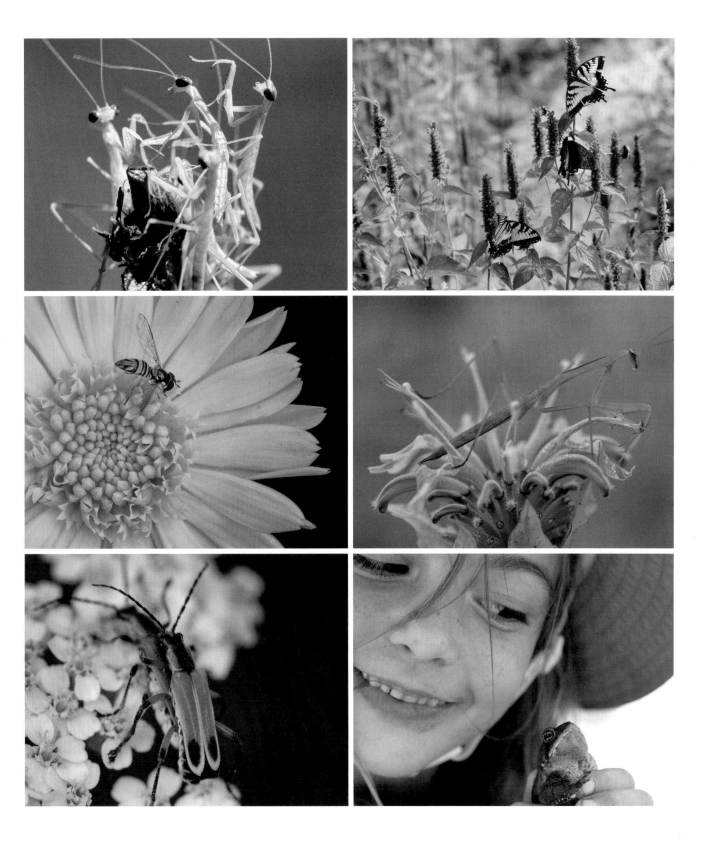

it's in full flower, and the leaves and flowers are used for medicine. But in my garden, by the time the bee balm is bold with crimson blooms, the leaves are covered with a white fuzzy coating from powdery mildew, making the plant unharvestable. I could vigilantly spray a natural fungicide on my bee balm plants to keep the fungal disease at bay, but honestly, in my hot and humid climate, it's hard to control. So instead, I simply harvest the plant earlier in the season, before the powdery mildew has crashed the party. The flowers aren't affected by the powdery mildew, so I harvest them separately and combine them with the dried leaves.

**4** PLANT HEALTHY STARTS. Plants that are stunted, root-bound, or runty often stay that way, and they are at higher risk for disease and predation. Healthy plants look perky: they fit their container, are compact, and possess a vital-looking green hue. Plant vibrant starts in the late afternoon, and water them frequently until they're established.

**5** REMOVE DISEASED PLANT MATERIAL. Walk through your garden in the early morning, taking in the beauty and also noting any diseased plants. When plants show an affliction, cut off the diseased portions or even pull out whole plants, if necessary, before the problem spreads. Don't throw these compromised plants onto the compost pile, though, as many pathogenic organisms can survive the temperatures of home compost piles. Instead, "solarize-murderize" the plant material by placing it in a black plastic bag, securing the bag tightly, and leaving it in the sun for a few weeks. The high temperatures will kill any spores, viruses, or bacteria. You can then compost or burn the plant material. Alternatively, you can place small amounts of diseased plants in the garbage.

**6** ROTATE CROPS. Change up the annuals you plant in one area to minimize the transfer of disease and pest problems that may be lingering from previous years in the form of insect eggs, soil larvae, or microbes.

**7** PLANT FOR DIVERSITY. When plants are grouped with only their kind, they are easy targets for pathogens and problem insects. Conversely, when plants are interspersed with other species, it's more challenging for diseases and insects to spread. Read more about interplanting in Chapter One.

**8** COMPANION PLANTS ARE NEIGHBORLY. Some plants are extraordinary companions— exemplary neighbors to the other plants in your garden. Their helpful qualities include deterring potential garden pests through aromatic compounds, creating habitat for beneficial insects that prey on problem pests, attracting and feeding beneficial insects with their flowers, and luring pollinators to the garden, which help to increase fruit set in vegetable and fruit crops. You'll find many of these herbs are in the carrot, mint, and aster families. Beneficial herbal companion plants include dill, fennel, cilantro, angelica, khella seed, calendula, feverfew, chamomile, borage, goldenrod, boneset, basil, tulsi, anise hyssop, bee balm, wild bergamot, and yarrow.

# Attracting & Nourishing Garden Beneficials

Rather than spend our energy on killing problem insects whose numbers have gotten out of hand, we can call in their predators to do the job for us. The dazzling array of predatory insects in the garden includes ladybugs, tachinid flies, parasitoid (or parasitic) wasps, damsel bugs, minute pirate bugs, soldier bugs, lacewings, and praying mantises. You can attract—and keep—these critters in your garden in a number of simple ways. The first and foremost step you can take is actually a nonaction: avoid using pesticides (chemical and organic alike), which kill both beneficial insects and pest insects with impunity.

We can provide a safe harbor for our friendly minions by planting a variety of shrubs, herbs, and trees, giving them plenty of nooks and crannies to serve as hiding places from their own predators. Beneficial insects also need water, which you can provide through small ponds or birdbaths with little rock perches so they can safely land and drink. Friendly garden insects aren't always exclusive carnivores: some species also sip nectar or munch on pollen. Some are predators in their larval form, while the adults take a more vegetarian view. Availability of nectar and pollen typically increase the life span—and voraciousness—of friendly predators, and in some cases, these plant nutrients are integral to their reproductive cycles. I've created a handy chart for attracting beneficial insects to the herb garden, which you can find in the Healing Garden Gateway. By planting herbs, shrubs, and trees that have long flowering periods and attract a wide variety of pollinators, we're feeding our tiny garden lackeys. These nectary plants are literally abuzz when they're blooming.

## My Favorite Companion Herbs

ANISE HYSSOP (*Agastache foeniculum*) has dense purple floral spikes that are pollinator magnets. This easy-going herb attracts honeybees, bumblebees, masked bees, digger bees, butterflies, moths, hummingbirds, and plenty of other pollinators.

ANGELICA (*Angelica* spp.) plants are large, striking members of the carrot family. Angelica's massive globes of minute flowers attract a legion of beneficials into the garden, including ladybugs, tachinid flies, syrphid flies, parasitoid wasps, and minute pirate bugs.

BEE BALM AND WILD BERGAMOT (*Monarda* spp.) are medicinal and culinary herbs native to North America. These showy bloomers are unparalleled for attracting hummingbirds, butterflies, bees, and the stupendous hummingbird moths.

BONESET (*Eupatorium perfoliatum*) is a fuzzy fluff monster in the late summer with its mass of creamy white blooms. It attracts tachinid flies, parasitic wasps, minute pirate bugs, damsel bugs, ladybugs, and many other beneficial insects.

FENNEL (*Foeniculum vulgare*) is a familiar carrot family member with a number of medicinal and culinary uses. The teensy-weensy flowers that make up fennel's yellow umbels are excellent for enticing lacewings, hoverflies, ladybugs, and parasitoid wasps. All fennel varieties are helpful as companion plants.

GOLDENRODS (*Solidago* spp.) are late bloomers, inviting a promenade of helpful insects into the garden late in the season, including soldier beetles, big-eyed bugs, minute pirate bugs, ladybugs, parasitoid wasps, damsel bugs, assassin bugs, and syrphid flies.

YARROW (*Achillea millefolium*) is a prime companion plant, providing shelter as well as nectar and pollen for a variety of beneficials, including ladybugs, lacewings, syrphid flies, parasitoid wasps, and damsel bugs. The ornamental cultivars and the straight species (the wild white) are equally helpful for attracting predatory insects.

## General Nectary Herbs

Alfalfa (*Medicago sativa*)
Angelica (*Angelica* spp.)
Anise hyssop (*Agastache foeniculum*)
Artemisia species (*Artemisia* spp.)
Bayberry (*Morella* spp.)
Bee balm and wild bergamot species (*Monarda* spp.)
Blackberry (*Rubus* spp.)
Boneset (*Eupatorium perfoliatum*)
Butterfly weed (*Asclepias tuberosa*)
Calendula (*Calendula officinalis*)
Chamomile (*Matricaria recutita*)
Chives (*Allium schoenoprasum*)
Cilantro/Coriander (*Coriandrum sativum*)
Comfrey (*Symphytum officinale*)
Common milkweed (*Asclepias syriaca*)
Dandelion (*Taraxacum officinale*)
Dill (*Anethum graveolens*)
Echinacea (*Echinacea* spp.)
Elderberry (*Sambucus canadensis*)
Elecampane (*Inula helenium*)
Fennel (*Foeniculum vulgare*)
Feverfew (*Tanacetum parthenium*)
Goldenrod (*Solidago* spp.)
Lavender (*Lavandula* spp.)
Lemon balm (*Melissa officinalis*)
Licorice (*Glycyrrhiza glabra*)
Linden (*Tilia* spp.)
Lovage (*Levisticum officinale*)
Marshmallow (*Althaea officinalis*)
Mint (*Mentha* spp.)
Oregano (*Origanum vulgare*)
Passionflower (*Passiflora incarnata*)
Prickly pear (*Opuntia* spp.)
Raspberry (*Rubus idaeus*)
Red clover (*Trifolium pratense*)
Red root (*Ceanothus americanus*)
Roselle hibiscus (*Hibiscus sabdariffa*)
Rosemary (*Salvia rosmarinus*)
Thyme (*Thymus vulgaris*)
Tulsi (*Ocimum tenuiflorum*)
Vitex/Chaste tree (*Vitex agnus-castus*)
White sage (*Salvia apiana*)
Wild cherry (*Prunus* spp.)
Wild indigo (*Baptisia tinctoria*)
Yarrow (*Achillea millefolium*)

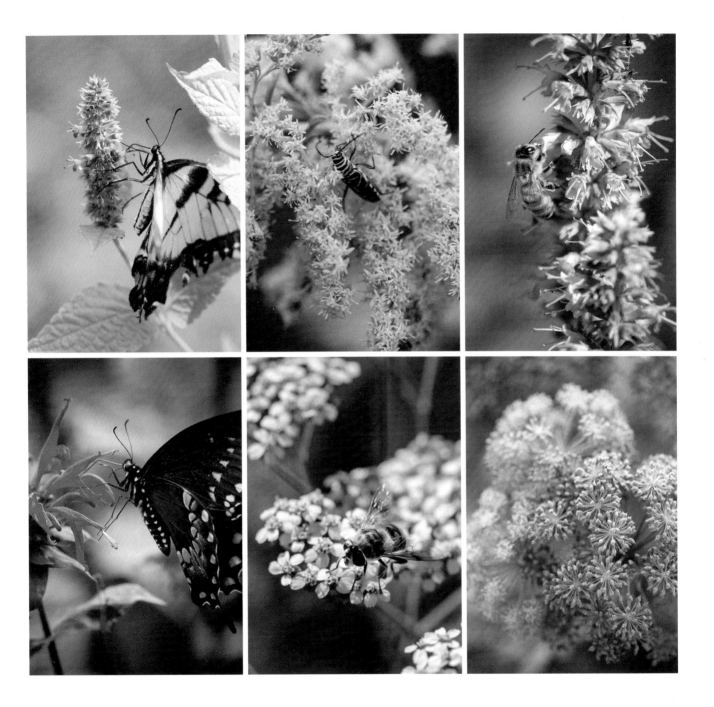

***From left to right:*** Anise hyssop (*Agastache foeniculum*) and nectaring Eastern tiger swallowtail; goldenrod (*Solidago* sp.) and a locust borer; honeybee pollinating licorice mint (*Agastache* sp.); Eastern black swallowtail pollinating a bee balm flower (*Monarda didyma*); hoverfly, or syrphid flies, on yarrow (*Achillea millefolium*); European angelica (*Angelica archangelica*)

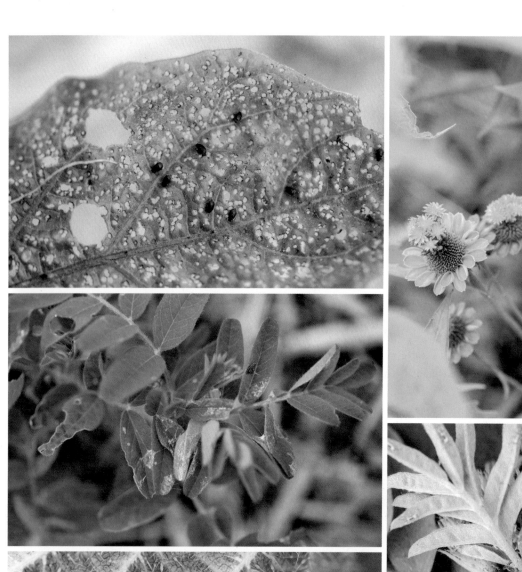
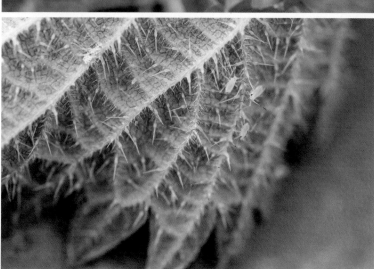
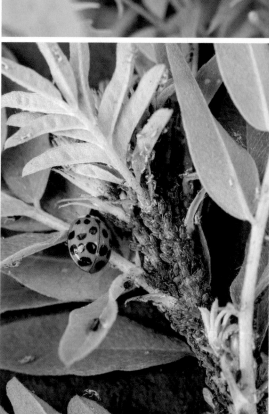

# Strategies for Plant Diseases & Problematic Insects

The first step in healing an ailing plant is identifying the cause, and the sooner you catch a budding problem, the easier it will be to control. Like humans, plants are subject to viral, bacterial, and fungal diseases. Common diseases in herbs include powdery mildew, damping-off, blights, and wilts. The most problematic herb garden pests include aphids, flea beetles, spider mites, scale, mealybugs, caterpillars, slugs, and furry wildlife. Pest and disease problems vary depending on your climate and location. Local experts will have the most knowledge about the likely culprits in your garden. If you live in the U.S., check your Cooperative Extension office or Master Gardeners Association. Other resources include municipal agricultural agencies and local universities.

ASTER YELLOWS. This disease is caused by a bacteria-like protozoan called a phytoplasma. Spread by aster leafhoppers, this nasty disease affects over 300 species of plants, including purple coneflower, calendula, and marigolds. Aster yellows disease causes a deformed appearance to the blooms of flowers (looks like mini flowers growing from a larger flower head) and causes the plant to eventually perish. Pull out any affected plants you find. There are no known cures, and the disease spreads quickly.

*Clockwise from top left:* Close-up of ashwagandha leaf being eaten by flea beetles; aster yellows disease on an Echinacea plant; black aphids feeding on an astragalus plant; green aphids feeding on the underside of a stinging nettle leaf; telltale iridescent slime track and munched leaves from slug activity on an astragalus plant

SLUGS AND SNAILS. Slugs have odd dietary preferences, turning their antennae up at sensible fare—kale, lettuce, and chard—and instead devouring the hairy and bioactive leaves of medicinal herbs such as elecampane, echinacea, and mullein. They also relish anise hyssop, culinary basil, tulsi, and spilanthes. You can identify slug and snail damage by the telltale iridescent sheen and the irregular "munching" holes on the leaves. Control slugs by handpicking at night with a flashlight, reducing mulch, and spreading diatomaceous earth (see page 75).

APHIDS. These minuscule, soft-bodied insects can have a beastly effect on many garden plants, including stinging nettles, gotu kola, calendula, white sage, garden sage, cayenne peppers, and more. Aphids are variably colored, but all have two little tubes protruding from their rear. They prefer to feed on tender young leaves, often on the undersides, and will cause a wrinkled or disfigured appearance to new growth. Wash aphids off plants by spraying with water repeatedly or use a homemade garlic-pepper spray or soap spray (see page 75). Lacewings and ladybugs are predators of aphids.

FLEA BEETLES. These shiny black insects hop like fleas and munch up some vegetable plants, including eggplants, tomatoes, peppers, and broccoli. They also like ashwagandha, belladonna, and henbane (these last two are toxic plants!). The best way to beat flea beetles is to plant large starts later in the season. You can also use a floating row cover with a plastic ground cloth to minimize their presence.

## Damage Control

After you've identified your pest or disease, you'll want to assess how extensive the damage is. If the problem seems isolated, removing afflicted plant parts or whole plants may be sufficient. However, if the problem is widespread, you can invoke some of these simple, natural measures. Mechanical methods of insect control include row covers, bird netting, handpicking, smooshing, trapping, and spraying with water. Nonmechanical means of insect control involve substances that are toxic, unpalatable, or otherwise deterring to problem insects. Organic sprays that repel insects can be purchased or made at home. Keep in mind that insecticide sprays often kill beneficial insects right along with the harmful ones.

Homemade sprays (such as the ones I describe on page 75) are generally safe and nontoxic, although they can be irritants, so protect eyes and tender mucosa when spraying, and keep out of the reach of children and animals. Spot-test and wait 48 hours before a full application to rule out any possible reactions. For smaller applications, use a household spray bottle; for larger areas, use a pressurized spray bottle and wear protective gear. Spray in the morning, and reapply every few days until the issue has cleared up. Alternatively, you can purchase manufactured sprays in garden centers that specialize in organic gardening. If you're not sure whether a product is organic and you live in the United States, look for the OMRI (Organic Materials Review Institute) seal on the label. Just be aware that some OMRI-approved plant-derived pesticides are potentially toxic, including rotenone and pyrethrum/pyrethrins, which I don't recommend using in the home garden.

ROW COVERS. These spun polyester cloths act as a physical barrier to pests. They come in a variety of

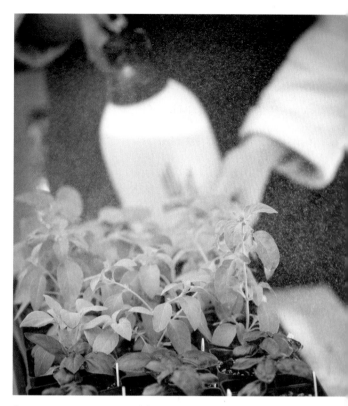

Spraying an organic insecticidal soap solution with a pressurized spray bottle

thicknesses and lengths and are often placed over a framework of wire, split bamboo, or PVC pipes. The loose weave allows for airflow, rainfall, and sunlight to reach the plants. Row covers can also protect plants from cold temperatures and wind, and they help warm the soil. Thicker row covers offer more of a temperature buffer at the cost of excluding more light. Covers can be used for multiple years if stored in a dry, dark location when not in use.

SMUSH OR SPRAY. This technique can help with small soft-bodied pests, such as aphids. Aphids tend to congregate on tender new leaves and are easy to smush. Often a spray of water is enough to dislodge small insects from plants. Repeated sprayings ensure that any returning freeloaders are given the boot.

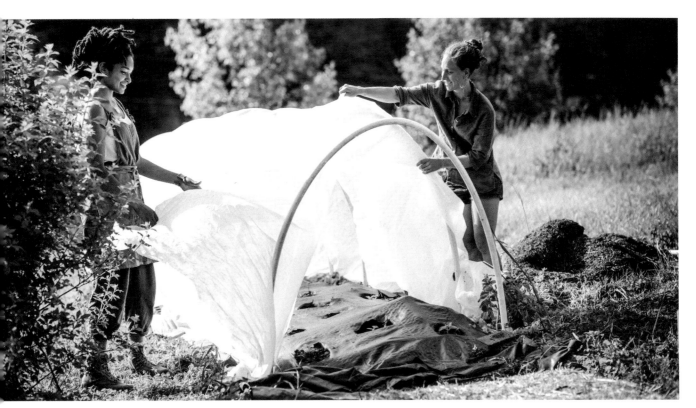

Spun polyester keeps problematic insects away from crops but lets in sunlight, air, and rain.

SOAP SPRAY. Commercially available sprays can be used to control insects such as aphids, whiteflies, mealybugs, spider mites, thrips, and fleas. To make your own, dissolve 3 tablespoons natural, liquid dish soap per 1 gallon of water, and spray as described above. Don't substitute dishwasher soap, and be sure to spot-test, as soap sprays can irritate some plants.

GARLIC AND HOT PEPPER SOAP SPRAY. This all-purpose insecticidal spray can be used to control aphids, thrips, leafminers, spider mites, whiteflies, and leafhoppers. Combine 1 quart of water, 2 fresh jalapeño or Serrano peppers, 7 peeled garlic cloves, and 2 teaspoons of natural dish soap in a blender. Blend and let the slurry infuse overnight. Strain and apply as described above. Refrigerate any unused portions for repeated applications.

DIATOMACEOUS EARTH. This white powder is mined from ancient marine deposits of microscopic sea creatures known as diatoms. Diatomaceous earth (DE) is completely natural and is used to control a number of household and garden pests. Diatoms are largely made up of silica dioxide, so DE acts on insects like teensy shards of glass. Harmless to human skin, it is razor-sharp to fleas, cockroaches, bedbugs, ants, aphids, silverfish, slugs, caterpillars, spider mites, and the newly hatched larvae of Japanese beetles, Mexican bean beetles, and Colorado potato beetles. DE kills beneficial and noxious insects alike. Follow the directions on the packaging for application.

CHAPTER FOUR

# Growing Medicinal Herbs in Containers

If you're tight on garden space, you'll be delighted to know there are bushels of healing plants that you can grow in pots. And even if you have heaps of soil, you'll be pleased to learn about the habitats you can create with containers. By choosing the appropriate planter, soil, and location, you can extend the growing season or simulate a drier or wetter environment, expanding the range of plants you can grow.

If you adorn your deck or porch with potted flowers every spring, there's a multitude of splashy herbs that can stand in for bedding plants. Herbs with edible flowers, such as calendula, pineapple sage, anise hyssop, chives, heart's-ease, and nasturtium, brighten up planters and can add contrast to leafy culinary herbs such as parsley, basil, or sage. I'm partial to the gray foliage of artichoke and the silvery lavender and thyme cultivars. The classic Mediterranean culinary herbs—basil, thyme, sage, parsley, chives, rosemary, and lavender—happily hop into most any container. Place them close to the front or back door to make them easy to reach for when you're cooking. Mint, stinging nettles, bee balm, horsetail, calamus, and jiaogulan are just a few plants that can overtake their surroundings in the garden; rein in these spreading botanicals with a container.

# A Tour of Containers

When selecting a planter, consider its size, shape, and construction. Larger vessels hold in moisture and need to be watered less frequently. In contrast, smaller containers sometimes need to be watered daily. You'll also want to think about how heavy it will be when filled with soil. Shallow, broad pots provide a homey environment for low-growing, spreading herbs like gotu kola, sweet violet, and thyme. Taller planters offer easy access to plants when mobility is a consideration.

BATHTUBS, WASHTUBS, AND SINKS: Retired tubs and sinks are some of the greenest options available, as they're destined for the landfill. They are long-lived, resistant to cracking from temperature fluctuations, and can provide a sizable growing area that holds moisture quite effectively. Know that cast-iron tubs covered with porcelain glazes manufactured before 1995 can contain lead. Reproduction washtubs are a fun option, and many come with a stand, putting the plants in easy reach.

PLASTIC POTS: Plastic nursery pots and food-grade buckets are lightweight, affordable, and sometimes free. The downside of plastic vessels includes their shorter life span and environmental toll. However, landscapers and nurseries often throw out plastic pots, so reuse helps keep them out of landfills. There is a possibility that chemicals, some of which are endocrine disruptors, might leach from the plastic into the soil and enter the plants via their roots, but I haven't found any studies researching this topic.

TERRA-COTTA POTS: Terra-cotta, or clay, pots wick away moisture quickly, so plants in terra-cotta pots need to be watered frequently. Unglazed terra-cotta will crack and break if left outdoors and filled with soil during freezing temperatures.

GLAZED CERAMIC PLANTERS: Offered in a variety of colors and textures, glazed ceramic pots retain more moisture than terra-cotta pots and are less likely to crack during the winter. But they are heavy, expensive, and I suspect some of the glazes may contain lead; however, I haven't been able to verify this, despite extensive research.

FIBER POTS: These natural pots are compostable and made from peat, manure, or pulp by-products. They typically last one season or less. Many people prefer using these over plastic because they are biodegradable, but unfortunately most are manufactured overseas and carry the environmental impact of transportation.

WOODEN CONTAINERS: Wine and whiskey barrels offer charm, a considerable planting area, and superior water retention due to their size. Tall wooden planters (like the one pictured here) also fall into this category; these offer easy access for folks in wheelchairs or with limited mobility. Avoid pressure-treated wood as it contains toxins that leak into the soil.

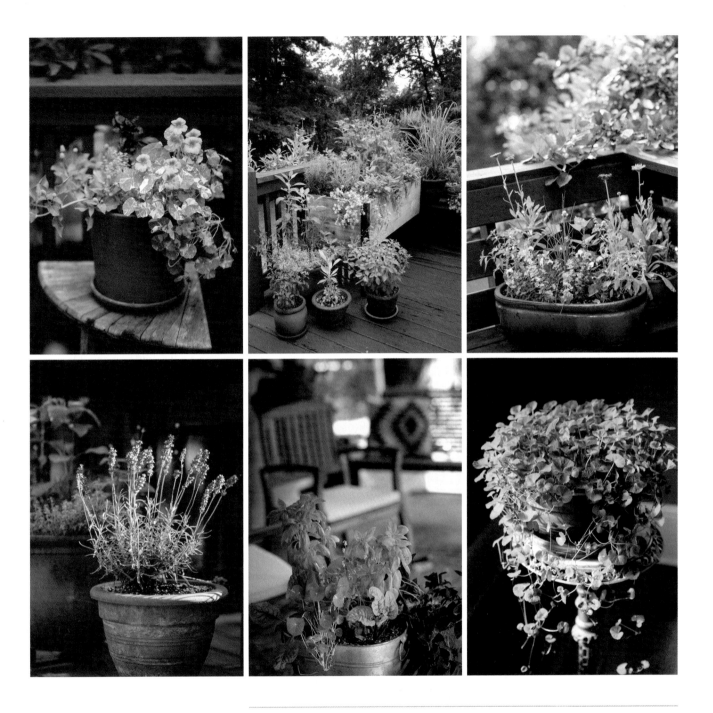

***From left to right:*** Alaska mix nasturtium, yellow spilanthes, hi-ho silver thyme, and amethyst purple basil growing in a terra-cotta pot; large raised wooden planters are helpful for easy access to herbs; lime basil, Oregano 'Kent Beauty', pansies, chives, and calendula growing in a glazed terra-cotta pot; Hidcote lavender 'Super Blue'; Swiss chard, nasturtium, basil, anise hyssop, and European vervain growing in a galvanized steel planter; gotu kola makes a lovely houseplant in the winter and can be brought outside in the summer

## Soil & Drainage Considerations: Keep It Fluffy, Friends

Large containers quickly become waterlogged and heavy through soil compaction. To encourage drainage, add a thick layer of criss-crossed sticks (not rotted) to the bottom of larger pots before adding soil. You'll also want to elevate the pot from the ground with bricks or flat rocks. Garden soil and topsoil are too heavy for container culture. Pine bark fines, when added to soil or potting mix, offer porosity *and* water retention, with a near-neutral pH.

For an optimal all-purpose potting mix, combine 3 parts pine bark fines with 1 part composted manure and ¼ part worm castings, plus organic fertilizer (use the quantity listed on the label). You can reuse the soil from large pots for three seasons by sprucing up the mix annually. Come springtime, I remove and compost the upper fourth layer of potting mix and then freshen up the remaining soil with compost, organic fertilizer, and worm castings.

## Container Culture: Habitat Creation

By altering your soil, type of container, and siting, you can create a variety of habitats and thus invite more herbs into your life. Say you live in a humid climate, but you want to grow a desert medicinal, like white sage. Plant the herb in a terra-cotta planter, and add coarse sand to your soil mix to keep the soil dry. Settle the planter under the roof's eaves—to keep out the rain—on a south-facing deck that receives plenty of sunshine. If you'd like to grow wetland herbs, encourage moisture retention by using a larger planter and a soil mix that's rich in organic matter. What if you want to grow woodland herbs, like goldenseal and blue cohosh, but you don't have any shade? Plant those coveted medicinals in a whiskey barrel with a soil mix full of decomposed leaves, and place it on an east-facing porch that receives a few hours of morning light. The plant lists aren't exhaustive but include the plants I've found to thrive in pots. For a full lineup of suspects, see the siting charts starting on page 38.

## Arid-Climate Herbs

To create a welcoming environment for herbs native to arid climates, add coarse sand, pea gravel, or pine bark fines to your potting mix to increase drainage. Wait to water until the soil dries out. If your climate receives high rainfall, keep these plants under cover but in a sunny spot. Water the plants directly at the soil level and avoid wetting the foliage.

### Arid-climate herbs for containers:

Aloe vera (*Aloe vera*)

Garden sage (*Salvia officinalis*)

Lavender (*Lavandula angustifolia*)

Lemongrass (*Cymbopogon citratus*)

Lemon verbena (*Aloysia citriodora*)

*Ma huang,* or ephedra (*Ephedra sinica*)

Prickly pear, or *tunas* (*Opuntia* spp.)

Rosemary (*Salvia rosmarinus*)

Thyme (*Thymus* spp.)

White sage (*Salvia apiana*)

## Shade/Part-Shade Herbs

If you're growing cooler-climate medicinals in an especially hot climate, provide the plants with afternoon shade. In the absence of a forest in your landscape, you can grow woodland herbs in planters on a shaded porch or deck. Research each plant's ideal level of shade by looking at the chart on page 39, and site accordingly.

### Shade-loving herbs for containers:

Aloe vera (*Aloe vera*)

Black cohosh (*Actaea racemosa*)

Blue cohosh (*Caulophyllum thalictroides*)

Goldenseal (*Hydrastis canadensis*)

Gotu kola (*Centella asiatica*)

Jiaogulan, or southern ginseng (*Gynostemma pentaphyllum*)

Lady's mantle (*Alchemilla mollis*)

Wild geranium (*Geranium maculatum*)

## Cold-Sensitive Herbs

Tender perennials can be grown outdoors in a pot during the warmer months and then brought indoors or to a sheltered location when the weather chills.

### Cold-sensitive herbs for containers:

Aloe vera (*Aloe vera*)

Citrus (*Citrus* spp.)

Ginger (*Zingiber officinale*)

Gotu kola (*Centella asiatica*)

Hibiscus, roselle (*Hibiscus sabdariffa*)

Lemon verbena (*Aloysia citriodora*)

Lemongrass (*Cymbopogon citratus*)

Mexican sage (*Salvia leucantha*)

Olive (*Olea europaea*)

Prickly pear, some varieties (*Opuntia* spp.)

Tea (*Camellia sinensis*)

Turmeric (*Curcuma longa*)

White sage (*Salvia apiana*)

## Wetland Herbs

Create a moister microclimate for herbs that appreciate the damper side of life by selecting a large vessel with slow drainage. Add aged compost or small amounts of clay to the soil to increase water retention, but still watch out for waterlogging, which can promote rot. Hydration requirements for water-loving plants range from slightly damp to fully submerged in water; research each herb's predilections by consulting the chart on page 38.

**Wetland herbs for containers:**

Blue vervain (*Verbena hastata*)

Boneset (*Eupatorium perfoliatum*)

Calamus (*Acorus calamus*)

Horsetail (*Equisetum* spp.)

Marshmallow (*Althaea officinalis*)

Meadowsweet (*Filipendula ulmaria*)

Skullcap (*Scutellaria lateriflora*)

Yellowroot (*Xanthorhiza simplicissima*)

Yerba mansa (*Anemopsis californica*)

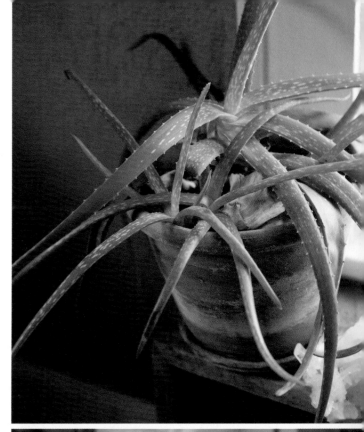

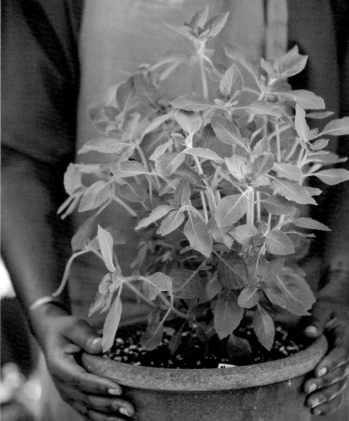

*From left to right:* Aloe vera prefers indirect light and makes a lovely houseplant; culinary herbs growing in a tall wooden planter, golden sage in the front and tricolor sage and purple sage in the rear; lemongrass grows well in terra-cotta pots; tulsi thrives in containers; potted lavender, aloe vera, yellow spilanthes, white sage, and tulsi; jiaogulan can be invasive but is contained in a pot

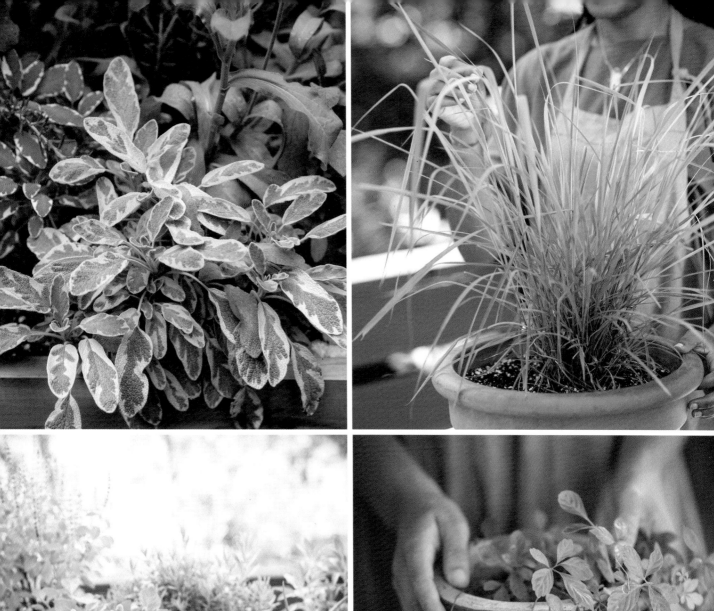
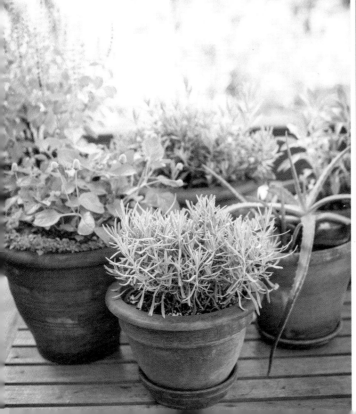
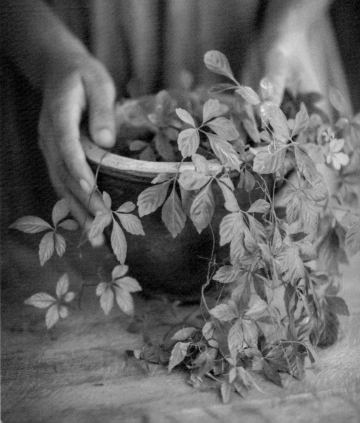

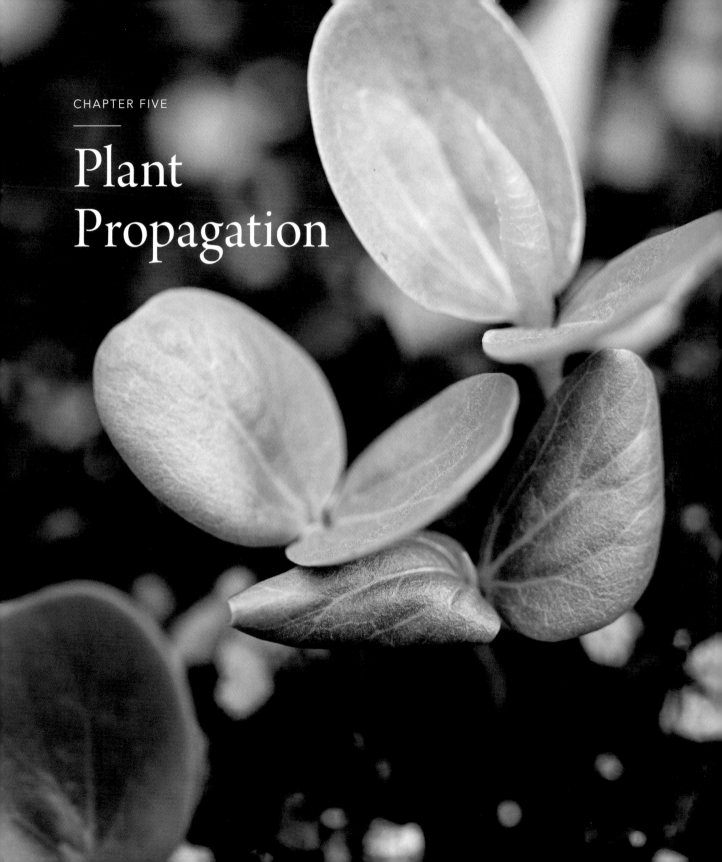

CHAPTER FIVE

# Plant Propagation

No matter how many years I plant seeds and watch them grow into full-grown plants, I'm still overcome by wonder and awe whenever I see a sprouting seed poking out of the soil. In a world growing more complicated and technological by the day, it's a comforting pleasure to witness this simple, yet miraculous, emergence of life.

Plant propagation involves making new plants from other plants. This ancient craft of the gardener is pure alchemy: coaxing roots from a severed stem; midwifing dozens of plants from a single plant's roots; conjuring forth a seedling after an extravagant germination saga beginning with scraping the seed from its fleshy cradle, then fermenting, scarifying, and hibernating the seed in dark, moist sand for three moons in an undergarment drawer. Propagating plants allows you to save money and grow varieties that might not be available from your local nursery. You can obtain free plant material from neighbors or friends or grow more plants from those already in your garden. Propagating plants requires us to slow down and think like a plant—imagining its needs and wants, putting ourselves in its roots, so to speak. It helps us to have an understanding plant heart, making us more skillful gardeners and better herbalists. The tips and tricks in this chapter were gleaned from the years I owned a medicinal herb nursery, where I grew thousands of plants every year from seed, root, and stem. When I first started growing herbs three decades ago, I floundered with seed starting in the absence of a reliable guide. I can't even begin to tell you how many pitiful mistakes I made in the first years of my nursery. I want it to be easier for you. So, when I designed this chapter, I created an Herb Propagation Chart covering the propagation basics so you can have roaring success and more plant babies. I hope you have as much fun as I do watching my plant progeny grow up. I've also created a few video tutorials on the propagation techniques contained in this chapter; you can find them in the HealingGardenGateway.com.

This chapter first focuses on starting plants from seed and then covers the most common forms of vegetative propagation: root division and stem cuttings. Propagating plants from seed involves the reproductive exchange of DNA from the two parent plants through pollination and fertilization. Vegetative propagation results in exact clones of the parent plant. If you've ever started a succulent from a leaf or rooted a philodendron from its stem, then you've engaged in vegetative, or asexual, propagation. *And please don't tell me that you did not enjoy it!*

You're likely aware of the fact that sexual reproduction strengthens the gene pool through increasing diversity, so you might be wondering why making plant "clones" is advantageous. If a plant is a named variety, or cultivar (cultivated variety), vegetative propagation is the best way to ensure that its unique traits, such as height, flower color, flavor, and aroma, are carried over to its progeny. How do you know if a plant is a named variety, or cultivar? If you buy a plant with a second name (typically enclosed in single quotation marks after the common or scientific name), then it's a cultivated variety, such as yarrow 'Cerise Queen' or *Achillea millefolium* 'Apricot Delight'. These plants typically won't come true to type if planted from seed—that is, their specific traits may not carry over—especially if they have an opportunity to reproduce with other members of their species. There are exceptions, however. Sometimes a cultivar will come loosely true to type if planted from seed. An additional benefit to vegetative reproduction is that mature plants can be obtained sooner than when grown from seed.

# Strategies for Germinating Herbs: Stratification, Scarification, & Light-Dependent Germination

Vegetables have been bred for countless generations for uniform and quick germination. Medicinal and culinary herbs, which typically have a longer germination period and sprout erratically, are a different story. Many medicinal herbs are perennials, which have a more selective strategy for germination. While some herbs, especially annuals, don't require any special seed treatments, many herb seeds benefit from coaxing, cajoling, and an ear pointed toward their needs. If you want to grow medicinal herbs from seed (either store-bought or home-saved), you'll need to give them some extra attention in the form of stratification, scarification, and surface sowing. These seed treatments aren't too hard to master, and the skills you'll learn will come in handy for germinating the seeds of most trees, shrubs, and perennial wildflowers. Check the Herb Propagation Chart on page 108 for each herb's germination requirements.

## Stratification, or Cold Conditioning

The seeds of temperate perennial plants have a built-in alarm clock that lets them know winter has passed, spring has arrived, and it's safe to begin life. Stratification—also called cold conditioning—is the process of replicating this seasonal rhythm. There are two primary methods for stratifying seeds: the first involves using outdoor conditions, and the second involves the refrigerator. Both strategies have their merits and drawbacks. In general, I prefer stratifying seeds in the fridge because I have more control over variables and a higher rate of success. However, there are plenty of instances where outdoor cold conditioning makes more sense. If you don't have the time to stratify seeds for the entire recommended period, try a minimum of two weeks—your seeds may sprout but with a lower germination rate or they may take longer to come up. Some perennial herbs whose seeds benefit from stratification include angelica, arnica, blue cohosh, ginseng, goldenseal, goldenrod, marshmallow, mullein, and wild yam. For a full list, including the ideal stratification period, consult the Herb Propagation Chart on page 108.

IN THE EARTH, OUTDOORS: Stratifying seeds outdoors is easy and low-tech, and you can even plant seeds right where you want the plants to grow. So, why wouldn't you go this route? Stratifying seeds outdoors often results in fewer seedlings because of predation by seed-eating animals and loss from disease and rot. Additionally, if you're not familiar with the appearance of the seedlings, they can get lost in the riot of weeds in spring garden beds. For garden herbs, plant seeds in prepared garden beds in the fall, and mulch lightly. Woodland herb seeds can be planted in prepared shade beds under the forest canopy in the fall.

DEEP SEED TRAYS, PLACED OUTDOORS: This method involves planting in deep seed trays in the fall. The trays are placed outdoors on a ground cloth or in an unheated greenhouse, cloche, or hoop house. This method is especially suitable for herbs like goldenseal and blue cohosh that have a long germination period—on the order of two to three years! Make sure the trays are at least 8 inches deep with drainage holes, and fill the trays with soil almost to the top; the soil will decompose and compact over time. Cover the trays with fine-mesh window screens (the kind that comes in rolls) to keep out squirrels and chipmunks (who will dig up your seeds and replace them with their own) and cats (who make their own special deposits). Weigh down the screen with rocks so critters can't crawl under the screen into the trays. If rodents are a problem where you live, consider placing your seed trays in an enclosure fitted with a heavy-duty metal screen, as they can eat through the fine-mesh kind. Make sure your trays don't dry out during dry weather.

IN THE REFRIGERATOR: You'll need seeds, a small bag of play sand, snack-sized ziptop bags, a fine-tip permanent marker, a label, clear packing tape, and a paper bag. I recommend using play sand (available at hardware stores) because it is fine, clean of organic matter (which may harbor fungal spores and seed-eating bacteria), and generally light in color (the better to see little seeds with, my dear). Don't use repurposed ziptop bags because they are likely to introduce microbes that will eat your seeds!

STEP 1: Wet the play sand slightly so it's visibly damp but no water comes out when squeezed (*opposite, top left*).

STEP 2: Place 2 to 3 tablespoons of the wet sand in a small ziptop bag with the seeds (*opposite, top right*). Mix the sand and seeds so that the seeds are evenly distributed; you want each seed to be surrounded by moist sand. Seal the bag.

STEP 3: Label your bag with the herb name and date, and then cover it with clear packing tape (don't write directly on the ziptop bag because the ink can dissolve over time) (*opposite, bottom right*).

STEP 4: Place your bagged seeds in a paper bag to keep out the light, and store them in the refrigerator for two weeks to three months, depending on the species (see the Herb Propagation Chart on page 108). If you're not sure about the optimal stratification period for a plant, try one month as a general guideline. Check your seeds every two weeks. Open the bag to see whether any have sprouted (this is rare), and check for signs of spoilage or mold. If you find any sprouted seeds, plant them right away; they won't survive long in the bag.

STEP 5: When it's time to plant your seeds, there's no need to separate the sand from the seeds— plant them both together unless the seeds are exceptionally large. The sand will help prevent damping-off—the most common disease that seedlings face. If a seed is a light-dependent germinator (see page 90), plant the seeds in their moistened sand directly on the surface of the soil; the sand will let in enough light to enhance germination.

## Multicycle Germinators

These seeds are the trickiest to germinate because they take two years, or even sometimes three, before they emerge (some grow a root the first year and exist as a subterranean "sprout," only to appear above ground the subsequent year!). They typically need warm, moist stratification for a few months and then cold, moist stratification for another few months. This slower germination strategy is common with woodland perennial herbs such as black cohosh, blue cohosh, and ginseng. Some seeds sprout the first year

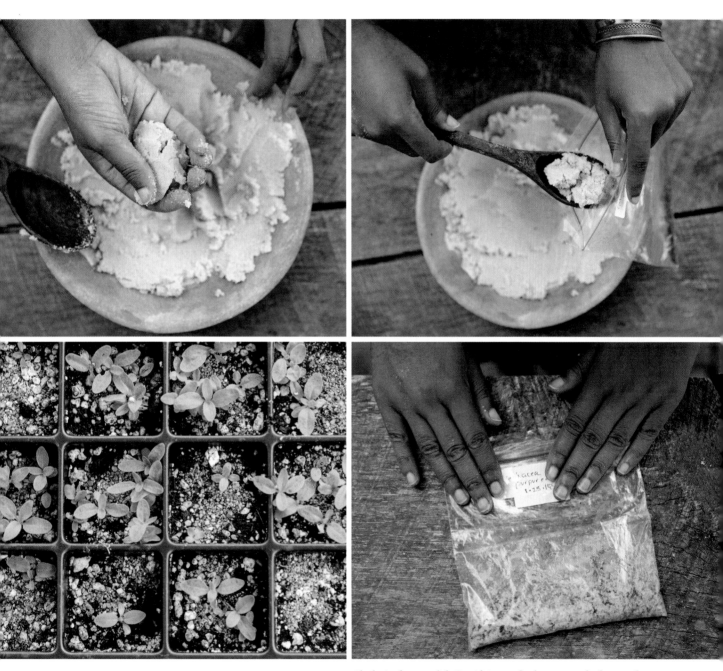

***Clockwise from top left:*** Stratifying seeds: dampen sand; place sand in a ziptop bag with the seeds; label and date the bag before refrigerating; arnica seedlings that have been stratified in sand and then surface-sown

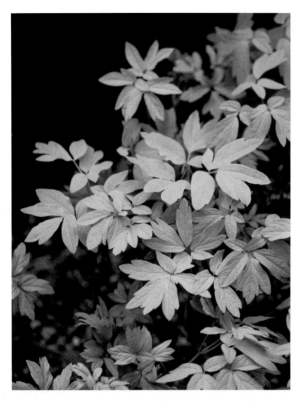

Blue cohosh is an example of a multicycle germinator. The seeds sprout two to three years after planting.

and others the following year. Most growers opt to plant these seeds in outdoor deep seed trays or prepared woodland garden beds because keeping track of stratifying seeds that need differing temperature schemes can prove tricky. If you plant the seeds outdoors in the summer or fall, they may come up the following spring or the subsequent spring. Prepare your ziptop seed bags as outlined above. Place them in a paper bag, and hide them away for the first period of warm, moist stratification. I think the back of the undergarment drawer is the perfect locale—there's a singular mojo found in that environment. Mark your calendar with the day you need to transition the seeds to cold, moist stratification. Once you're ready, keep them in the same bag and place them in the refrigerator. If you're using the outside environment for this two-phase conditioning, just make sure to plant the seeds in the summer, when they can receive ample warmth and moist weather before the cold sets in.

## Light-Dependent Germination and Tiny Seeds

Seeds have formidable patience and can lie in the soil for decades, or even centuries, waiting for their opportunity. Sunlight is often the big break. In a natural setting, extra light may be brought about by wildfire, storm, or tree fall. You've probably witnessed a flush of weed seedlings after tilling or digging; this is because many weeds are light-dependent germinators, and you've brought them to the surface of the soil. To plant light-dependent germinators, sow the seeds directly on the surface of premoistened soil, and very gently press them down. Tiny seeds are planted in the same manner as light-dependent seeds because they need to be close to the surface to be able to grow toward the light. Seeds that should be surface-sown include ashwagandha, bee balm, arnica, mullein, yarrow, goldenrod, boneset, and elecampane. Water the seeds gently by misting or bottom watering so they are not washed off the surface of the soil or driven deep into the soil mixture. See page 96 for more information on watering seedlings.

## Scarification

Some seeds have a thick, impervious seed coat that must be nicked or cracked before the seed can germinate. In nature, fire or the digestive enzymes of seed-dispersing animals sufficiently damage the seed coat. You can mimic these processes by rubbing the seed between two pieces of medium-grit sandpaper until you see a bit of the seed's guts poking through. This is the *endosperm,* the seed's nutrient reserves. The endosperm is usually a lighter color and a different texture from the seed coat. It can be tricky to know when to stop. But you'll catch on quick. If you start to crush any seeds, lighten up your pressure, and check the seeds for any signs of nicking. You'll inevitably scarify some seeds to the point of no return and underscratch others. Aim for the middle ground. If you need to scarify and stratify a seed, scarify *before* stratification. Examples of seeds that germinate better after scarification include astragalus, hibiscus, licorice, marshmallow, passionflower, prickly pear, rose, and uva-ursi.

## Planning Your World Germination Takeover

Whichever method you choose, it's good to spend some quality time with all your seeds in the fall and make a master plan. Take stock of all the seeds you saved over the growing season, including any leftover stash from previous years, and figure out which seeds you may want to order. After you receive your seeds, sort which ones need to be stratified for two weeks, one month, two months, and three months. I like to write on the seed bags if they are light-dependent germinators or need stratification. Then I mark my calendar for the stratification dates by counting backward from my ideal planting date. It's more efficient to stratify seeds in a batch, mixing up a large bowl of damp sand and assembling all your seed baggies in one sitting.

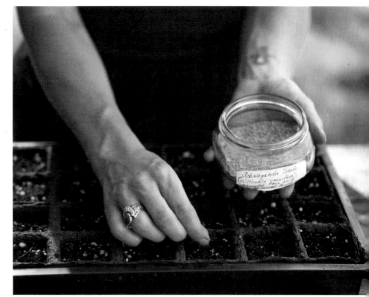

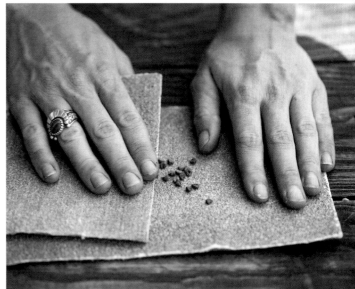

Surface sowing ashwagandha seeds; scarifying seeds between two pieces of sandpaper

# Preparing Seed Trays & Sowing Seeds

## Direct Seeding versus Sowing in Containers

Before we discuss planting seeds in trays, let's take a moment to explore the alternative: direct seeding into the soil. There are two main reasons you might bypass containers when planting seeds. First, sowing seeds directly into the garden is straightforward and requires fewer resources. And second, some herbs just don't like to be transplanted. You may want to plant seeds that need stratification directly in the garden in the fall to let the elements work their magic. Some plants with high survival rates after direct seeding include calendula, basil, tulsi, feverfew, German chamomile, borage, garden sage, skullcap, echinacea, boneset, and anise hyssop. These herbs can also be planted in seed trays if you prefer. The downside to direct seeding is the higher attrition rates when tender seedlings are left to fend for themselves in the face of frost, competition, herbivory, drought, and disease. Weed competition can be fierce, and if you aren't familiar with the appearance of the seedlings, you may have a hard time distinguishing them. For these reasons, I rarely direct sow, with the exception of cover crops and herbs that don't transplant well, such as oats, California poppy, opium poppy, cilantro, parsley, khella, red clover, alfalfa, and fenugreek.

## Germination Setups for Seed Trays

Where you choose to germinate depends on a few factors, including how many seedlings you'll be growing and how much time and money you have to invest in your setup.

SUNNY WINDOWS: A south-facing window with direct light is the simplest seed-starting setup, requiring little to no initial investment. This can be an excellent choice for folks who live in a sunny, warm climate but not so great for those living in a cloudy or cold climate, as seedlings typically need more light than a window can provide. If you live in a warm climate with sunny spring days, you can put your seedlings outside on warm days in a sheltered spot that receives direct sunlight. Slowly increase "outdoors time" an hour or two in the morning, so the wind and sunlight don't shock the seedlings. If you live in an area with cloudy or cold spring days, you'll need to add some grow lights to augment the direct light from the window.

GROW LIGHTS: This germination setup requires a start-up investment but can last for many years. You can build your own system with LED grow lights over a movable metal shelving unit (see the example of my indoor setup on page 93). Assemble the lights with wire so they can be moved farther from the plants as the plants grow.

GREENHOUSES: Available in a wide variety of sizes and materials, greenhouses are typically made from glass or thick UV-resistant plastic. Airflow in a greenhouse is paramount, both for lowering temperatures on sunny days and for minimizing fungal diseases. Some features you'll want to consider include fans, side openings, doors, and heating systems.

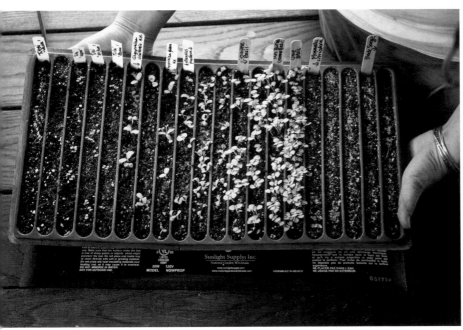 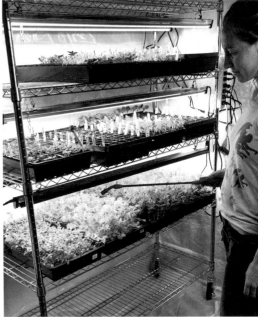

Seedlings germinated next to a south-facing sunny window with a heat mat to enhance germination; my LED grow light setup

## Bottom Heat for Enhancing Germination

Many herb growers apply bottom heat as a way to nudge sleeping seeds toward the sun. Warmth improves the speed of germination, which is important because herb seeds typically have lengthier germination periods than vegetable seeds. Seeds emerge based on the temperature of the soil, not the temperature of the air, so heating soil directly is more efficient than is heating a larger air space.

The easiest and most popular method for applying bottom heat is the seedling heat mat. When using a mat, place it directly under the seed tray with the soil in it, and forgo the additional flat tray that typically goes underneath it. It's helpful to have a soil thermometer and keep the soil temperature between 60°F and 80°F. Don't let the nighttime soil temperature dip too low, or germination will slow down. Yet you don't want to overheat the soil, because tender seedlings are easily damaged by excessive heat. If you're starting seeds indoors and you keep the space consistently warm, there's no need for bottom heat.

## Containers for Seedlings

PLASTIC SEED TRAYS: These come in a variety of sizes and are cheap or even free. My nursery got its start with discarded mismatched seed trays, which I reused for years. I recommend trying a few different kinds of seed trays before you heavily invest in a system, especially considering many of the low-end seed trays are flimsy and aren't built to last many seasons. Harder plastic seed trays are more expensive but can last for a decade, perhaps even longer, if stored properly (out of the elements) during the off-season.

BIODEGRADABLE POTS: Recently, biodegradable pots made from peat and manure have entered the market, and although more expensive, they're better choices environmentally than plastic pots. However, many aren't domestically manufactured, so they carry the environmental cost of long-distance transportation.

SOIL BLOCKS: These are blocks of soil prepared using soil block makers, which are specialized metal forms with handles. You use the metal forms to shape and press out a row of freestanding soil cells, which you can arrange on a wooden or plastic tray. The individual blocks are open to the air, so plant roots that reach the edge of the block are naturally "air pruned." Because plants aren't root-bound, they take off more quickly after transplanting. Another distinct advantage of soil blocks is the absence of plastic. Soil block makers require an initial investment but can last for many years if cared for properly.

## Sterilization

I don't sterilize my seed trays for several reasons. One, it is a pain in the derriere, and, two, my soil is alive with mycorrhizal fungi and beneficial soil bacteria from compost, worm castings, and mycorrhizal inoculants. Plants with a healthy diet and environment, including beneficial soil microbes, have more vitality to fend off pathogens. Creating a healthy terrain is much easier than combating disease. I recommend spray-cleaning seed trays of soil residue and placing them in the sun for a few days before using. However, if you've had problems with diseased seedlings, including damping-off, you may choose to sterilize. (You can use a hydrogen peroxide sterilizing solution or powder, available online and sold for various sterilizing needs.)

## Seed-Starting Soil Mixes

I recommend using a very fine seed-starting soil mix, one with a smaller particle size than your standard vegetable starting mix. It's all too easy for teensy herb seeds to fall into the large air pores of a coarse soil blend. Look for a mix containing organic fertilizer.

FILLING TRAYS: Premoisten your seed-starting soil mix in a bucket so it's slightly damp but not dripping water. Fill your trays or pots to the top, and tap on a table, bench, or the ground, compacting the soil a bit so there aren't any air pockets, which can pose a problem when transplanting. If the soil level is more than a smidgen below the top of the tray, add a little more but not too much. Overfilling trays makes them harder to water and may cause seeds to be washed away.

SEEDING AND LABELING: There are about as many tricks to planting seeds as there are growers. Some people like to make a crease in the paper of a seed packet and tap the seed packet to slowly release its contents. Try mixing tiny seeds with a teaspoon of fine sand to avoid seedling clumps. Use a pencil to make your seed holes, and plant one to two seeds per hole. A good general rule for seed depth is to plant the seed two times as deep as the seed is wide. (Seeds that must be surface-sown are an exception—see page 90 and the Herb Propagation Chart on page 108 for more information.) Label your seedlings with wooden or plastic tags using either a pencil or ultra-permanent markers (regular permanent markers aren't so permanent when exposed to light and water over time).

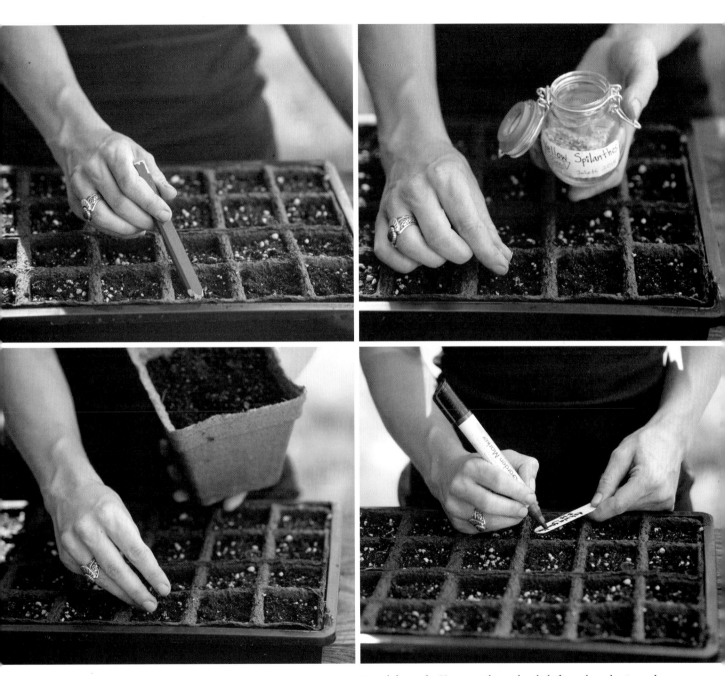

***From left to right:*** Use a pencil to make a hole for each seed twice as deep as the seed is wide; place one to two seeds in each hole; lightly cover the seeds with dirt, taking care to not bury tiny seeds too deep; label each tray with a pencil or garden permanent marker

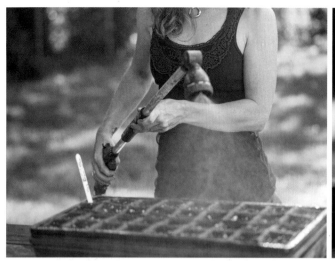

Water surface-sown seeds with a fine mist

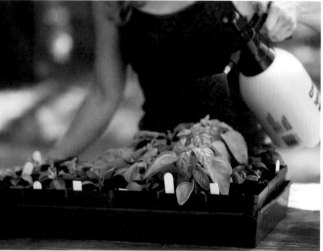

Foliar feed seedlings with diluted fish emulsion and seaweed

## Watering

Watering herb seeds requires more attention than watering vegetable seeds, because a heavy spray easily dislodges tiny herb seeds or surface-sown seeds. You can use the mister setting on a watering wand as long as it's a fine spray. Or use a pressure sprayer with a hose nozzle, like the one pictured in the photo above. This is helpful for an indoor setup, as you have more control over the spray. Be prepared to spend a good bit of time watering—thoroughly wetting the soil via a fine mist is a slow-going process. Once the seedlings develop true leaves (the second set of leaves that emerge—these are usually shaped differently from the cotyledons, or "seed leaves"), they are ready for the hard-knock school of regular watering. Let the soil dry out a tad in between watering to decrease the chances of rotting or damping-off (a common disease of seedlings), yet don't let it get so dry that your seedlings wilt. Watering is a dance, requiring you to respond to your dance partners—the plants—as well as the musicians: light, airflow, and temperature.

## Fertilizing Seedlings

Be sure your potting mix contains a small amount of organic fertilizer for optimal growth and vigor. You can also foliar feed your seedlings after they develop their true leaves. Foliar feeding directly applies nutrients to leaves, where they are rapidly absorbed and put to work, and it's one of the best ways to encourage vigor and growth in seedlings. On a cloudy morning, water the plants, and then, with a pressure sprayer, spray a diluted mix of fish emulsion and seaweed (available at garden supply centers). Because plants can be burned from the nitrogen in the foliar feeding solution, especially on sunny days, you'll want to start with a highly diluted mixture and slowly increase the concentration over time as you observe the plants' response. Some plants are more sensitive to nitrogen than others are. Begin with a more diluted solution than the manufacturer suggests (unless they have suggestions for small seedlings), and apply it every 3 days. If plants are yellow or slow-growing after a handful of foliar feedings, you may need to increase the concentration of your solution.

## Common Problems with Seedlings

***Seedlings are spindly, yellowish, and stretching toward the light.***

Get these babes to more light; you may need to put them under grow lights or adjust their placement.

***Seedlings are keeling over, pinched at the level of the soil, and now it's spreading like wildfire.***

You've got yourself a case of damping-off, a commonly encountered seedling disease caused by a number of fungi. Increase ventilation with fans and increase sunlight, if possible. Take care not to overwater. To prevent damping-off, add a small amount of sand to the soil mix or a fine layer of coarse sand on top of the soil, both of which discourage fungal activity. In addition, look for an organic biological fungicide, labeled for the prevention of damping-off in seedlings.

***Seedlings are slightly yellow and just don't seem to be growing very fast.***

Your seedlings probably need more nitrogen. See the notes above on foliar feeding.

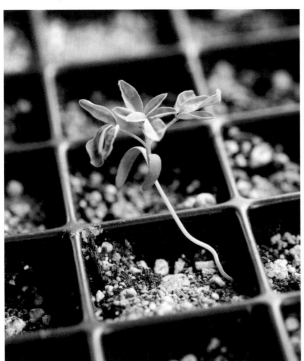

Seedlings that don't receive enough light are spindly and leaning toward the light.

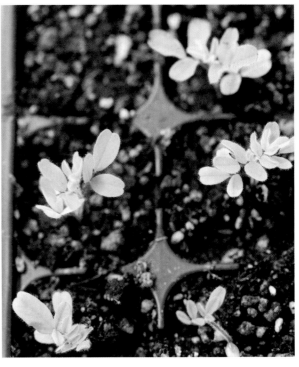

Nitrogen deficiency causes seedlings to become stunted and yellow.

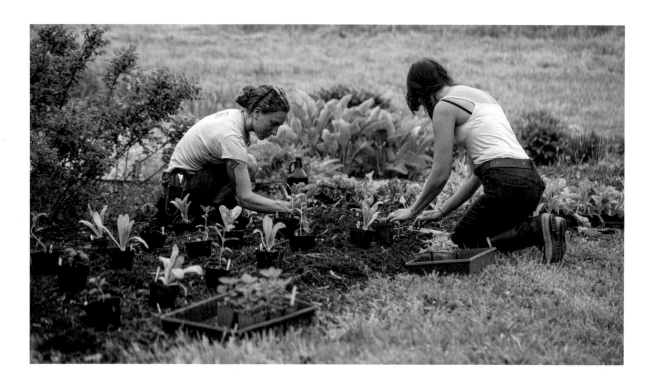

## Hardening Off

If your seedlings have been coddled in the greenhouse or the warm indoors, they won't appreciate sudden exposure to sunshine, wind, and lower nighttime temperatures. You'll want to habituate them to the elements slowly—a process called hardening off. For a week, place the seedlings outside—when it's not too windy—for a few hours in the morning.

## Transplanting

The big day! There's immense satisfaction in sending forth seedlings that you've nurtured from seed. The best time to transplant is in the late afternoon on a still day. If the plants are root-bound (the roots travel in a tight circle around the edge of their pot), break up the root system by teasing apart the roots and spreading them out. Sometimes you need to cut the roots so they don't get stuck in a vicious cycle of growing around and around, even after being planted in good soil, which would limit growth. This can feel a little scary and counterintuitive the first time you do it, but it will genuinely help your plants. Plant your starts at the same soil level that they were growing in in their pots—in other words, don't bury the stems in the soil. Water your transplants in and continue to water your seedlings when the soil gets dry, as often as every day or two, for a few weeks.

---

*Above:* Transplanting seedlings after they've been hardened off
*Opposite:* (A) Thin or divide seedlings that are growing densely and transplant into larger cells; (B) step up seedlings into trays with larger cells; (C) dig a hole as deep as the pot and loosen the soil; (D) if the seedling is rootbound, break up the roots; (E) plant the start at the same soil level it was growing in its pot; gently tuck it in and replace the mulch

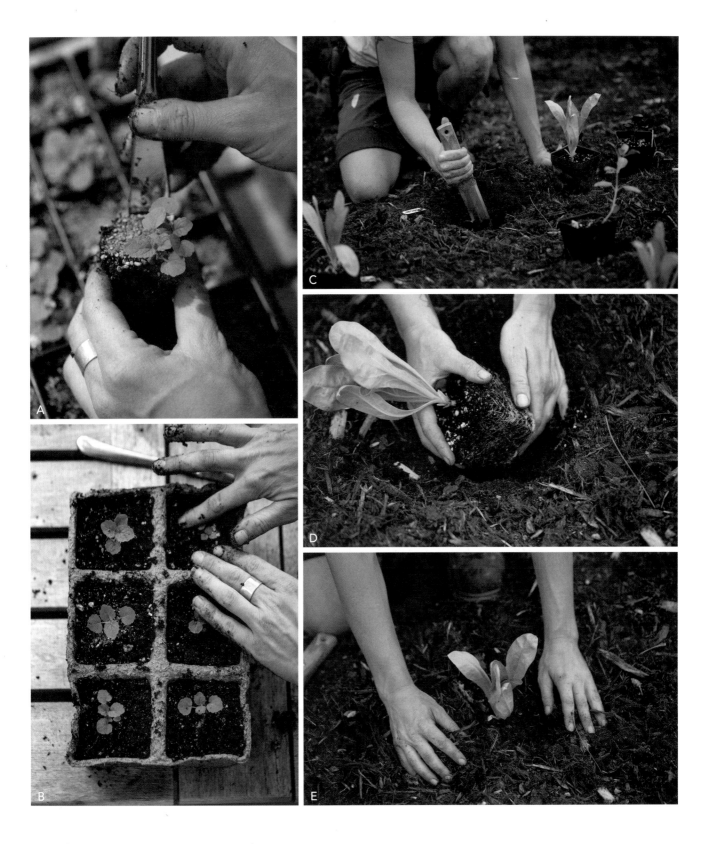

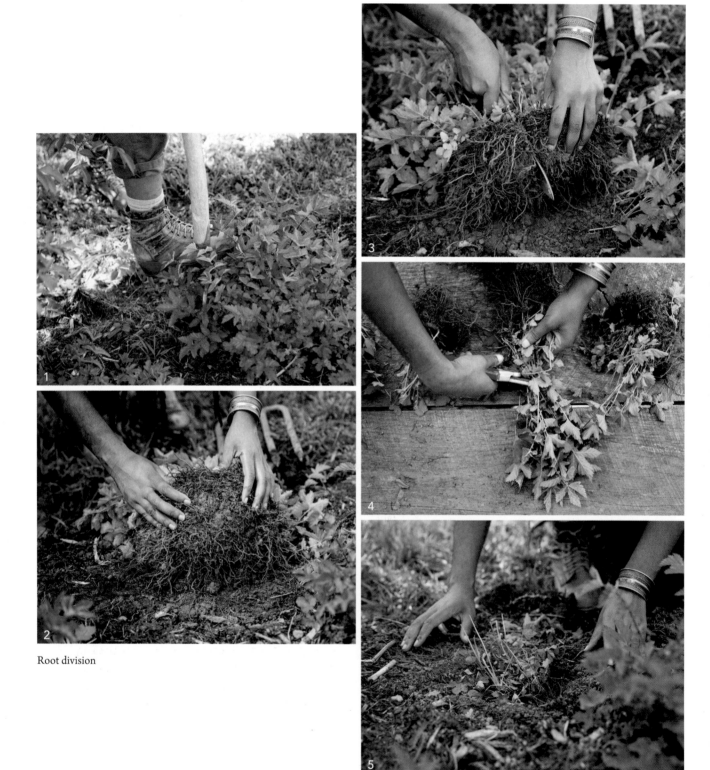

Root division

# Root Division

This vegetative form of plant propagation involves digging up and separating part of the root system of a plant to form new plants. The daughter plants, or divisions, may be planted directly in the garden or potted up in preparation for moving to a new location. Depending on the plant species, age, and size of the divisions, 1 to 20 divisions can be made from one mother plant. Early fall and early spring are the best times to divide roots because plants are dormant, or soon to be dormant, with little aboveground growth present. I prefer to propagate roots in the early fall, before the hard freezes, as there are fewer garden responsibilities at the end of the growing season. Divide roots when the ground isn't too wet, otherwise the soil will be clumpy and adhere to the root system, making the task challenging. Most perennial herbs can be propagated this way, especially plants that run or clump; the exception is plants with taproots. (Taproots are elongated central roots, like a carrot.) Several tools are useful for dividing roots, including a digging fork, a set of pruners, a flat-edged shovel, and a Japanese digging knife, or hori-hori.

## Directions for Root Division

STEP 1: Choose a vigorous, large plant that can withstand losing some of its roots. Using a digging fork or shovel, gently loosen the soil in a circle around the plant, excavating any side roots, and then free the roots from the earth (*opposite, top left*).

STEP 2: Shake off excess dirt from the roots so you can see what you're working with (*opposite, bottom left*). If your soil is clayey or damp, you may need to thump the root system in its hole to dislodge any adhering soil clumps. Size up your root system by looking at how many buds or shoots it has, and decide how many cuts you want to make. Depending on your needs and the plant at hand, you may want a few large divisions or many small divisions. The larger the size, the higher the chance the divisions will take. Meadowsweet, yarrow, comfrey, and mint are all plants that survive well with small divisions. You'll want to have at least one shoot or bud per division and an attached root system that is large enough to sustain the growth of the bud.

STEP 3: Divide your roots into the desired number of divisions (*opposite, top right*). If the roots are growing loosely and aren't too tough, you may be able to pry apart divisions with your hands or gently snap the roots. If the root system is denser, try turning it upside down or placing it sideways and sawing it into segments with a hori-hori. If the root system is too tough for this, use a sharp, flat-ended shovel to sever the root system. A shovel offers the least amount of precision, but it gets the job done. If you want the mother plant to continue growing in its original location, replant the largest division back in the hole.

STEP 4: If your plant is an herbaceous perennial that is getting ready to be dormant for the winter, you can completely cut back the aboveground growth. If it's spring, and the plant is actively growing with many stems, cut the stems back by half (*opposite, middle right*). If it just has emerging leaves, remove half the leaves. (When you disturb the root system, the plant can't support the original amount of vegetation.)

STEP 5: Directly transplant your divisions into their forever home (*page 100, bottom right*) or plant them up in a pot. Plant them bud side up and at the same soil depth they were originally growing. Water your divisions. You can also use a natural rooting preparation from willow or seaweed (see below).

## Natural Rooting Preparations: Willow and Seaweed

Willow twigs contain a high concentration of indolebutyric acid (IBA), which is a natural plant hormone that encourages rooting. In nature, willow twigs readily break in storms, fall into nearby waterways, travel downstream, and become lodged in the riverbank. The stems—filled with rooting compounds—then take root in the riverbank. Making a willow rooting "tea" to nourish your divisions, cuttings, and transplants capitalizes on this nifty adaptation. Use any species of willow, including ornamentals, to make the tea. Cut a bunch of switches (about 10 to 20), about an arm's length long, strip the leaves off, and place the twigs in a 5-gallon bucket with water. After a few days of soaking, water the plants with the willow soak water to encourage rooting. Use the soak water every few times you water, rotating with regular watering. Replace the water in the bucket as needed, until it becomes aromatic from fermentation; if needed, start a new batch at that time.

Seaweed extracts contain a large number of natural plant growth hormones. Seaweed extracts are often sold as concentrates, which are diluted and used to water in cuttings, divisions, layered twigs, and transplants. Follow the instructions on the packaging.

# Stem Cuttings

Stem cuttings are one of the simplest ways to propagate new plants. Stems are cut from existing plants and are encouraged to form roots, resulting in a clone of the parent plant. Many herbs, fruit trees, shrubs, conifers, and vines can be propagated by stem cuttings. Not all plants are candidates, however. Consult the Herb Propagation Chart on page 108 to see which plants can be rooted by cutting and the preferred method of cutting for that species. Semi-ripe cuttings are the easiest method for beginning propagators. To learn how to perform other cuttings, I highly recommend *Making More Plants: The Science, Art, and Joy of Propagation* by Ken Druse.

HARDWOOD CUTTINGS are taken from woody (brown) stems of deciduous and evergreen shrubs and trees when they are dormant in the fall to early winter.

SOFTWOOD CUTTINGS are taken from the green growing tips (softwood) of plants when the leaves are full grown yet still tender.

SEMI-RIPE SOFTWOOD CUTTINGS are softwood cuttings that are taken later in the season (summer to early fall as opposed to spring).

LAYERING involves bending a flexible low-growing branch into a hole and pinning a portion of the stem under the soil (with the leafy tip of the branch above ground). The buried section eventually forms roots. The growing tip and its newly rooted stem (a clone of the parent plant) can then be severed from the parent plant and transplanted. While not technically a type of cutting because you don't sever the branch from the parent plant until it forms roots, I think of layering as a "living cutting."

## Directions for Semi-Ripe Softwood Cuttings

STEP 1: In summer or early fall, select the most vital plants for your cuttings. The optimal stage of plant growth for semi-ripe cuttings is the green new growing tip; it should be hard but not yet woody. The best time of day to take cuttings is in the early morning. Using sharp, sterilized pruners, cut stems that have three to five nodes, are 4 to 8 inches in length, and are free from flower buds and blossoms (A). Take more than you'll need, as not all the cuttings will survive.

STEP 2: Gently strip the leaves and any side shoots from the lower nodes, leaving only a few leaves at the upper tip (B). For larger-leafed plants, cut in half to reduce water loss—leaving too much foliage will cause the plant to desiccate before it has a chance to root.

STEP 3:. Dip the ends of your cuttings in an organic rooting promoter; you can use a store-bought one or try willow tea or seaweed extract as described on

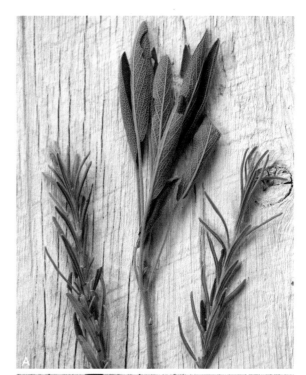

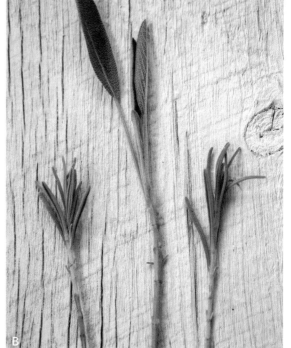

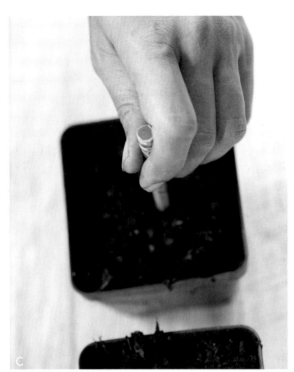

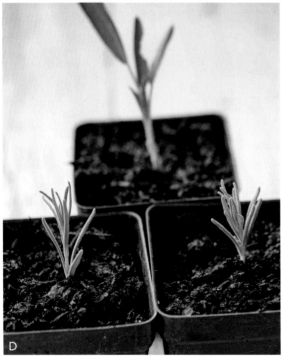

page 102. Fill pots with a potting soil that preferably does not contain fertilizer, and make a hole in the soil using a pencil (C). Plant the cuttings with the lower nodes in the soil, making sure the leaves don't touch the planting medium, and tamp the soil securely around each cutting.

STEP 4: Warmth, moisture, and diffuse sunlight are key for encouraging semi-ripe cuttings to take root (D). The light should be as bright as possible yet indirect and the soil consistently moist but not waterlogged. Cuttings can be kept in a greenhouse, a cold frame, or a warm room by a window that receives indirect light. You can also rig up a makeshift mini-greenhouse using wire and a clear plastic bag over each pot. Commercial rooting chambers, with a plastic lid, are an affordable option. Mist the cuttings daily with a household spray bottle or pressurized spray bottle and remove any dead or dying cuttings.

STEP 5: After one to two months, check to see if roots have formed by giving each cutting a gentle tug. If you meet with resistance, you've got roots. New green growth is another indicator that roots have developed.

STEP 6: Because you've been keeping your cuttings out of direct sunlight, they'll need to be hardened off for two or three weeks before transplanting. This is simply a process of acclimating them to the full sun and wind. Begin by placing your plants outside for an hour in the morning and gradually lengthening the amount of time they spend outside.

STEP 7: Transplant the rooted cuttings to the garden and water them well. If it's late in the season, pot them up in good-quality potting soil and overwinter indoors or in a greenhouse; plant them the following spring.

## Medicinal Plants That Can Be Propagated through Semi-Ripe Cuttings

Blackberry and Raspberry species (*Rubus* spp.)
Blueberry (*Vaccinium* spp.)
Butterfly weed (*Asclepias tuberosa*)
Catnip (*Nepeta cataria*)
Cinnamon (*Cinnamomum verum*)
Citrus (*Citrus* spp.)
Elderberry (*Sambucus nigra, S. nigra* var. *canadensis*)
Forsythia (*Forsythia suspensa*)
Ginkgo (*Ginkgo biloba*)
Hawthorn (*Crataegus* spp.)
Honeysuckle (*Lonicera japonica*)
Hops (*Humulus lupulus*)
Juniper (*Juniperus* spp.)
Lavender (*Lavandula* spp.)
Lemon verbena (*Aloysia citriodora*)
Mimosa (*Albizia julibrissin*)
Oregon grape (*Mahonia* spp.)
Passionflower (*Passiflora incarnata*)
Prickly pear (*Opuntia* spp.)
Red root (*Ceanothus americanus*)
Rose species (*Rosa* spp.)
Rosemary (*Salvia rosmarinus*)
Sage species (*Salvia* spp.)
St. John's wort (*Hypericum perforatum*)
Tea, green and black (*Camellia sinensis*)
Thyme (*Thymus vulgaris*)
Vitex, Chaste berry (*Vitex agnus-castus*)
Witch hazel (*Hamamelis virginiana*)
Wormwood (*Artemisia absinthium*)

# Saving Seeds of Medicinal Herbs

Saving your own seeds is economical and satisfying, bringing the kinship with your herbs full cycle. Watch your plants closely as their seeds ripen—there's a narrow window for gathering the seeds. After the plants are done flowering, the blooms will develop into fruit, seedpods, or capsules. When the capsules or seedpods are starting to dry out and open up and the seeds fall out easily when tapped, they are ready to be harvested for seed saving. If a plant produces fruits, they'll look ripe or fall when you shake the plant. Press your nail into a seed. If the seed easily gives way to your nail, it's probably not ripe. However, if the seed coat is hardened and won't yield to your nail, it's likely to be ready for saving. Harvest seed from the strongest, or most productive, plants in your garden.

## Harvesting Seeds

The easiest and most common way to save seeds involves tapping or shaking seeds into a bowl. This method works well for dozens of herbs, including stinging nettles, lemon balm, anise hyssop, echinacea, tulsi, and garden basils. You can also place seed heads in paper bags to dry; after a few days, the seeds will mature and loosen, and you'll significantly increase your yield. Using either method, you'll end up with seeds and chaff (seed husks, or unwanted reproductive parts) and need to clean your seeds. Some seeds require more attention from your fingers—calendula, fennel, and sunflower seeds, for instance, can easily be pulled from their base but won't necessarily shake free.

## Seed Cleaning

Home-gathered seed has more chaff than store-bought seeds do, which isn't an issue as long as everything is dry. You can plant the chaff right with the seed or even stratify it (see page 87) with the seed and in most cases it won't pose a problem. However, it's easier to store and plant seeds when they're clean, so I like to spend a little time cleaning seeds without going overboard. An assortment of screens is super handy, as seeds vary in size. Set a screen over a bowl. Take a handful of dried plant material and rub it over the screen to crunch up any hard bits and pieces. The seeds will fall through to the bowl below while the screen catches any chaff. You can also remove the chaff from your seeds by blowing it away, a process known as *winnowing*. Place your plant material in a small bowl and swirl it around as you gently blow the chaff away. Or pour seeds slowly from one bowl to another while blowing. Winnowing seeds requires a bit of finesse

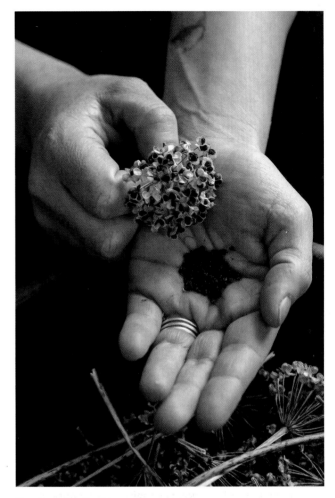

Tapping out garlic chive seeds

and practice. Place a sheet underneath your winnowing to catch the whole shebang, seeds and all, when you're a little overzealous.

Fermentation is the easiest method I've found for cleaning the seeds from fleshy fruits, such as passionflower, prickly pear, ashwagandha, and woodland herbs, like ginseng, goldenseal, bloodroot, blue cohosh, wild ginger, partridgeberry, and trillium. Many plants with fleshy fruits have compounds surrounding the seed that inhibit germination. In nature, a seed-dispersing animal eats the fruit, and its digestive juices effectively dissolve these germination-inhibiting compounds. To mimic this process, ferment the fruit, allowing bacteria to dissolve the pulp along with the germination inhibitors. Break up the fruit if possible and add it to water in a small jar; place it in a warm, dark environment; and stir daily. If there's bubbling action, the bacteria are doing their job. After a few days, pour off the upper layer of floating pulp and nonviable "floater" seeds, and then wash the seeds in a strainer that will retain the seeds but allow the pulp to be discarded. Work the seeds and pulp with your fingers to loosen any particles. Repeat the fermentation and washing process until the seeds are cleaned from their pulp.

## Seed Storing and Viability

Seeds must be completely dry before storage, or they can mold and decay. Store them in small glass or plastic jars in a cool, dark location. A space-saving option is to store your seeds in envelopes in an airtight container. Most herb seeds will last two to five years if they're stored properly, but I've seen impressive germination rates with seeds that are seven to ten years old! If you have aging seeds, consider sowing heavier than usual—you'll be surprised with how many sprouts come up. Hydrophilic seeds are the exception; they can't withstand extended periods of dry storage and instead should be planted fresh soon after developing on the plant. Some hydrophilic seeds include bleeding heart, bloodroot, blue cohosh, ginseng, goldenseal, partridgeberry, trillium, and wild ginger.

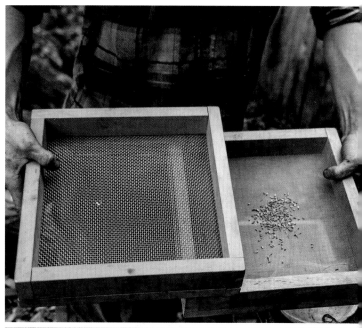

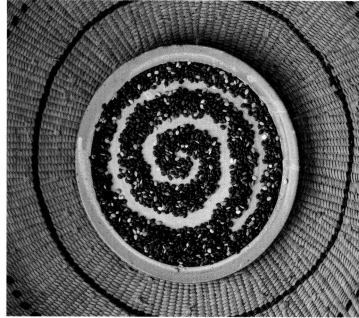

Cleaning seeds with different-sized screens at Mountain Gardens in Celo, North Carolina; passionflower seeds that have been cleaned through fermentation

# Herb Propagation Chart

## KEY

**Notes**

**Surface-sown** = Plant seeds on the surface of the soil; tiny seeds or light-dependent germinators; mist to water

**Scarify** = Seed coat must be nicked with sandpaper

**WM** = Warm, moist stratification at 70°F

**CM** = Cold, moist stratification at 36–40°F

**H** = Seed is hydrophilic; must be kept moist

**GI** = Seed contains germination inhibitors; clean seed from pulp before sowing

**MCG** = Multicycle germinator; seed needs alternating periods of warmth and cold before it will sprout

**EPA** = Easiest to propagate asexually; cuttings or root division are quicker than planting seeds

**CVA** = Cultivars (named varieties) should be propagated asexually (cuttings or root divisions) to maintain desired characteristics

**\*** = May be highly invasive in your region; research before planting

| PLANT | SCIENTIFIC NAME | SURFACE SOWN | SCARIFY | STRATIFICATION (COLD, MOIST UNLESS SPECIFIED) | NOTES | DAYS TO GERMINATION/ OPTIMAL TEMPERATURE | ROOT DIVISION | LAYERING | CUTTINGS | LIFESTYLE |
|---|---|---|---|---|---|---|---|---|---|---|
| Angelica | Angelica archangelica | ✓ | | 1 month | SS, seed should be fresh | 7 to 14 days at 70°F (prestratified seed) | ✓ | | | Bi |
| Anise hyssop | Agastache foeniculum | ✓ | | | SS | 7 to 14 days at 75°F | | | Softwood | HP |
| Arnica | Arnica chamissonis, A. montana | ✓ | | 2–4 weeks | | 9 to 21 days at 65°F (prestratified seed) | ✓ | | | HP |
| Ashwagandha | Withania somnifera | ✓ | | | Start indoors at the time you plant tomatoes | 7 to 14 days at 77°F | | | | An to WP (in tropics) |
| Astragalus | Astragalus propinquus (formerly A. membranaceus) | | ✓ | | Scarify and soak seed overnight, cover lightly | 6 to 21 days at 65–70°F | ✓ | | | HP |
| Basil | Ocimum basilicum | | | | | 5 to 10 days at 70–80°F | | | | An |
| Bay | Laurus nobilis | | ✓ | 2 months | EPA, fresh seed, low germination rates | 1 to 12 months at 65–70°F (prestratified seed) | | | Semi-ripe, hardwood | WP to Sb |
| Bayberry/ Wax myrtle | Morella spp. (formerly Myrica spp.) | | ✓ | 3 months | GI | 9 months to 2 years (from sowing nonstratified seed outdoors in the fall) | ✓ | ✓ | Root cuttings with suckering shoot in early spring | Sb to ST |
| Bee balm/ Wild bergamot/ Horsemint | Monarda spp. | ✓ | | | EPA (except M. citriodora), CVA, SR | 6 to 21 days at 65–70°F | ✓ | | Softwood, root cuttings | CP |
| Black cohosh | Actaea racemosa (formerly Cimicifuga racemosa) | | | 1 month WM + 3 months CM | H, GI, EPA, MCG, best started outdoors in late summer or early fall | 6 months to 2 years (from sowing fresh, nonstratified seed outdoors in early fall) | ✓ | | | HP |

## KEY

**CW** = *Cosmopolitan weed (already weedy, or invasive, in disturbed areas throughout the globe)*
**SS** = *Self-sows; may spread throughout the garden*
**SR** = *Spreads by runners, will expand if not contained*

### Cuttings
**Softwood** = *Softwood cuttings*
**Semi-ripe** = *Semi-ripe cuttings*
**Hardwood** = *Hardwood cuttings*

### Lifestyle
**An** = *Annual*
**Bi** = *Biennial*
**HP** = *Herbaceous perennial*
**CP** = *Creeping perennial*
**WP** = *Woody perennial*
**Sb** = *Shrub*
**ST** = *Small tree*
**T** = *Medium to large tree*
**WV** = *Woody vine*
**HV** = *Herbaceous vine*

| PLANT | SCIENTIFIC NAME | SURFACE SOWN | SCARIFY | STRATIFICATION (COLD, MOIST UNLESS SPECIFIED) | NOTES | DAYS TO GERMINATION/ OPTIMAL TEMPERATURE | ROOT DIVISION | LAYERING | CUTTINGS | LIFESTYLE |
|---|---|---|---|---|---|---|---|---|---|---|
| Blue cohosh | *Caulophyllum thalictroides* | | | Best started outdoors in summer with fresh seed | H, GI, MCG, EPA | 1½ to 3 years (from sowing seed fresh, nonstratified seed outdoors in summer) | ✓ | | | HP |
| Black haw | *Viburnum prunifolium* | | | 5 months WM + 3 months CM | GI, MCG | 1 to 3 years; 2 years average (from sowing nonstratified seed outdoors in summer) | ✓ | ✓ | Root cuttings, hardwood<br><br>Semi-ripe cuttings from non-flowering suckers | Sb to ST |
| Bloodroot | *Sanguinaria canadensis* | | | 5 months WM + 3 months CM | H, EPA, MCG, best started by sowing fresh seed outdoors in early summer | 1 to 2 years (from sowing fresh, nonstratified seed outdoors in early summer) | ✓ | | Root cuttings | HP |
| Boneset | *Eupatorium perfoliatum* | ✓ | | 1 month | | 10 to 25 days at 60–65°F (prestratified seed) | ✓ | | | HP |
| Borage | *Borago officinalis* | | | | SS, lightly cover | 5 to 14 days at 60–65°F | | | | An |
| Burdock | *Arctium lappa, A. minus* | | | | CW, SS, direct sow (*Arctium minus* native to N. America) | 5 to 14 days | | | | Bi |
| Butterfly weed | *Asclepias tuberosa* | | | 1 month | | 7 to 21 days at 65–70°F (prestratified seed) | ✓ | | Semi-ripe, root cuttings | HP |
| Calamus/ Sweet flag | *Acorus calamus, A. americanus* | | | 1 month WM + 2 months CM | MCG, EPA, barely cover seed, SR | 10 to 21 days (prestratified seed) | ✓ | | | HP |
| Calendula | *Calendula officinalis* | | | | SS | 5 to 14 days at 65–70°F | | | | An |

| PLANT | SCIENTIFIC NAME | SURFACE SOWN | SCARIFY | STRATIFICATION (COLD, MOIST UNLESS SPECIFIED) | NOTES | DAYS TO GERMINATION/ OPTIMAL TEMPERATURE | ROOT DIVISION | LAYERING | CUTTINGS | LIFESTYLE |
|---|---|---|---|---|---|---|---|---|---|---|
| California poppy | Eschscholzia californica | ✓ | | | SS, direct sow in early spring, barely cover seed | 5 to 14 days at 65–70°F | | | | An |
| Catnip | Nepeta cataria | ✓ | | | SS | 7 to 20 days at 65–70°F | | ✓ | Semi-ripe | HP |
| Chamomile, German | Matricaria chamomilla, syn. M. recutita | ✓ | | | SS, direct sow in early spring | 10 to 14 days at 65–70°F | | | | A |
| Chamomile, Roman | Chamaemelum nobile | ✓ | | | | 10 to 12 days at 70°F | ✓ | ✓ | Softwood | HP |
| Chickweed | Stellaria media | ✓ | | | CW, SS | 3 to 12 days at 53–65°F | ✓ | | | An |
| Chives | Allium schoenoprasum | | | | SS, direct sow in early spring, lightly cover seed | 10 to 14 days at 60–70°F | ✓ | | | HP |
| Cilantro/ Coriander | Coriandrum sativum | | | | Direct sow | 7 to 10 days at 60–70°F | | | | An |
| Cleavers | Galium aparine | | | 1 month | CW, SS, cover seed | 15 to 60 days at 60–65°F (prestratified seed) | ✓ | | | HP |
| Comfrey | Symphytum officinale | | | 1 month | EPA, SR (if roots are disturbed) | 15 to 30 days (prestratified seed) | ✓ | | | HP |
| Cramp bark | Viburnum opulus | | | 5 months WM + 3 months CM | Sow fresh seed when ripe outdoors in earth or pots. Or stratify as outlined. | 20 months (from sowing fresh, nonstratified seeds outdoors in summer) | | ✓ | Softwood, hardwood | Sb |
| Culver's root | Veronicastrum virginicum | ✓ | | 1–2 months | EPA | 14 to 21 days at 65–70°F (prestratified seeds) | ✓ | | | HP |
| Dandelion | Taraxacum officinale | ✓ | | 1 week | CW, SS | 10 to 21 days at 50–75°F | | | | HP |
| Dill | Anethum graveolens | | | | SS, direct sow in early spring | 5 to 21 days at 70–80°F | | | | An |
| Echinacea (pale purple, narrow-leafed) | Echinacea pallida, E. angustifolia | | | 3 months | SS | 10 to 28 days at 70°F (prestratified seed) | ✓ | | | HP |
| Echinacea (purple coneflower) | Echinacea purpurea | | | 2 weeks | CVA, SS | 10 to 21 days at 70°F (prestratified seed) | ✓ | | | HP |
| Elderberry | Sambucus nigra, S. nigra var. canadensis | | | 3 months | EPA, GI, best started outdoors in late summer or fall | 9 months plus (from sowing nonstratified seed outdoors in early fall) | ✓ | ✓ | Semi-ripe, hardwood, transplant wayward shoots | Sb |
| Elecampane | Inula helenium | ✓ | | | SS (in temperate climates only) | 4 to 15 days at 65–70°F | ✓ | | | HP |

| PLANT | SCIENTIFIC NAME | SURFACE SOWN | SCARIFY | STRATIFICATION (COLD, MOIST UNLESS SPECIFIED) | NOTES | DAYS TO GERMINATION/ OPTIMAL TEMPERATURE | ROOT DIVISION | LAYERING | CUTTINGS | LIFESTYLE |
|---|---|---|---|---|---|---|---|---|---|---|
| False unicorn root | *Chamaelirium luteum* | ✓ | | 2–3 months | H, best started outdoors in summer, cover seeds lightly with coarse sand | 9 months (from sowing fresh, nonstratified seed outdoors in summer) | ✓ | | | HP |
| Fennel | *Foeniculum vulgare* | | | | SS, direct sow in early spring | 7 to 14 days at 65–70°F | | | | HP |
| Feverfew | *Tanacetum vulgare* | ✓ | | | SS | 4 to 14 days at 65–70°F | ✓ | | Softwood | HP |
| Gentian | *Gentiana* spp. | ✓ | | 3 months | Cover seeds lightly with coarse sand | Varies by species | ✓ | | | HP |
| Ginkgo | *Ginkgo biloba* | | | 2 months WM + 2 months CM. Or sow seeds outdoors in early fall | H, soak overnight, low germination rate, dioecious (male + female plants), MCG | 9 months (from sowing nonstratified seed outdoors in early fall) | | | Semi-ripe, hardwood | T |
| Ginseng | *Panax* spp. | | | 9 months CM (35°F) + 3.5 months WM (60°F) at 15 percent humidity | H, GI, MCG, best started outdoors in fall from prestratified seeds (available commercially) | Fresh, nonstratified seeds sown outdoors in the fall will germinate in 16 to 22 months whereas 1 year prestratified seeds planted in the fall will germinate the following spring | | | | HP |
| Goldenrod | *Solidago* spp. | ✓ | | 3 months | SS | 7 to 21 days at 70°F (prestratified seed) | ✓ | | Softwood | HP |
| Goldenseal | *Hydrastis canadensis* | | | Best started outdoors in summer or early fall | H, GI, MCG (sometimes), EPA | 10 to 22 months (from sowing fresh, nonstratified seed in the summer) | ✓ | | Root cuttings | HP |
| Gotu kola | *Centella asiatica* | ✓ | | | EPA, low germination rates | 21 to 28 days at 70°F | ✓ | ✓ | | HP |
| Hawthorn | *Crataegus* spp. | | ✓ | 3 months WM + 3 months CM | EPA, GI, MCG, poor germination common | 1 to 2 years (from sowing nonstratified seed outdoors) | | | Semi-ripe | Sb to ST |
| Heart's-ease | *Viola tricolor* | ✓ | | | SS | 4 to 7 days at 62–68°F | ✓ | | | An |
| Hibiscus, Roselle | *Hibiscus sabdariffa* | | ✓ | | Start indoors at the time you plant tomatoes | 5 to 14 days at 75–85°F | | | Softwood, semi-ripe | An to WP |
| Hops | *Humulus lupulus* | | | 1 month | CW, EPA, SR, sow in the fall, dioecious (male + female plants; only female plants produce hops) | 7 to 21 days at 70–75°F (prestratified seed) | ✓ | ✓ | Semi-ripe, transplant wayward shoots (vegetative methods ensure sex of plants) | HV |

| PLANT | SCIENTIFIC NAME | SURFACE SOWN | SCARIFY | STRATIFICATION (COLD, MOIST UNLESS SPECIFIED) | NOTES | DAYS TO GERMINATION/ OPTIMAL TEMPERATURE | ROOT DIVISION | LAYERING | CUTTINGS | LIFESTYLE |
|---|---|---|---|---|---|---|---|---|---|---|
| Horehound | Marrubium vulgare | | ✓ | | CW, SS | 10 to 21 days at 65–70°F | | | | HP |
| Hyssop, true | Hyssopus officinalis | ✓ | ✓ | | Cover seed lightly with coarse sand | 7 to 21 days at 60–65°F | | ✓ | Softwood | HP to WP |
| Jiaogulan* | Gynostemma pentaphyllum | | | | EPA, SR | Not recommended | ✓ | ✓ | | HP |
| Lady's mantle | Alchemilla vulgaris | ✓ | | 2 months | SS (temperate climates), best started outdoors in fall or early spring | 20 to 28 days at 65–70°F (prestratified seed) | ✓ | | | HP |
| Lavender | Lavandula angustifolia | ✓* | ✓ | 1 month | EPA, CVA, *cover seed with a fine layer of sand | 5 to 21 days at 70–85°F (prestratified seed) | | ✓ | Semi-ripe | WP |
| Lemon balm | Melissa officinalis | ✓ | | 2 weeks | SS | 7 to 14 days at 65–70°F (prestratified seed) | ✓ | ✓ | Softwood | HP |
| Lemon verbena | Aloysia citrodora | | | | EPA | | | ✓ | Softwood, semi-ripe | WP to Sb |
| Lemongrass | Cymbopogon citratus | ✓ | | | EPA, cover seed lightly | 8 to 14 days at 65–70°F | ✓ | | | HP |
| Licorice, Chinese and European | Glycyrrhiza uralensis and G. glabra | | ✓ | | Scarify and soak overnight | 5 to 30 days at 70°F | ✓ | | Softwood | HP |
| Lobelia | Lobelia inflata | ✓ | | 2 months | | 7 to 21 days at 70°F | | | | An to Bi |
| Lovage | Levisticum officinale | | | | | 10 to 20 days at 70°F | | | | HP |
| Marshmallow | Althaea officinalis | | ✓ | 1 month | | 5 to 21 days at 60–65°F (prestratified seed) | ✓ | | | HP |
| Meadowsweet | Filipendula ulmaria | | | 3 months WM + 3 months CM | MCG, EPA, cover seed lightly | 14 to 35 days at 70°F (prestratified seed) | ✓ | | | HP |
| Milk thistle* | Silybum marianum | | | | CW, SS | 5 to 14 days at 65–70°F | | | | An, Bi |
| Milkweed, common | Asclepias syriaca | ✓ | | 1 month | SR | 10 to 25 days (prestratified seed) | ✓ | | Root cuttings | HP |
| Mimosa* | Albizia julibrissin | | ✓ | | SS, EPA, scarify and soak overnight | 7 to 14 days at 70–75°F | | | Semi-ripe, root cuttings | Sb to ST |
| Mints | Mentha spp. | ✓ | | | EPA, CVA, SR, not recommended from seed for most varieties | 10 to 14 days at 70–75°F | ✓ | ✓ | Softwood, root cuttings | CP |
| Motherwort | Leonurus cardiaca | | | 2 weeks | SS | 7 to 21 days at 65–70°F (prestratified seed) | ✓ | | | HP |

| PLANT | SCIENTIFIC NAME | SURFACE SOWN | SCARIFY | STRATIFICATION (COLD, MOIST UNLESS SPECIFIED) | NOTES | DAYS TO GERMINATION/ OPTIMAL TEMPERATURE | ROOT DIVISION | LAYERING | CUTTINGS | LIFESTYLE |
|---|---|---|---|---|---|---|---|---|---|---|
| Mullein | Verbascum thapsus, V. olympicum | ✓ | | 1 month | CW, SS | 7 to 15 days at 65–70°F (prestratified seed) | | | | Bi |
| Oats | Avena sativa | | | | Direct sow in early spring | 7 to 10 days | | | | An |
| Oregon grape | Mahonia aquifolium | | | 3 months WM + 3 months CM | EPA, MCG, GI, SS | 9 months (from sowing nonstratified seed outdoors in early fall) | ✓ | | Semi-ripe | WP to Sb |
| Oregano | Origanum vulgare | ✓ | | | EPA | 7 to 21 days at 65–70°F | | | Softwood | HP |
| Parsley | Petroselinum crispum | | | | Direct sow in early spring or fall | 2 weeks to 3 months at 65–70°F | | | | An to Bi |
| Passionflower | Passiflora incarnata | | ✓ | 2–3 months | GI, SR, sporadic germination | 7 to 28 days, sometimes longer, at 70–80°F (prestratified seed) | ✓ | ✓ | Semi-ripe, transplant wayward shoots | HV |
| Prickly pear* (some species) | Opuntia spp. | | ✓ | 3 months (depending on species) | EPA, CVA, plant seed shallowly and cover seed with a fine layer of sand | 1 to 2 years (from sowing nonstratified seed) | | | Root cactus pads | Perennial Cactus |
| Raspberry and blackberry species | Rubus spp. | | | 3 months | GI, EPA, CVA, SR | 9 months (from sowing nonstratified seed outdoors in fall) | ✓ | ✓ | Semi-ripe, hardwood | WV |
| Red clover | Trifolium pratense | | | | CW, SS, direct sow | 7 to 10 days | | | | HP |
| Red root/ New Jersey tea | Ceanothus americanus | | ✓ | 3 months | EPA | 4 to 21 days at 65–70°F (prestratified seed) | | | Semi-ripe, root cuttings | Sb |
| Rhodiola/ Roseroot | Rhodiola rosea | | | 6 weeks | EPA, lightly cover seed | 5 to 28 days at 65–70°F (prestratified seed) | ✓ | | | WP |
| Rose | Rosa spp. | | ✓ | 3 months WM + 3 months CM | H, GI, EPA, CVA, research if species need scarification | 10 to 18 months (from sowing nonstratified seed outdoors in late summer) Prestratified seed (warm + cold treatment) germinates in 7 to 21 days | | ✓* | Semi-ripe, hardwood, *vining species can be layered | Sb, WV |
| Rose of Sharon | Hibiscus syriacus | | | | SS, EPA, CVA, soak overnight | 7 to 14 days at 70–75°F | | | Hardwood | Sb |
| Rosemary | Salvia rosmarinus | | | | EPA, CVA | 14 to 28 days at 65–70°F | | | Semi-ripe | WP |
| Rue | Ruta graveolens | | ✓ | | | 10 to 14 days at 60–70°F | | | Semi-ripe, root cuttings | WP |
| Sage, common | Salvia officinalis | | | | CVA | 7 to 20 days at 70–85°F | | | Semi-ripe | WP |

| PLANT | SCIENTIFIC NAME | SURFACE SOWN | SCARIFY | STRATIFICATION (COLD, MOIST UNLESS SPECIFIED) | NOTES | DAYS TO GERMINATION/ OPTIMAL TEMPERATURE | ROOT DIVISION | LAYERING | CUTTINGS | LIFESTYLE |
|---|---|---|---|---|---|---|---|---|---|---|
| Sage, white | Salvia apiana | | ✓ | | Poor germination rates, barely cover seed, EPA | 7 to 21 days plus at 70–85°F | | | Semi-ripe | WP |
| Saint John's wort* | Hypericum perforatum | ✓ | | 2 months | SS | 4 to 21 days at 65–70°F (prestratified seed) | ✓ | ✓ | Semi-ripe | HP to WP |
| Schisandra | Schisandra chinensis | | | 1 month WM + 3 months CM | SR, MCG, GI, soak overnight, EPA, dioecious (male + female plants; only females bear fruits), poor germination rates | 7 to 18 months (from sowing nonstratified seed outdoors in early fall) | | ✓ | Semi-ripe, transplant wayward shoots (Vegetative methods ensure sex of plants) | WV |
| Shiso* | Perilla frutescens | | | | SS | 7 to 14 days at 70–85°F | | | | An to HP |
| Skullcap | Scutellaria lateriflora | | | 1–2 months | EPA | 5 to 25 days at 65–70°F (prestratified seed) | ✓ | | Softwood | HP |
| Solomon's seal | Polygonatum biflorum | | | Best started outdoors when seed is fresh | H, GI, MCG | 2 years from sowing (seed germinates underground first spring but won't sprout until the second spring) | ✓ | | Root cuttings | HP |
| Spikenard | Aralia racemosa | | ✓ | 2 months WM + 4 months CM. Or start outdoors in late summer/ early fall | MCG, poor germination rates | 7 to 18 months (from sowing nonstratified seed outdoors in early fall) | ✓ | | | HP |
| Spilanthes | Acmella oleracea | ✓* | | | SS, *lightly cover seed | 5 to 10 days at 70–85°F | ✓ | ✓ | Softwood | An to HP (in tropics) |
| Stinging nettles | Urtica dioica | ✓ | | 1–2 months | CW, EPA, SR | 7 to 14 days at 65–70°F (prestratified seed) | ✓ | | Root cuttings | HP |
| Sweetfern | Comptonia peregrina | | ✓ | | MCG, EPA | Up to 2 to 3 years | | ✓ | Root cuttings, semi-ripe from young shoots | WP to Sb |
| Sweet woodruff | Galium odoratum | | | | | 3 weeks to 9 months at 60–65°F | ✓ | | | HP |
| Tea, green and black | Camellia sinensis | | | | EPA, seed needs to be fresh, soak overnight | 1 to 2 months plus at 65–75°F | | | Semi-ripe, hardwood | Sb |
| Thyme | Thymus vulgaris and other Thymus spp. | ✓ | | | EPA, CVA | 5 to 21 days at 60–70°F | ✓ | ✓ | Semi-ripe | WP |

| PLANT | SCIENTIFIC NAME | SURFACE SOWN | SCARIFY | STRATIFICATION (COLD, MOIST UNLESS SPECIFIED) | NOTES | DAYS TO GERMINATION/ OPTIMAL TEMPERATURE | ROOT DIVISION | LAYERING | CUTTINGS | LIFESTYLE |
|---|---|---|---|---|---|---|---|---|---|---|
| Tulsi | *Ocimum tenuiflorum*, formerly *O. sanctum* | ✓* | | | SS, *barely cover seed | 5 to 21 days at 70–85°F | | | Semi-ripe | An to WP |
| Valerian | *Valeriana officinalis* | ✓ | | | EPA, low germination rates | 5 to 21 days at 65–70°F | ✓ | | | HP |
| Vervain, blue | *Verbena hastata* | ✓ | | 2–4 weeks | | 5 to 21 days at 65–70°F (prestratified seed) | ✓ | | | HP |
| Vervain, European | *Verbena officinalis* | ✓ | | 2–4 weeks | SS (tropical and subtropical climates) | 6 to 21 days at 65–70°F (prestratified seed) | ✓ | | | HP |
| Violet, common and sweet | *Viola sororia, V. odorata* | ✓ | | 2 months | H, SS, EPA, lightly cover seed, low germination rates | 10 days to 1 year at 65–75°F, sporadic germination | ✓ | | | HP |
| Vitex/chaste tree | *Vitex agnus-castus* | | ✓ | | Low germination rates | 14 to 40 days at 65–75°F | | ✓ | Semi-ripe, hardwood | Sb |
| Wild geranium | *Geranium maculatum* | | | 3 months / Best started outdoors in summer | H, EPA | 1 to 2 years (from sowing nonstratified seed outdoors in summer) | ✓ | | | HP |
| Wild indigo | *Baptisia tinctoria* | | ✓ | | Scarify and soak overnight | 7 to 15 days at 65–75°F | | | | HP |
| Wild yam | *Dioscorea villosa* | | | 3 months / Best started outdoors in fall | EPA | 9 months (from sowing nonstratified seed outdoors in fall) | ✓ | | Root cuttings | HV |
| Willow | *Salix* spp. | ✓ | | | H, EPA, CVA | 14 to 28 days at 70°F | | ✓ | Semi-ripe, hardwood | Sb to ST |
| Witch hazel | *Hamamelis virginiana* | | | 2 months WM + 3 months CM | MCG | 9 months (from sowing nonstratified seed outdoors in early fall) | | ✓ | | Sb to ST |
| Woad | *Isatis tinctoria* | | | | | 10 to 14 days at 65–70°F | | | | Bi to HP |
| Wormwood | *Artemisia absinthium* | ✓ | | 1 month | | 5 to 10 days at 55–65°F (prestratified seed) | | ✓ | Semi-ripe | WP |
| Yarrow | *Achillea millefolium* | ✓ | | | SS, EPA, CVA | 10 to 14 days at 70–80°F | ✓ | | | HP |
| Yellow dock | *Rumex crispus, R. obtusifolius* | | ✓ | | CW, SS, direct sow, sporadic germination | 2 weeks to several years | ✓ | | | HP |

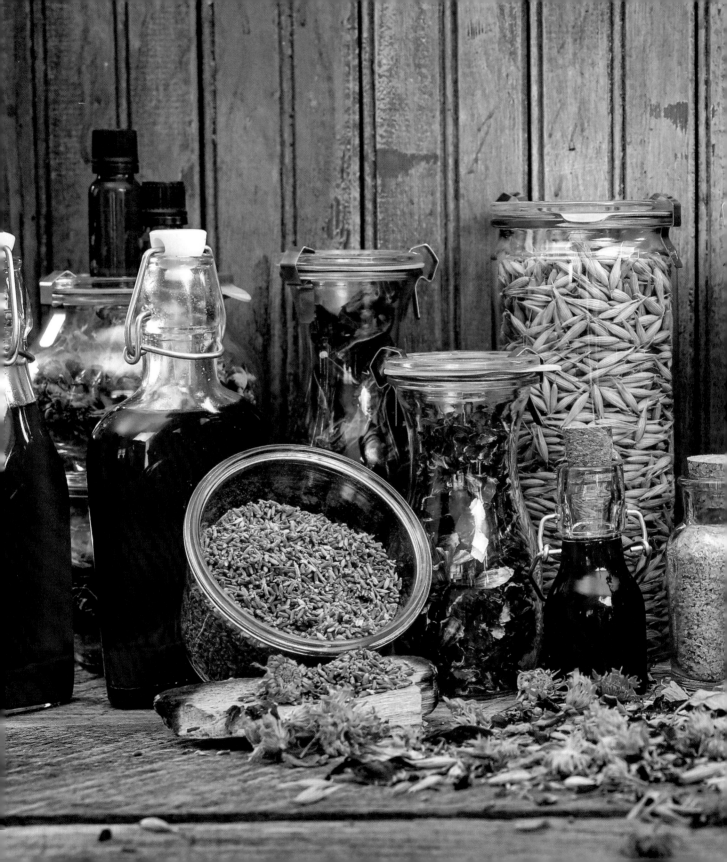

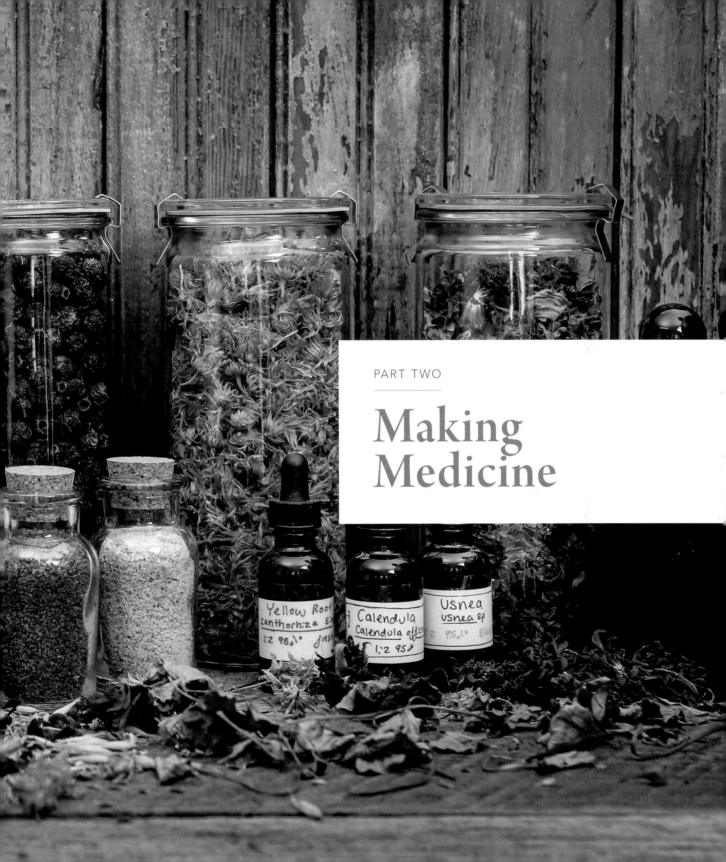

PART TWO

# Making Medicine

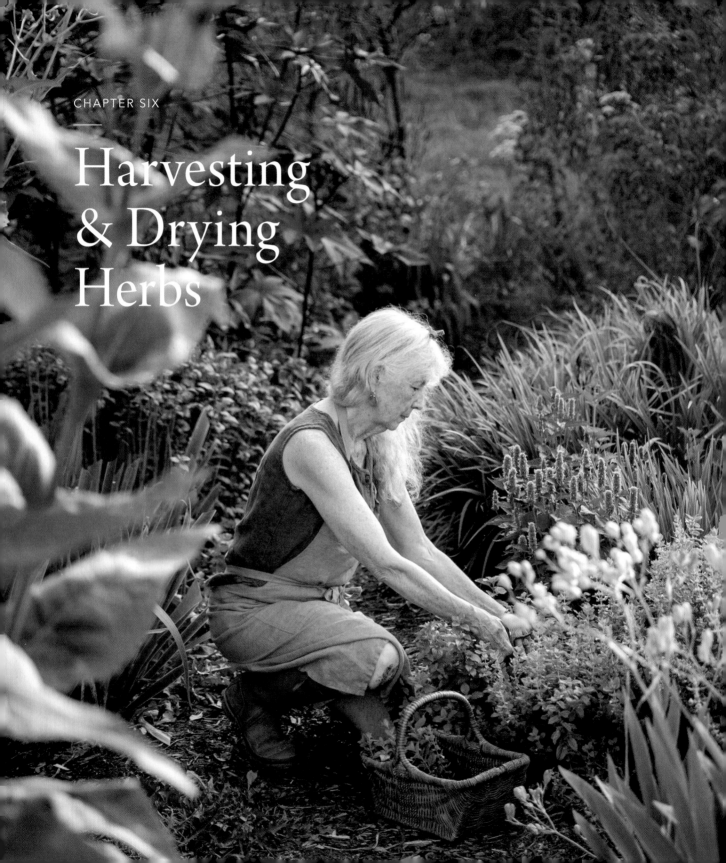

CHAPTER SIX

# Harvesting & Drying Herbs

Silently a flower blooms,
　　In silence it falls away;
Yet here now, at this moment, at this place,
　　The world of the flower, the whole of
　　the world is blooming.
This is the talk of the flower, the truth
　　of the blossom;
The glory of eternal life is fully shining here.
　　　　　　　　　　　~ Zenkei Shibayama

When you go to harvest an herb, you're provided with an opportunity to slow down and connect with the plant and its medicine. Every one of us lives in a body sustained by the sun and the earth. Take a moment to pause before the plant, taking in its beauty and your surroundings. Center yourself in gratitude—appreciating your ability to garden and grow this medicine. Think about how the herb has enriched your life with its medicine, flavor, or flowers. Give thanks to the land with a song, a prayer, a token of your appreciation, or a simple acknowledgment of how it brings you joy and sustenance. As you inhale and exhale, know that you are bound to the green world, your union sealed by exchanged oxygen and carbon dioxide.

# Harvesting Leaves & Flowers

Harvest the aboveground parts of an herb—leaves and flowers or both—in the morning after the dew has evaporated. See the "Harvesting" section in the herbal profiles starting on page 208 for harvesting tips for each herb. A good pair of sharp pruners is indispensable for harvesting plants with woody or thicker stems; use kitchen or garden scissors for tender herbs such as mint, lemon balm, violet, dandelion, or chickweed. With one hand holding the leaves or stems upright, give the plants a haircut close to the base of the plant, leaving some foliage intact. As long as it's early in the growing season, most herbs will regrow, often giving you a second or even a third harvest. Gently stack your harvest in a basket without bruising or piling too high—one to two layers deep at most. Bring your bounty indoors or into the shade as soon as possible, and inspect it for dirt, diseased parts, fungal growth, or insects. Remove damaged parts, and if necessary, wash off any dirt or insects. If your harvest is clean and free of insects, there's no need to wash it before processing. Picking through your herbs and removing undesirable portions is called *garbling*. At this point, you're ready to prepare the harvest into medicine or dry it using one of the methods described starting on page 124.

# Harvesting & Processing Roots

The best time to harvest the roots of perennial herbs is while plants are dormant, in the fall or early spring, because they store much of their energy, including medicinal compounds, belowground when they aren't actively growing and photosynthesizing. If you take only part of the root system, as described below, the plants will continue to grow. You can even harvest roots throughout the winter if the ground isn't frozen and you're still able to identify the plant. With biennial herbs—plants like burdock and angelica, with a lifespan of just two years—harvest the roots in the fall after their first year's growth or in the spring of their second year. Perennial garden herbs typically need to grow for two to three years before their roots are sizable enough to harvest. While dormant harvesting is preferable, if you need a root immediately for medicine, go ahead and harvest a small amount out of season. Dig that burdock in July. I won't tell!

I harvest roots with a digging fork, but a sharp shovel will also do. First, dig a circle around the plant, gently prying the root from the soil by rocking your digging fork back and forth. You're loosening the root without actually digging it from the ground. (Lift a root prematurely, and you'll snap off precious parts that are still buried.) I kneel near the plant after loosening the root, sizing things up using my

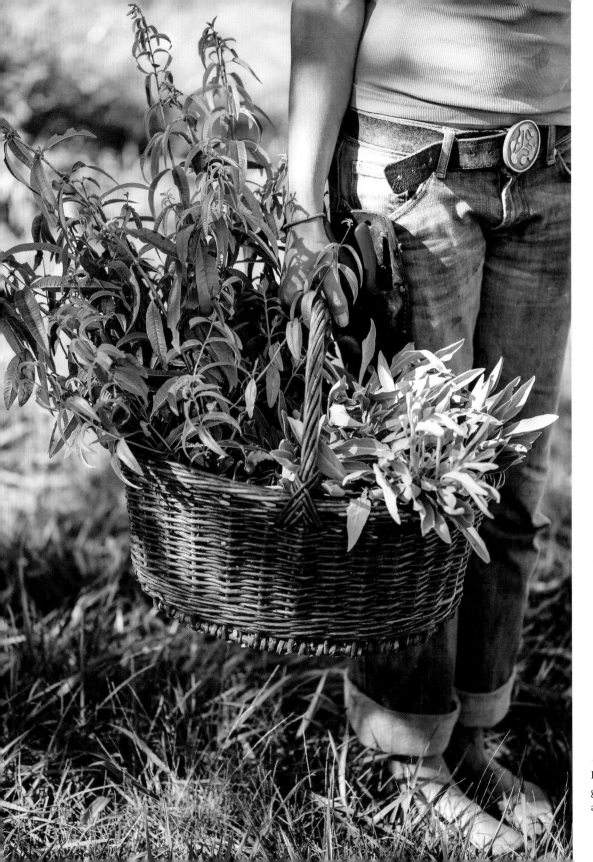

Harvesting home-grown white sage and lemon verbena

hands and cajoling side roots free from the dirt. After you've located and liberated the entire root system, you can fully unearth the plant. Be careful not to accidentally harvest the roots of neighboring plants, which is quite easy to do, as root systems become intertwined. If I find a cut-off piece of root and can't positively confirm its identity, I give it back to the earth, erring on the side of caution.

## Regenerative Root Harvesting

For perennial herbs, you can harvest their entire roots or only part of their root systems, allowing them to continue growing. Using this second method, I rotationally harvest my garden herbs, taking only a portion of each plant's root system every three years. Similar principles apply to the regenerative harvesting of wild plants.

STEP 1: Dig the plant's entire root system, as described above (*top right*).

STEP 2: Harvest half to three-fourths of its root system (*middle right*).

STEP 3: Replant the remaining root crown at its original soil depth, with the buds pointing up (*bottom right*). Cut back a proportional amount of stems and leaves so that the diminished root system can nourish the remaining parts of the plant. This goes for woody plants in any season or herbaceous perennials that aren't dormant; however, if a plant is dormant or has no woody growth, you can skip this step without unduly stressing the plant.

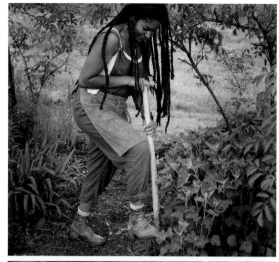

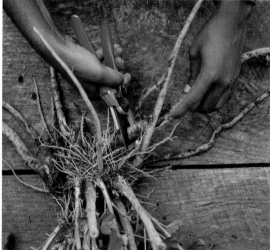

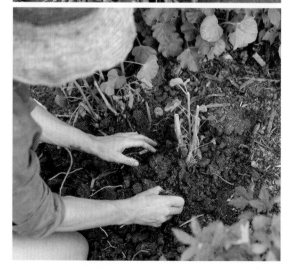

Harvesting roots in a regenerative fashion

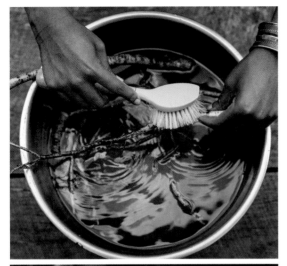

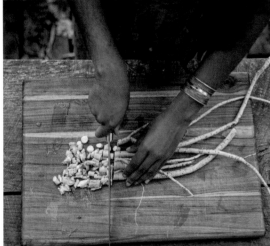

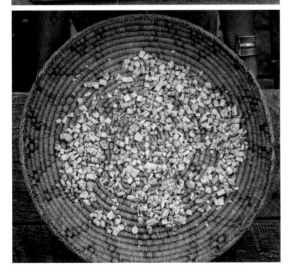

## Washing and Chopping Roots

After your roots are harvested, process them as soon as possible. Scrub them with a vegetable brush to remove all the soil *(top left)*. If the root is in a tight or convoluted mass, use pruners to cut it apart so you can clean every nook and crevice. After the roots are squeaky clean, chop them immediately *(middle left)*. They become substantially harder to cut once they are dried. Use sharp pruners or a large, sharp knife to process woody roots into smaller pieces. At this point, you're ready to dry the chopped roots on screens or baskets *(bottom left)* or prepare them as medicine.

Washing and chopping marshmallow roots

# Drying Methods

Two crucial factors for drying herbs at home are heat and airflow. Look for a space in your home that gets moderately hot but has plenty of air movement or can be helped along with a fan. A little heat speeds the drying process, but too much heat degrades plant material. Direct sun will also lessen the quality of your harvest. If you have an area in your home where you use an air conditioner or a dehydrator, that's an ideal space to dry herbs.

## Bundling and Hanging Herbs

Hanging bundled leafy stems or flowering stalks is one of the easiest ways to dry harvests, especially herbs with long stalks. In a quiet spot out of direct sunlight, hang a string between two nails from which to hang the bundles. Or use a foldable wooden clothes rack as an impromptu drying setup. I prefer bundling herbs with rubber bands instead of twine. As herbs dry, they shrink. If you use string to bundle your harvest, some stalks will fall to the floor, but with rubber bands, the bundles hold.

STEP 1: Harvest your plant material, removing any undesirable portions. Gather up smallish bundles, typically with 5 to 10 stems per bundle, depending on the herb (A). If your bundle is too large, it won't dry in the middle.

STEP 2: Split each bundle into two, and loop your rubber band around one of the halves (B).

STEP 3: Encircle the entire bundle with your folded rubber band until it is taut (C).

STEP 4: Take one end of the rubber band and loop it over a few stems to hold the band in place (D).

STEP 5: Pry open the bundle into two halves and place on top of the hanging string or drying rack (E).

## Dehydrators

Home dehydrators work fine for drying small amounts of loose plant material. Make sure you have the dehydrator temperature set on low, as excess heat can degrade the quality of the herbs.

## Screens and Baskets

Dry loose plant materials—flowers, roots, bark, or free leaves—on screens or in wide baskets. The looser the basket's weave, the more air can circulate, helping to dry the herbs. You can make your own drying rack out of wood and screen material. Hanging commercial drying racks, like the one pictured on page 126, are inexpensive and have a loose enough mesh weave to allow for good airflow and rapid drying. To speed the drying process and prevent molding, place a single layer of your plant material on the basket or screen, and periodically tousle the herb. *Schluffle* is a word I made up for the tussling of drying herbs. Here's an example of how you, too, might use the term at home: "No honey, I can't wash the dishes right now—I must go schluffle my calendula flowers instead."

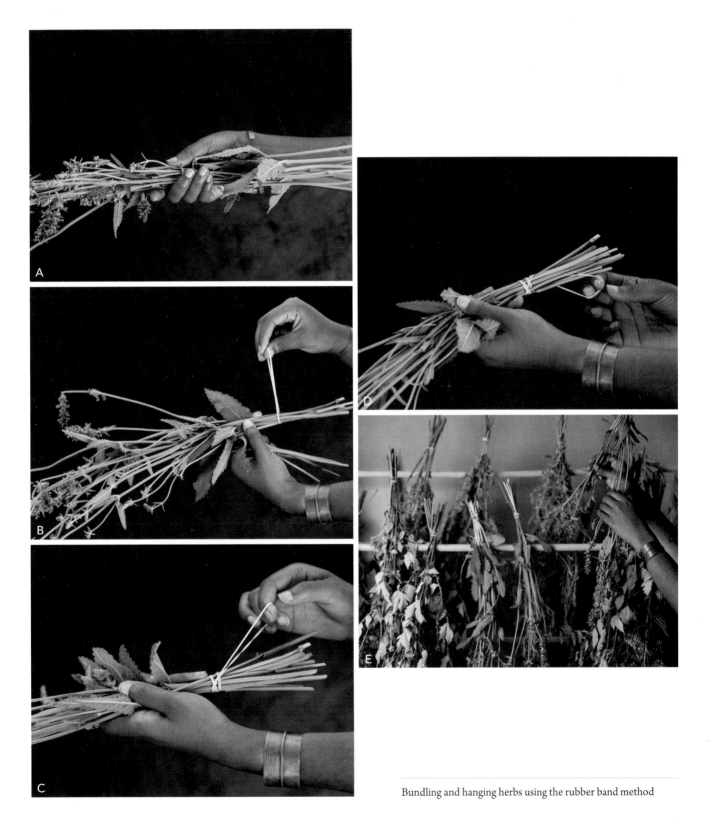

Bundling and hanging herbs using the rubber band method

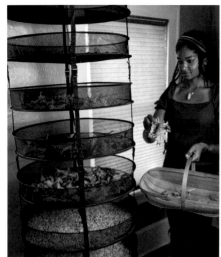 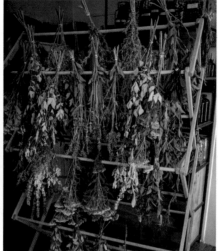 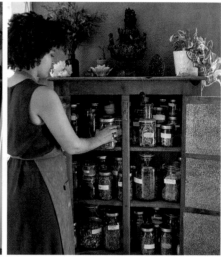

A commercial hanging drying rack; a foldable clothes rack is handy for drying herb bundles; store dried herbs in a dark cabinet or hutch

### Car-as-Greenhouse Method

This is a helpful technique if you live in a humid climate or are on a road trip. Park your car in a sunny spot, roll down the windows a few inches, and suspend a sheet between the front and rear seat. Rest your harvest baskets on the rear seat, under the shade of the sheet. When the car heats up, the moisture inside the plant material escapes, leaving the car through the open window. Close the windows at night to prevent the reabsorption of moisture. Depending on the humidity and plant material, the herbs may take two to three days to dry.

## Testing for Dryness

It's crucial that your harvest is thoroughly dried before storage, because any moisture in stored herbs will allow for mold growth, rendering the herb unusable. Use the crunch test to determine if an herb is dry enough to store. Rub a leaf between your fingers. If it crumbles, it's dry enough; if it bends but doesn't feel crisp, it probably needs a little more drying. With roots, it's harder to figure out if they're fully dry. If the root pieces are brown on the outside and shriveled, cut open a few pieces and see how they look on the inside. If they look dry all the way through, then it's time to put them up.

# Storing Herbs

If you're putting up a large harvest, bring your work outside and wear a mask and/or goggles to keep the small particles from irritating your respiratory passages and eyes.

FOR LOOSE HERBS THAT HAVE BEEN DRIED ON SCREENS OR BASKETS, put the herb in a jar whole, or if the leaves are in larger pieces, crumble them a tad before storing.

FOR BUNDLED MEDICINAL HERBS, strip the leaves from the stem using broad strokes. Store the leaves whole or crumbled.

FOR CULINARY HERBS, take special care to break up the plant material into finer pieces, pulling out little stems or woody parts, which can be unpleasantly pokey in food.

Store your herbs in glass jars inside a cabinet, hutch, pantry, or dark shelf. Label the jars with the name of the plant, the part gathered, and the date they were stored. I organize my herbs alphabetically so they're easy to find and keep beverage herbs in the kitchen cabinet close to the stove to make teatime easier. Herbs that are more medicinal and are used less frequently are stored in a hutch away from the kitchen's prime real estate. Dried leaves and flowers will typically last one to two years, and roots can last two to three years. To determine if an herb is still vital, use your senses—if the herb looks, smells, and tastes vibrant, it's still good medicine! Additionally, check for signs of spoilage: mold, insect webs, or off-smells are all signs that the herb should be composted.

Stripping dried meadowsweet leaves from the stem; jarring dried violet leaf and flower; labeled and jarred dried violet leaf

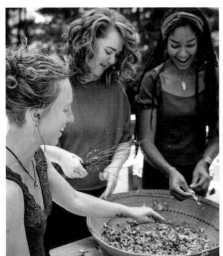 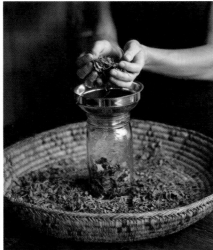 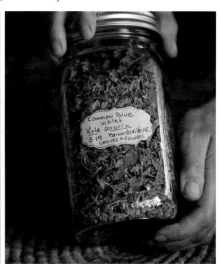

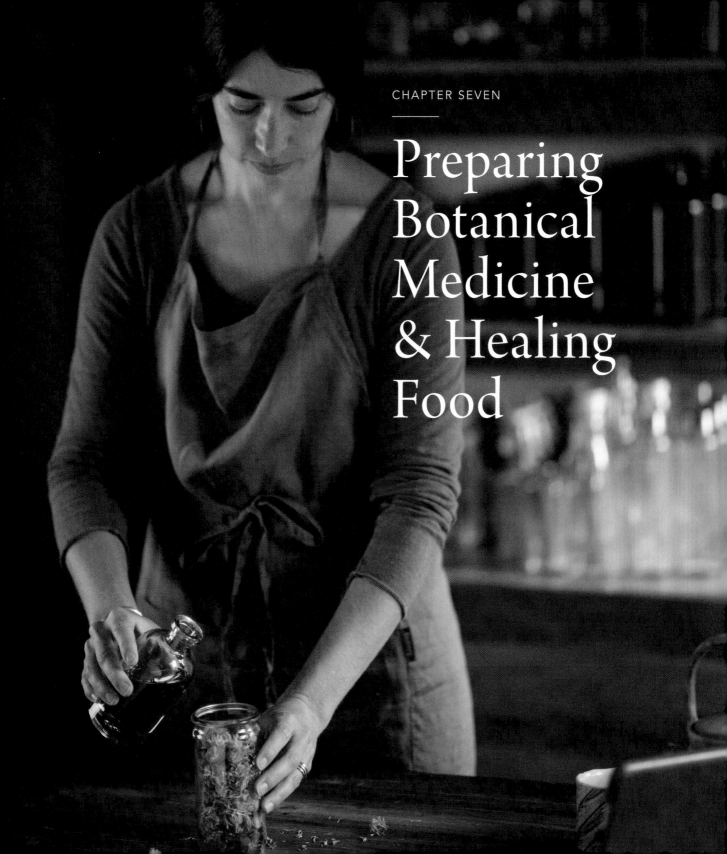

CHAPTER SEVEN

# Preparing Botanical Medicine & Healing Food

**Spring Tea Poem**
To you I would serve cedar tea
mixed with a touch of April
distilled from shy green stems,
the frosted perfume of spring
rain along with a dollop
of honey and ice

~ Keewaydinoquay Peschel

# Introduction to Medicinal Preparations

When I was first learning about herbs, I was downright smitten. I was intrigued by their folklore and enchanted by each botanical's aroma and texture. Three decades later, I'm still amazed by how effective and safe herbs are as medicine. And my daily life is that much richer for herbs—from the tasty teas that bring comfort to my afternoons to my herbal tonics that keep me feeling vital as I grow older. I can't imagine a kitchen without herbs! The zestiness of herbal dishes and drinks simply makes life that much sweeter.

Herbal medicine has been my primary form of health care for the past three decades—my plant allies help me feel vital and calmer, and I feel equipped to handle life's bumps and bruises. I feel more grounded to the elements, my ancestors, and the earth through my plant connections. As preventive medicine, herbs reign supreme. If you're looking to weather cold and flu season like a champ, immunomodulating herbs can bolster your immune system. Immune-stimulating and antimicrobial herbs are also effective for addressing minor infections and can help reduce antibiotic overuse and misuse.

Over the years, I've seen botanical remedies help countless people with insomnia, mood, stress, infertility, pain, infections, autoimmune conditions, colds, flu, arthritis, skin conditions, and many other problems. At times, herbal medicine mends an ailment completely, but often it gives ease by lessening pain or discomfort. Other herbal remedies might shorten the duration of sickness or assuage the severity of the condition and thereby improve a person's quality of life.

Plant medicines aren't always the only healing we need. Our medicine can come in the form of additional therapies, which might include acupuncture, massage, chiropractic adjustments, talk therapy, human connection, time in nature, rest, hydrotherapy, physical therapy, supplements, nutritional changes, pharmaceuticals, surgery, or other conventional medical approaches. My own journey has included surgery and many of the above strategies. Herbs have enriched my life and health, but they haven't been the only medicine I've needed to thrive, or even stay alive!

Disease and healing are complex and mysterious, and both are part and parcel of having a body. None of us lives in a vacuum. Our health is affected by genetics, epigenetics, trauma, environmental health, and cultural stressors like racism, homophobia, sexism, and other forms of discrimination and bias. These stressors can sometimes limit our access to healthy food, housing, safety, freedom, and health care, which in turn has obvious consequences on health. Our water, air, and food are becoming more contaminated every day with human-made chemicals and microplastics. People of color and lower-income folks are more affected by pollution. Environmental chemicals significantly affect our endocrine system (hormonal regulation) and stress the eliminative channels of the body (the liver, kidneys, and skin). Now more than ever, humans need herbs for their antioxidant, anti-inflammatory, and hormone-balancing qualities.

The goal is to feel better. Sometimes that means eradication of the disease or disorder, and sometimes the healing will be in the ease you find when your mood, energy, or vitality is improved or your pain or discomfort is lessened. Profound healing can occur even when a health challenge is here to stay. Wellness is not an all-or-nothing affair. It's about feeling *your* best, or sometimes, your "better."

Foundational wellness measures—sleep, rest, exercise, nutrition, hydration, and stress relief—are key to staying healthy and feeling vital and are even more critical than herbal therapies in the prevention and healing of disease. Think of botanicals as the icing on the cake. In my decades of helping people feel healthier with plant medicine, I've seen firsthand how much better herbs work when a person gets enough sleep, nourishes their body with healthy food, reduces stress, and surrounds themselves with loving relationships.

One of the best ways to ensure that your herbal remedies are high quality is to prepare them yourself with vital homegrown herbs. With careful attention to cleanliness and plant identification, you'll know that your medicine is pure and unadulterated. (Store-bought, conventionally grown herbal products, especially lower-quality preparations from large manufacturers, can be contaminated with herbicides and pesticides. Products sometimes contain adulterated herbs, which means another herb is intentionally or accidentally substituted for the herb listed on the label.) You can also save money by preparing medicine at home, especially if you use homegrown or gathered herbs. Many of the recipes in this book showcase beverages or food that double as preventive medicine for overall vitality and wellness. You won't find these preparations on the shelf of the health food store or on any menu—you'll need to make them at home to enjoy them on a regular basis.

In this chapter and throughout the herbal profiles, you'll find culinary and medicinal preparations, along with herbal dishes and beverages that are both therapeutic and delectable. We'll start with the most familiar herbal medicines: tinctures, infusions, decoctions, honeys, and syrups. Tinctures are concentrated alcohol-based preparations that are usually sold in dropper bottles.

Because they are potent, small doses are used—usually a few dropperful to a teaspoon. Depending on the herb, tinctures can be tonic (daily, long-term) remedies or they may be a remedy used short term for a specific illness or condition. Infusions and decoctions are forms of herbal teas that can be tasty, enjoyed purely for pleasure, or therapeutic, taken primarily for their medicinal virtues; sometimes they are both. Herbal honeys are prepared from honey that has been infused with herbs. They can be used to flavor or medicate teas or be taken by the spoonful. Herbal honeys can also be combined with other ingredients to make herbal syrups. Both herbal honeys and syrups have an affinity for soothing sore throats and assuaging respiratory conditions.

Then we move on to topical preparations. Herbs can be applied to the skin in water-based or in oil-based preparations. Infused herbal oils can be used to calm inflamed skin or as massage oils to soothe achy joints or sore muscles, or they can be used as the base of natural body care products. Herbal oils can be prepared into herbal salves to soothe dry, inflamed skin conditions by adding wax to harden the oil. Water-based topical preparations include poultices, compresses, washes, and soaks. These are helpful for easing muscular and joint pain and inflammation and addressing infections and weepy skin conditions like poison ivy, acne, or weeping eczema.

Next we turn to culinary concoctions like herbal butters, salts, vinegars, simple syrups, pestos, and broth. Some of these are enjoyed purely for their flavor and others are a base for medicine. After preparing a number of these recipes—and reading their descriptions—you'll find the line between medicine and food is not often hard and fast.

If you enjoyed conjuring up potions as a child, medicine making will bring out your inner alchemist. You may remember the following concepts from high school chemistry. A solvent is a substance that dissolves a solute, resulting in a solution. For our purposes, the solutes are the medicinal constituents within herbs, and the solution is the finished medicine. The solvent is the liquid that's extracting, or pulling out, the medicinal compounds from the plant. Common solvents in medicine making include honey, alcohol, water, vinegar, and oil.

Water and alcohol are near-universal solvents—they are both excellent at extracting the majority of constituents from medicinal plants. However, alcohol can extract compounds that water cannot, and vice versa. In general, honey, oil, and vinegar are weaker solvents, but they still have an essential place at the medicine-making table. Honey in particular has its own medicinal qualities and is quite palatable, which can make all the difference in someone taking their medicine. The information listed below can help as a guide in deciding which solvent to choose. You'll also find more information in the instructions for each medicinal preparation.

| SOLVENT (EXTRACTING LIQUID) | HERBAL PREPARATIONS | NOTES |
|---|---|---|
| Water | Infusions, decoctions, soaks, baths, compresses, poultices, syrups, and broths | Strong solvent; especially effective at extracting mucilage, minerals, and long-chain polysaccharides; ineffective at extracting resins; best solvent for external infections and weepy skin conditions; shortest shelf life |
| Alcohol | Tinctures and syrups | Strong solvent; effective at extracting essential oils, resins, and alkaloids; ineffective at extracting minerals, mucilage, and long-chain polysaccharides; long shelf life |
| Vinegar | Culinary and medicinal infused vinegars, oxymels, fire cider, and shrubs (drinking vinegars) | Medium solvent, effective at extracting minerals, shorter shelf life |
| Oil | Infused culinary oils and infused topical oils, salves, serums, body butters, lotions, and creams | Weaker solvent; heat extraction optimal, especially with resin-containing herbs; readily dissolves essential oils; shorter shelf life |
| Honey | Infused honey, syrup, topical treatment | Weaker solvent; long shelf life if not diluted with water |

### When to Choose Herbal Teas over Tinctures

**1.** When you want to hydrate or drink a hot and comforting beverage.

**2.** When you need to or want to avoid alcohol.

**3.** When you want to extract minerals. Teas are a better choice than alcohol-based tinctures for extracting the minerals from mineral-rich herbs, such as nettles, chickweed, violet, red clover, alfalfa, and dandelion leaf.

**4.** When you want the slime. Teas are a better choice than alcohol-based tinctures for extracting mucilage from mucilaginous herbs such as slippery elm, marshmallow, corn silk, violet, linden, cinnamon, and licorice. (Mucilage is a thick and slimy therapeutic substance that herbalists use to soothe inflammation internally and topically. It is a type of soluble fiber and is biochemically comprised of a polar glycoprotein and an exopolysaccharide.)

**5.** When you want the immunomodulating compounds from medicinal mushrooms and herbs such as astragalus, maitake, shiitake, turkey tail, lion's mane, and reishi. These compounds are best extracted in water through long decoctions of a few hours or longer, as high alcohol levels destroy long-chain polysaccharides—key compounds involved in immunomodulation.

### When to Choose Herbal Tinctures over Teas

**1.** When you're short on time and need a convenient and easily transportable medicine. You can even fly with tinctures in your carry-on luggage, as long as they are in a 3-ounce bottle or smaller.

**2.** When you want to take a medicinal that is bitter or yucky-tasting.

**3.** When you want to extract resin from resinous herbs. Alcohol is more effective than water at extracting resins. Examples of resinous herbs include balm of Gilead, grindelia (rosinweed), pine, propolis, spruce resin, and cannabis (note that the medicinal use of cannabis, or marijuana, is illegal in some countries and/or municipalities).

4. When you want to extract sizable quantities of essential oils. Essential oils are slightly soluble in water but more soluble in mid- to-high-percentage alcohol. Examples of medicinal herbs with a high essential oil profile are garden sage, lavender, rosemary, thyme, and white sage.

## Giving Medicine to Children

You'll want to be extra careful in choosing herbs for young children under the age of three. (See "Herbal Safety" on page 198.) A good resource to determine if an herb is safe for infants and toddlers is Aviva Jill Romm's *Natural Healing for Babies and Children: A Commonsense Guide to Herbal Remedies, Nutrition, and Health*. After determining that a remedy is safe for a child, there are several methods for delivering the medicine. For starters, breastfeeding parents can take an herbal medicine and then breastfeed, effectively passing along the medicine. Herbal teas can be given to infants by the dropperful or mixed into formula. After the child is over two years old, I feel comfortable giving *very* small amounts of alcohol-based tinctures because they're taking such a minute amount of alcohol, usually 5 to 10 drops. You'll want to dilute tinctures in a small amount of juice, tea, water, or honey, as the high alcohol can irritate and "burn" the mouth. To evaporate half of the alcohol from a tincture, add the tincture to a small amount of just-boiled water or hot tea and let it stand, uncovered, for 10 minutes. If you prefer to completely avoid alcohol, tincture alternatives include teas, vinegars, syrups, oxymels, honeys, or herbal powders in food.

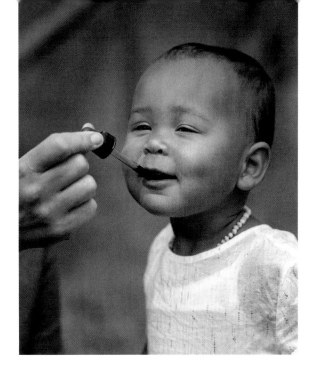

**Don't give honey to babies under the age of one, as it may contain botulism spores, which can result in severe illness or fatality.**

### Determining Dosage in Children by Weight

A typical adult dosage assumes a 150-pound adult. To determine a child's dosage, divide the child's weight by 150. Take that number and multiply it by the recommended adult dosage. For example, if a child weighs 50 pounds, they will need one-third the recommended dose for a 150-pound adult. Here are some example calculations for different medicinal preparations:

**If the adult dosage is 3 droppersful of a tincture, a 50-pound child should take ⅓ of that dose, or 1 dropperful.**

**If the adult dosage is 1 cup (8 fluid ounces) of tea, a 50-pound child should take ⅓ cup.**

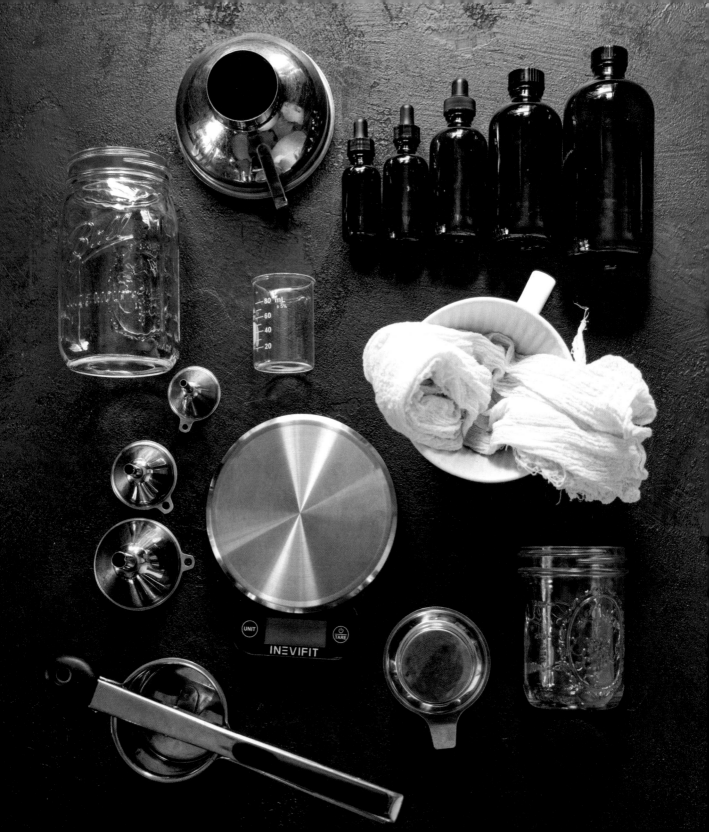

# Medicine-Making Tools & Techniques

Here are my tried-and-true methods and tools for preparing herbal medicines. You likely already have many of these tools and can slowly build up a cache of essential supplies, most of which are reusable. Choose glass, ceramic, and stainless steel over all types of plastic, as heat and solvents can degrade plastic and leach chemicals into your medicine.

## Medicine-Making Supplies

### Essential Tools and Supplies
*(listed clockwise, starting at 11 o'clock)*

**STAINLESS-STEEL FUNNEL:** Useful for filling canning jars.

**ASSORTED AMBER BROWN GLASS DROPPER BOTTLES AND AMBER BROWN GLASS BOTTLES WITH POLYSEAL CAPS:** 1- and 2-ounce dropper bottles are handy. Larger brown bottles are helpful for storing and dispensing tinctures, infused oils, syrups, and vinegars. The polyseal cap is resistant to solvents. (More on these dispensing bottles on page 138.)

**CERAMIC COFFEE DRIPPER:** Convenient for straining when lined with a straining cloth. A stainless-steel strainer is a fine alternative but is less stable.

**STRAINING CLOTH:** Look for unbleached cotton cloth, sold for straining nut milk, coffee, or cheese. Cut pieces of the fabric to size, depending on your needs.

**ASSORTED WIDE-MOUTH CANNING JARS:** It's useful to have a few of each size: half-pint (8 ounce), pint (16 ounce), and quart (32 ounce).

**STAINLESS-STEEL TEA STRAINER:** Convenient for preparing single cups of tea and straining small quantities of medicine.

**POTATO RICER:** Sold for making mashed potatoes, this is a useful tool for small-scale straining and pressing. These can easily warp, so invest in a quality version.

**ASSORTED SMALLER FUNNELS:** Handy for filling smaller bottles.

**GLASS BEAKER:** Useful for measuring small quantities of liquid ingredients.

**DIGITAL KITCHEN SCALE:** Weighing ingredients is important for achieving success with medicine making. Choose one that has a tare function and a metric option.

### Other Useful Tools *(not pictured)*

**LABELS, FINE-POINT PERMANENT MARKER, AND CLEAR PACKING TAPE**

**GLASS-JAR BLENDER:** You'll use a blender when making infused oils, salves, tinctures, body care products, and many herbal foods. Glass is resistant to heat, aromatic compounds, and solvents, unlike plastic. You can use your regular kitchen blender for medicine making as long as it's super clean.

**FOOD PROCESSOR:** Useful for preparing poultices and herbal finishing salts, hummus, pesto, and pâté, and grinding herb/solvent mixtures into a slurry.

**KITCHEN THERMOMETER:** Used for preparing herbal honeys and infused oils.

SALVE AND CREAM JARS: As needed.

GLASS OR STAINLESS STEEL FRENCH PRESS: Sold for making coffee, a French press can also be used for making herbal infusions.

GLASS MEASURING CUPS

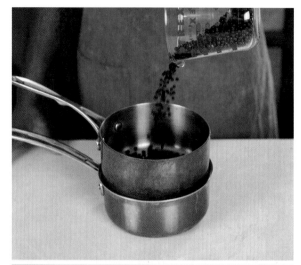

## Double Boilers and Homemade Versions

You'll often want to apply gentle heat in the extraction process of an herbal medicine. When making herbal-infused oils and honeys, for example, you need to maintain a low, steady temperature over time. A double boiler consists of a pot or bowl nested tightly over a lower pot, containing a few inches of water *(top right)*. When heated on a stovetop, the water in the lower pot releases steam that gently heats the ingredients in the upper pot. You can purchase a double boiler or fashion one with kitchen items you already have on hand. Use a stainless-steel or glass bowl that fits snugly over your saucepan but doesn't touch the bottom. Alternatively, nest a smaller pot in a larger pot, taking care that the pots won't stick. To avoid burns, be careful of the steam when handling the pot, and watch the water content in the lower pot, replenishing as needed.

## Weight versus Volume Measurements

My recipes often include both weight and volume measurements. The weight measurement (measured in grams) is more accurate and will yield the best results. If I only give a volume measurement (cups, teaspoons, fluid ounces, etc.), there's no need to weigh ingredients because they are uniform in density or texture.

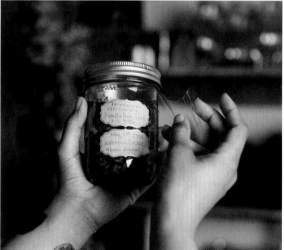

## Sterilizing Jars and Bottles

Some of the recipes in this book mention sterilizing canning jars or glass bottles before making medicine or storing an herbal remedy. A dishwasher set on the "sanitize" setting or a pressure cooker will do the trick for our purposes. To be on the safest side and fully sterilize your glass canning jars, place them on a rack in a water-bath canner and boil for 10 minutes. Don't do this to jars with rubber gaskets, or they may melt.

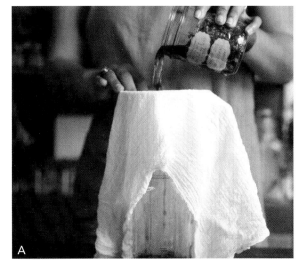
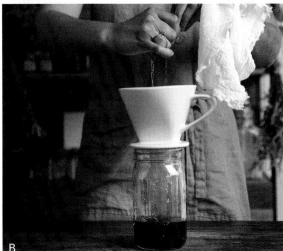
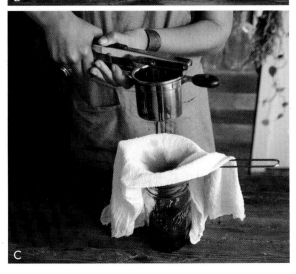

## Labeling

Add a label to your medicinal preparations with the name of the herb(s), part used, date, extracting liquid, and proportions, if applicable. Write down where you sourced the herb, whether gathered, grown, or purchased. If you purchased a dried herb in bulk, record the lot number on the label in case you ever need to track down the source of the herb. Use a fine-point permanent marker, and place clear packing tape over the label so that alcohol, vinegar, essential oils, and oils—which act as solvents—won't dissolve the ink and cause your label to run.

## Straining and Pressing

It's helpful to have several straining options available, including stainless-steel strainers, a potato ricer, and a tea strainer. You'll also need a loose-weave fabric for straining out finer herb particles when preparing herbal honeys, tinctures, oils, syrups, and vinegars. Look for unbleached cotton cloth—sold for straining nut milk, coffee, or cheese—and then cut pieces of the fabric to size. If the weave's too tight, straining is a chore, and if it's too loose, your medicine won't be properly strained.

Straining medicine is a two-step process. First, place a straining cloth in a ceramic coffee dripper or stainless-steel tea strainer, nested over a glass mason jar or measuring cup (A). Pour over the liquid to strain. After most of the liquid has passed through the cloth, the remaining saturated herb needs to be pressed or wrung out (B). You can use your hands in a pinch, but some solvents are irritating. The best straining tool for home medicine making is a stainless-steel potato ricer. Place the plant material in the ricer and use the handle to express the liquid (C). After straining, the herb residue may be composted.

## Storing and Organizing Your Medicine

I store tinctures, syrups, vinegars, oxymels, infused oils, serums, and simple syrups in amber glass dispensing bottles (sold as amber Boston round glass bottles) with polyseal caps. These bottles have several helpful attributes. The brown glass excludes light, which can degrade medicine over time. The inside of the polyseal cap is resistant to solvents, as it is manufactured for chemical storage. I don't like that the inside of the cap is plastic, as I am concerned about the plastic compounds leaching into the medicine, but I haven't yet found a better system. These bottles are easy to pour. You can pour directly from a dispensing bottle into a tincture bottle without a funnel. The bottles are a small investment, but they are washable and reusable—I have dozens that have been with me over a decade. As an alternative, people often store their medicine in glass canning jars, but alcohol and vinegar will corrode canning lids over time, contaminating the medicine with plastic compounds. To prevent this, use natural waxed paper as a barrier on the inside of the lid.

An *apothecary* is a collection of herbal medicines, which can include tinctures, dried herbs, medicinal honeys, syrups, and the like. You can store your apothecary in a cupboard, cabinet, or hutch, as long as it's some distance from the stove and potential kitchen fires (alcohol-based tinctures are very flammable). Keep your medicines out of the reach of small children and always label each bottle, as it's all too easy to forget the contents of an unmarked bottle over time. I store my dispensing bottles in alphabetical order in a wooden cabinet with doors.

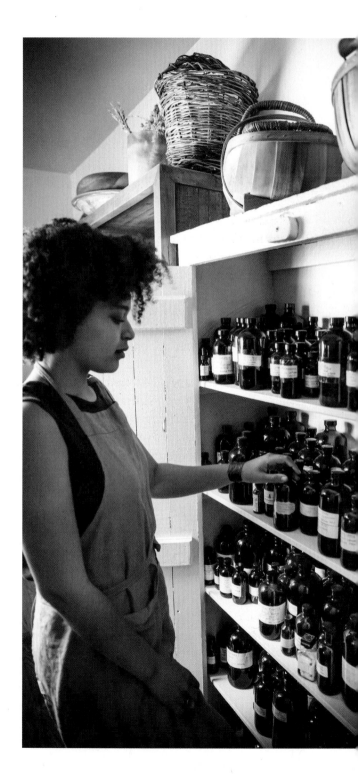

My apothecary consists of tinctures and syrups stored alphabetically in amber Boston round glass bottles, also called amber glass dispensing bottles.

# Herbal Tinctures

Herbal tinctures are surprisingly easy to prepare, and if you grow your own herbs, they are quite affordable compared to store-bought tinctures. When I was first learning about herbs, I made elaborate labels for my tinctures, which included drawings of the plants, along with color-coded lists of their medicinal actions and uses. Every time I shook my tinctures (part of their preparation), I would get to know the herb more, feeling connected to the plant and its medicine. In this visceral way, I learned more about each herb than I would have by sitting down with a book. If you're a hands-on learner, try this with all your medicinal preparations, and you'll literally soak in the knowledge.

Alcohol-based tinctures, if stored properly, maintain their potency for decades or longer. I have some tinctures that are three decades old, and they still taste and smell like their younger counterparts! Tinctures are handy for travel and offer a convenient way to take medicine, especially when it's bitter in flavor. Alcohol is excellent at extracting most medicinal constituents. It's a good solvent for alkaloids, essential oils, and resins but ineffective at extracting minerals, mucilage, or long-chain polysaccharides. See below for a more detailed discussion on this topic.

Keep your tinctures out of the reach of children's curious hands, and always label each bottle. Don't store tinctures in dropper bottles for more than two years, as the alcohol will dissolve the dropper's rubber, contaminating the tincture with plastic compounds. If the rubber has gone soft, it's time to discard the medicine. Along that same vein, don't be tempted to use canning jars or flip-top glass jars with rubber gaskets for your tincture making. I tried this, and in less than a month, the alcohol had dissolved part of the gasket, and there were visible orange rubber parts in the tincture from the gasket.

## Alcohol Variety and Percentages

In the United States, "proof" is a measure of alcohol concentration, expressed as two times the alcohol percentage. For instance, 100-proof vodka consists of 50 percent alcohol. I prefer to use 95 percent organic ethanol (180-proof alcohol) derived from corn, grapes, or cane sugar because of its long shelf life and superior capacity for extracting the widest array of constituents. When I need 50 percent alcohol, I dilute it with water.

The upper level of alcohol percentages available varies by state, including what you can buy in a store or order online. If you need to order high-percentage spirits, it can require a bit of paperwork; you may decide it's not worth the hassle for home medicine-making purposes. (Visit the HealingGardenGateway.com for links to online sellers of organic alcohol.) Vodka (100 proof, or 50 percent) is a fine option for home tincture making and is probably the most popular for the home herbalist because of its efficacy and availability. If you're using fresh plant material (herbs that haven't been dried), I recommend using 50 percent alcohol or higher. Fresh plant juices dilute the alcohol, resulting in a lower alcohol percentage, which ultimately shortens the tincture's shelf life. Gluten-free options include gluten-free vodka and the other high-percentage alcohols mentioned (check with the manufacturers).

Professional herbalists and tincture manufacturers vary their alcohol level for each herb, based on its unique molecular profile and optimal extraction of desired constituents. This isn't necessary for the home herbalist, but if you like, you can check out the tincture labels from larger herb companies and copy the proportions and percentages at home. For the herbs covered in this book, look in the "Medicinal Preparations" section (starting on page 210) for each herb's optimal alcohol percentage as well as specific ratios of herb to alcohol.

## Tincturing Methods

There are two ways to make an alcohol-based tincture: the folkloric method or the weight-to-volume method. The folkloric method is the simplest, but it's less exact, so you won't know the potency of the final product. The advantage of the weight-to-volume method is that it uses precise measurements; a tincture's strength can be quantified and duplicated. Herbal manufacturers and professional clinical herbalists use this method. All you need is a kitchen scale and measuring cup and the ability to do simple multiplication.

I conducted an informal trial of the two methods in my lab (kitchen) with several herbs and found that the folkloric tinctures made from fresh or dried leaves were generally half as potent as those made with the weight-to-volume method. This means that you would be ingesting half the medicine in a folkloric tincture for the same dosage as a weight-to-volume tincture. Tinctures made from fresh or dried roots, using either method, were fairly similar in potency. If you can stomach the extra work (weighing, measuring, and doing simple math), I think it's worth going the weight-to-volume route. However, if the additional steps feel so daunting that it would make the difference between you making a tincture or not, go ahead and make folkloric tinctures. They may be weaker, but if they are made with home-grown or home-gathered herbs, their quality and vitality will be excellent. When possible, I prefer to use fresh plant material for my tinctures and skip the drying process. That said, for most herbs, it's fine to start with dried plant material for tincture making if you don't have the fresh herb on hand.

## Directions for Folkloric Tinctures

**STEP 1:** Prepare your herbal material. If you're using fresh roots, they will need to be washed and scrubbed first; leaves may sometimes need to be cleaned, too. Chop your plant material finely (A); smaller pieces of plant material expose more surface area to the alcohol, resulting in a concentrated medicine. If you've harvested a large quantity of an herb, this is the time to consider if you really need that much tincture. If not, dry the excess. If you're using homegrown dried herbs, be sure they are in small pieces. Crumble dried leaves down to the finest consistency.

**STEP 2:** Add your plant material to the appropriately sized canning jar and pour the alcohol over the herbal material using the proportions listed below (B). Pick the smallest size jar for your plant material. For home use, a pint jar (16 ounces) is a good choice, as it will yield about 10 to 12 ounces of the finished tincture, depending on the herb. Keep the alcohol from touching the lid, and make sure your lid doesn't have nicks or scratches on the bottom.

**FOR FRESH OR DRIED FLOWERS, SEEDS, LEAVES, AND BARK:** Cover the herb completely, leaving 1 inch of alcohol over the plant material.

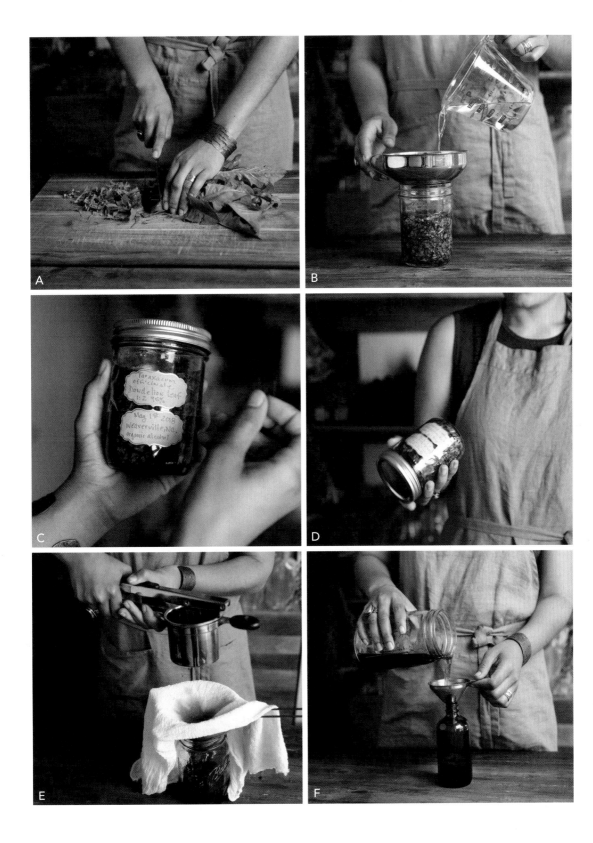

FOR FRESH ROOTS: Fill a jar two-thirds full with the roots, and then fill the jar almost to the top with the alcohol.

FOR DRIED ROOTS: Fill a jar halfway with the roots, and then fill the jar almost to the top with the alcohol.

STEP 3: Label the tincture (C, page 141). Include the common name, scientific name, date, ratios, alcohol type, and percentages, by following the directions on page 137. Mark your calendar for when you want to strain the tincture, after four to six weeks. It won't go bad after that time (it can stay good indefinitely in all that alcohol), but the alcohol will eventually dissolve the plastic compounds on the inside of the lid, resulting in contaminated medicine.

STEP 4: Place the tincture (D, page 141) in a dark cabinet for four weeks, shaking periodically. Here's a little secret: after a few days, your tincture will be plenty potent—if you need the medicine immediately, sneak off what you need, leaving the remainder to finish extracting.

STEP 5: Strain the tincture (E, page 141), following the directions on page 137.

STEP 6: Bottle the tincture in a glass amber bottle with a polyseal cap (F, page 141) and label it, following the directions on page 137.

## Directions for Weight-to-Volume Tinctures

STEP 1: Prepare your herbal material. Follow the directions in Step 1 in the Folkloric Method on page 140 (A).

STEP 2: Weigh your herb with a kitchen scale (B).

STEP 3: Determine the amount and percentage of alcohol you need, using the following proportions (C).

FOR FRESH HERBS: Multiply the weight of your herb by 2. For every 1 ounce of the herb by weight, use 2 fluid ounces of alcohol. This is written as a 1:2 extract (1 part weight of herb: 2 parts volume of alcohol). Use the highest alcohol percentage available, a minimum of 50 percent. Make a note of the alcohol percentage. If you use 95 percent alcohol, write this as 1:2 95%. If you use 50 percent alcohol (100 proof), record this as 1:2 50%.

FOR DRIED HERBS: Multiply the weight of your herb by four. For every 1 ounce of the herb by weight, use 4 fluid ounces of alcohol. This is written as a 1:4 extract (1 part weight of herb: 4 parts volume of alcohol). If you have a high-percentage alcohol, you'll want to dilute it with water to reach the desired alcohol percentage of 50 percent or 60 percent for dried herbs. Make a note of the percentage. For example, if you use 100-proof vodka (50 percent alcohol), record it as 1:4 50%

STEP 4: Combine the herbal material and alcohol in a canning jar and cap (D). Pick the smallest size jar that will accommodate your plant material and alcohol. Keep the alcohol from touching the lid, and make sure your lid doesn't have nicks or scratches on the bottom.

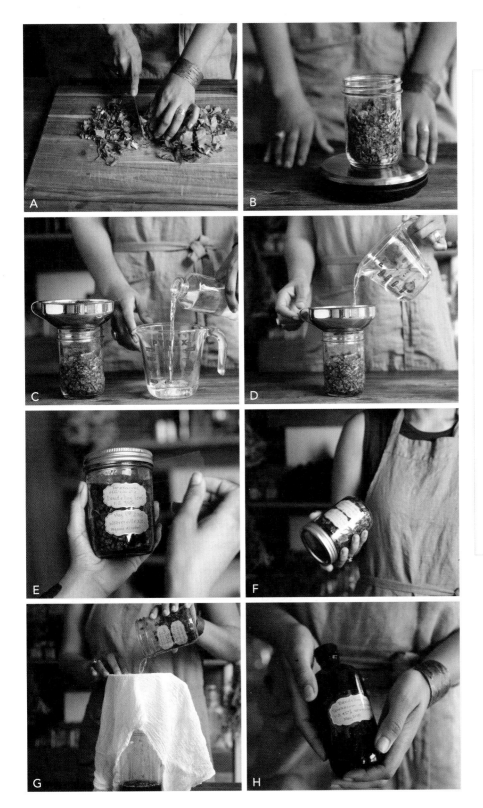

## What If I Can't Cover the Herb?

You most likely won't have a problem covering roots with liquid in the jar, whereas it's often hard to cover dried leaves using a 1:4 or 1:5 ratio. (Remember, 1 refers to the *weight* of the herbs not the volume. Dried herbs in particular are quite light.) Sometimes it's hard to cover fresh leaves with a 1:2 ratio. This freaks some people out, but it's not a big deal, I promise. If the alcohol doesn't completely cover the herb, push the plant material down with a stainless-steel spoon. If the herb is still uncovered, blend the alcohol-and-herb mixture in a glass blender, stirring as needed, until it reaches a slurry consistency. If the herb still isn't covered after blending, add enough alcohol to cover the herb, and use that high school algebra (finally!) to recalculate your proportions. Or, more simply, make a note on the label that you added extra alcohol, and know that you made your tincture as concentrated as humanly possible. And then give yourself and your tincture a pat on the back.

Preparing a weight-to-volume tincture

STEP 5: Label the tincture (E). Include the common name, scientific name, date, ratios, alcohol type, and percentages, by following the directions on page 137. Mark your calendar for when you want to strain (after four to six weeks). The tincture won't go bad after that time (it can actually stay good indefinitely in all that alcohol), but the alcohol will eventually dissolve the plastic compounds on the inside of the lid, resulting in contaminated medicine.

STEP 6: Place the tincture in a dark cabinet for four weeks, shaking every few days (F).

STEP 7: Strain the tincture, following the directions on page 137 (G).

STEP 8: Bottle the tincture in a glass amber bottle with a screw cap and label it, following the directions on page 137 (H).

> *Note for Metric Users (Sensible Folk):* **For fresh herbs:** *For every 1 gram of herb, use 2 milliliters of alcohol. This is written as a 1:2 extract (1 part weight of herb: 2 parts volume of alcohol). Use the highest alcohol percentage you can procure.* **For dried herbs:** *For every 1 gram of herb, use 4 milliliters of 50 percent to 60 percent alcohol. This would be written as 1:4 50% or 1:4 60%.*

## Combining Herbal Tinctures in Formulas

When preparing a tincture blend, tincture each herb separately rather than tincturing the herbs together. This allows you to use the proper ratios for each herb and you can reserve some of the single tinctures.

When I combine multiple tinctures for a formula, I measure the proportions in a small glass beaker and then pour the combination into a tincture bottle. Here's how to calculate formulas with different parts:

1. Figure out how much of the formula you'd like to make.

2. Add the total parts (the amount of herbs relative to each other) in a given formula.

3. Divide your formula quantity by the number of parts. This determines what one part is worth.

4. Multiply this number by each herb's part to determine how much of that herbal tincture you need to add to the formula.

5. Measure the quantity of each herbal tincture into the glass beaker and then pour it into your tincture bottle.

Let's see this in action. Here's a sample tincture formula:

2 parts hawthorn, flowers (*Crataegus* spp.)

2 parts rose, petals or buds (*Rosa* spp.)

1 part tulsi, leaves (*Ocimum tenuiflorum*)

Let's say we want to make 10 ounces of this tincture formula. We have 5 parts. We would divide 10 ounces by 5 parts, which equals 2 ounces for each part. Then, multiply 2 ounces by each herb's number of parts to determine how much of each herbal tincture to add. To make this formula, we would add 4 ounces of hawthorn tincture, 4 ounces of rose tincture, and 2 ounces of tulsi tincture.

# Infusions & Decoctions

If you've made a mug of tea with a teabag, you've made an herbal infusion. Preparing daily tea is soothing to the spirit, a ritual that promotes mindfulness and gratitude. Take a moment to close your eyes, breathe deeply, and feel gratitude for the herbs in your tea. Expand your attention to the elements sustaining all plants: the sunshine, fertile earth, air, and rainfall. These same elements make your life possible. Inhale the aroma wafting from your tea; the molecules now entering your lungs were once inside the plants. Sip the tea, contemplating how the compounds entering your digestive system were born from photosynthesis: fueled by the sun's benediction, the leaves of the plant converted rainfall and air into essential plant building blocks and the oxygen you're breathing—building blocks that gave life to the plant in your tea. In essence, you are now part raincloud, birdsong, sunshine, leaf, and root.

Tea is one of the simplest and most effective ways to ingest botanical medicine. Water extracts minerals, mucilage, long-chain polysaccharides, and most other medicinal constituents, but it doesn't effectively extract resins. Teas made from fresh herbs are delightful, but they are weaker than tea made from dried herbs. If you're drinking a tea for pleasure, use fresh or dried herbs as you prefer, but if you're drinking a tea for its medicinal qualities, use dried herbs. In the summertime, I prepare beverage teas

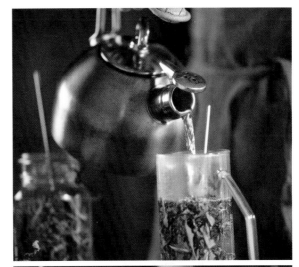
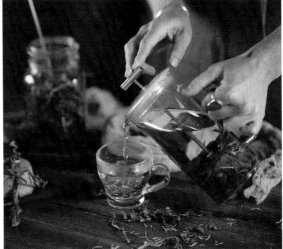
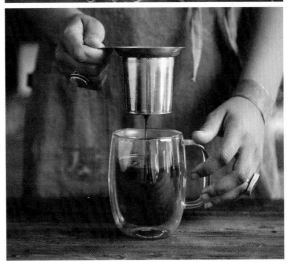

Preparing an infusion with a French press; pouring an infusion with a French press; preparing an infusion with a stainless-steel tea strainer or tea infuser

with fresh handfuls of mint, lemon verbena, and lemon balm, but most of my other teas are made with dried medicinals. Buying herbs in bulk is substantially cheaper than purchasing teabags, and if you grow or gather your own herbs, tea is free.

I prepare a quart of tea in the morning and slowly sip on it for the first part of the day. Tea stays fresh at room temperature for about six to eight hours before it will develop an off or stale flavor. It's convenient to make a larger batch of tea—three days' worth of tea at a time—and refrigerate it in a large jar or pitcher. Then, you can easily heat cups of the tea as needed. In the summer, iced herbal teas are refreshing.

## Directions for Herbal Infusions

An infusion is prepared by bringing water to a boil, pouring it over lightweight plant material such as leaves, flowers, and fruits, and letting it sit, covered, for 20 minutes. You can use a French press, stainless-steel pot, ceramic or glass teapot, or a stainless-steel or bamboo tea infuser. A stainless-steel tea infuser, also called a tea strainer, filled with loose herbs is the simplest method for infusing a single cup of tea. When the tea is finished steeping, lift the infuser out of the cup and compost the herbs. I use an insulated stainless-steel French press for larger batches of tea because it's sturdy, easily cleaned, and keeps my tea warm for hours. Covering the infusion as it steeps is essential for aromatic plants in order to trap the essential oils in the tea instead letting them evaporate. Some herbalists use canning jars for their infusions, but I strongly counsel against it. Jars can have invisible cracks, causing the glass to break upon contact with boiling water. I've seen tea jar accidents lead to second-degree burns. If you must use a canning jar, place it in the sink when you pour your boiling water into it.

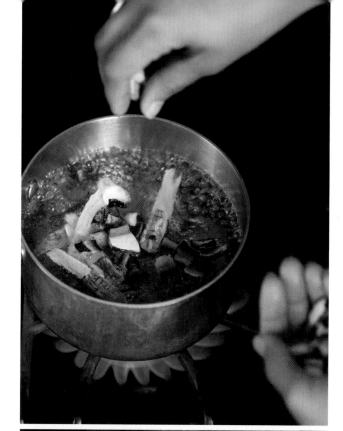

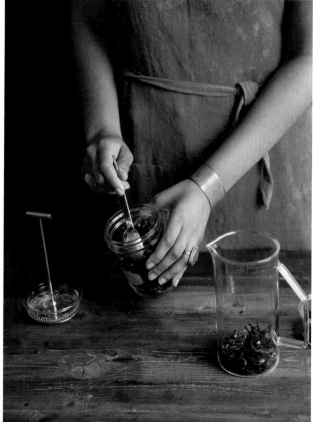

### Directions for Herbal Decoctions

A decoction involves simmering tea, covered, for 20 minutes. It is preferred for tougher botanical parts such as bark, roots, dried mushrooms, and hard seeds. Prepare your decoctions in a nonreactive glass or stainless-steel pot.

### The Two-Step Tea: Combined Infusions and Decoctions

What if your formula contains both leaves and roots—with some herbs needing an infusion and some a decoction? You can make a two-step tea in a single pot, a combined decoction and infusion. First, make a decoction with the roots, simmering them for 20 minutes, then turn off the heat and add the infusion herbs. Cover, let sit for 20 minutes, and strain.

### Tea Potency: How Much Herbs Should I Add?

Recommended proportions vary with the material you are using. See the notes below for a full discussion on tea dosage.

STORE-BOUGHT OR MAIL-ORDER, BULK DRIED HERBS (CUT AND SIFTED): Use 1 teaspoon of herb(s) per 8 ounces of water.

HOMEGROWN DRIED HERBS: Use 2 to 3 teaspoons of herb(s) per 8 ounces of water. In general, homegrown herbs are fluffier than machine-blended herbs, so you'll need more herbal material by volume to achieve the same dosage by weight. If you've broken down your homegrown plant material to a fine consistency—similar to cut and sifted dried herbs—you can use 1 teaspoon of herb(s) per 8 ounces of water.

FRESH, NOT DRIED HERBS: Fresh herbs are less concentrated than dried herbs. Use 1 to 2 tablespoons of chopped fresh herb(s) per 8 ounces of water.

### Tea Dosage

A typical dosage of a medicinal herb tea for adults is 1 cup (8 ounces) tea one to three times a day. (See page 133 for determining dosage for children.)

Each herb has its own dosage, depending on its medicinal strength and flavor. If an herb is covered in this book, look up the dosage in the "Medicinal Preparations" section beginning on page 210. If it's not covered here, you'll want to consider the herb's flavor and medicinal strength. Pungent herbs such as clove, cayenne, ginger, and black pepper have a smaller dosage. Astringent and bitter herbs are also consumed in smaller quantities. Herbs like dandelion leaf, violet, chickweed, and nettles can be taken in larger doses because they are food herbs—medicinals that are also eaten and thus can be consumed liberally. Beverage teas—herbs that are consumed for flavor and not just medicine—such as hibiscus, mint, chamomile, lemon balm, lemon verbena, and linden—can also be taken in higher doses.

Volume measurements, such as teaspoons and tablespoons, are less precise measurements than weight. For the home herbalist, it's perfectly fine to use volume measurements for most herbs, including all the medicinals featured in this book. But for the small minority of medicinals that are potent and tend to have more side effects, you'll want to use weight measurements, usually in grams. Herb dosage can vary from 0.5 to 5 grams for every 8 ounces of water. Obviously, this is an extremely wide range. Research each herb's dosage using one of the resources listed at HealingGardenGateway.com.

## Formulating Medicinal Tea Blends and Constitutional Considerations

It's quite satisfying to create herbal tea blends, and it's easy to do once you become familiar with each herb's flavor and medicinal qualities. If the blend is purely for enjoyment, flavor is paramount. If the tea is medicinal, consider its therapeutic qualities along with the taste. For example, if you want to make a warming tea that increases circulation, your blend is likely to be pungent, spicy, and stimulating. If you're preparing a tea intended to lessen inflammation in the gastrointestinal tract through astringent medicinals, don't skimp on astringent herbs like meadowsweet or raspberry leaf. But that's not to say you can't balance their astringency with other flavors. If you're concocting a mixture for someone who might not sip on a strong brew, go lighter with the strong-tasting herbs. It's better to take a smaller amount of medicinal herbs than none at all. Dogmatism yields yucky tea that may end up forever relegated to the cupboard.

You'll also want to consider a person's constitution. Folks with a sensitive nature need smaller quantities of medicinals. People who run cold benefit from warming herbs; those who run hot benefit from cooling herbs. If you have dry skin and sinuses, moistening herbs will be your allies. If you tend to have excess mucus in your sinuses and lungs or you have oily skin, look to drying herbs. You'll find each herb's energetics listed in the Medicinal Properties section starting on page 210. Experiment with each herb, getting to know its unique medicinal profile, flavor, and aroma. When determining the dosage for each medicinal, use common sense, research, intuition, and your senses to match the herb and the person.

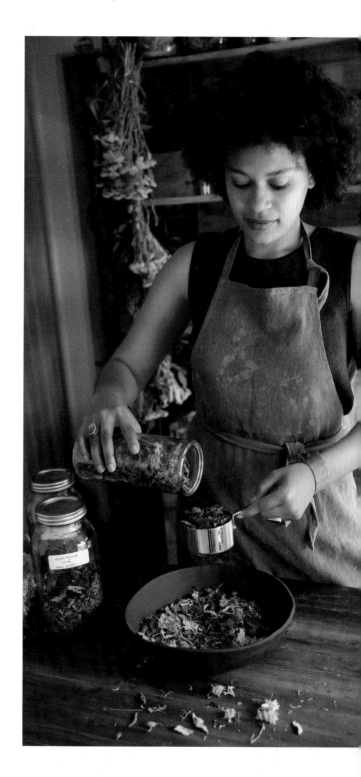

# Herbal Honeys & Syrups

Herbalists make syrups with honey, sugar, or glycerin. I prefer honey-based syrups because honey has medicinal qualities and can be sourced locally. Honey is an alchemical concoction, an ambrosial embodiment of the reciprocity between bloom and bee. With antimicrobial and anti-inflammatory attributes, honey helps soothe sore throats, eases the spasms of dry, hacking coughs, and tames nagging nighttime coughs. Children love honey and will eagerly take a medicinal syrup over a tea or tincture. (**Safety note:** Don't give honey to babies under the age of one as it may contain botulism spores, which can result in severe illness or fatality.)

Herbal honeys can be a stand-alone remedy, or they can be transformed into herbal syrups, which are thinner than honeys and often contain additional medicinal ingredients. Use herbal honeys to sweeten tea, or take them by the spoonful. They also make a handy base for diluting and flavoring tinctures. When made from dried herbs, infused honeys have a substantial shelf life—lasting decades to centuries. Some of my favorite botanicals for steeping into honey include angelica, elecampane, hawthorn, elderberry, and ginseng (cultivated only).

For a non-alcoholic syrup, combine tea and honey in equal parts. You'll need to refrigerate this syrup; it will only last a week. For another syrup on the fly, use equal parts herbal honey and tincture. Elderberry honey, with its fruity flavor and medicinal versatility, is my favorite here. See my two syrup recipes on page 154 for specifics on how to make honey-tincture syrups.

My syrup recipe begins with preparing an herbal honey. You may want to make extra honey so you can put some aside for another use.

## Directions for Herbal Honeys
*See the photos on page 150.*

STEP 1: Combine equal proportions, by volume, of your dried herb, or herbal mixture, and honey in a double boiler (A, B). For example, if you have ½ cup of herb(s), use ½ cup of honey. Don't use herbal powders as they can be impossible to strain. If the honey doesn't cover the herb by 1 inch or more, add more honey. I make an exception with elderberries, using fresh berries instead of dried, as I find fresh elderberries yield a fruitier-tasting honey that's more potent. Because the honey is diluted with the fresh juices from the elderberries, it must be kept refrigerated so it doesn't ferment or mold.

STEP 2: Heat the honey-herb mixture on low heat for 6 to 8 hours. Use a kitchen thermometer to make sure that the temperature of the honey mixture doesn't exceed 120°F. You'll likely need to take the pot off the burner from time to time to cool the honey. Stir the mixture periodically, and watch the water in the bottom pot of the double boiler, replenishing as needed.

STEP 3: Strain and press the honey while it's still warm yet comfortable to touch, following the directions on page 151 (C). Don't skimp on pressing the honey or you'll lose much of the goodness. The temperature of the honey makes all the difference here; room temperature honey is almost impossible to strain.

STEP 4: Store in a clean, dry jar (D). There's no need to refrigerate. Enjoy by the teaspoonful, add to tea, or proceed with the syrup recipe on page 151.

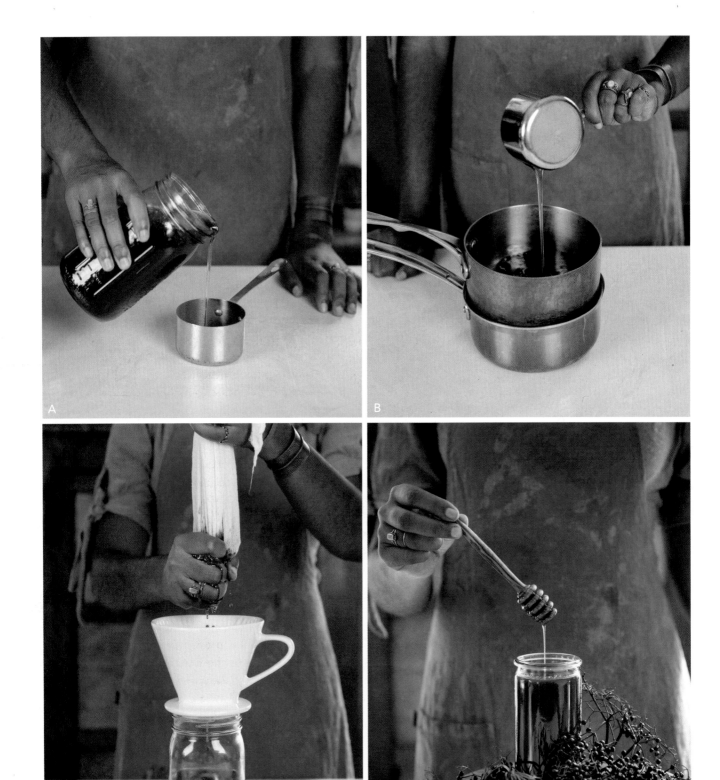

## Directions for Herbal Syrups
*See the photos on page 152.*

This triple-extraction herbal syrup (honey + water + alcohol) allows for the extraction of both alcohol-soluble and water-soluble constituents and has a long shelf life due to its high alcohol content. Use a single herb in this recipe or combine multiple herbs in each step. As long as you remember to maintain the proper proportions of honey, water, and alcohol, you can be creative with the botanicals. If you want to use homemade tincture(s) in your syrup, you'll need to make your tincture at least four weeks before making your syrup. See the directions on tincture making on page 139. You can always substitute store-bought tinctures for this step.

> The syrup contains equal parts by volume:
> - 1 part herbal honey infusion
> - 1 part concentrated tea (infusion or decoction)
> - 1 part tincture

STEP 1: Prepare your herbal tincture(s) as instructed on page 140.

STEP 2: Prepare your herbal honey infusion by following the directions on page 149. Be sure to start with more honey than you ultimately need, as you'll lose some of the honey when straining.

STEP 3: Prepare the concentrated tea via infusion or decoction. Use 1 part herb(s) to 1 part water by volume. For example, if you have ½ cup of herb(s), use ½ cup of water. Depending on the herb(s) you are working with, you will either make a concentrated decoction or an infusion. See page 146 for directions on infusions and decoctions, but be sure to use the extra concentrated proportions outlined in this recipe. Start with more water than you ultimately need for the syrup, as you'll lose some in the tea-making process.

STEP 4: Combine the honey infusion, herbal tincture(s), and concentrated tea. Combine in equal parts by volume: for example, 4 fluid ounces of honey, 4 fluid ounces of tincture, and 4 fluid ounces of concentrated tea. Label your syrup with the herb(s), date, and alcohol percentage. Depending on the alcohol percentage in your tincture, the alcohol level in your finished syrup will be anywhere from 10 to 30 percent. If you used a 50 percent alcohol tincture made from dry herbs, the syrup would be about 16 percent alcohol. If you used a 50 percent alcohol tincture made from fresh herbs, the syrup might be closer to 10 to 13 percent alcohol. If you used a 95 percent alcohol tincture made from fresh herbs, the syrup would be around 20 to 25 percent alcohol.

STEP 5: Store your syrup. If you used a tincture lower than 75 percent alcohol, keep the syrup refrigerated. It should last six months to one year. Watch for signs of spoilage, such as bubbling, off-smells, or mold. If you used a 75 percent alcohol or higher tincture, you can store your syrup unrefrigerated for one to two years. However, if you have the space in the fridge, keeping the syrup refrigerated will enhance its freshness and longevity, regardless of its alcohol percentage.

Syrup dosage varies by herb. A general dosage for a 150-pound adult would be 1 to 2 teaspoons (5–10 ml) of syrup up to three times a day. Pay special attention to the alcohol level. If the syrup is 30 percent alcohol, then 2 teaspoons of syrup will contain about 3 droppersful of alcohol. See the notes on page 133 for calculating dosage for children, paying particular attention to your syrup's alcohol level. If you prefer a nonalcoholic syrup, use the honey and concentrated tea method outlined on page 149.

# Warming Elderberry Syrup & Elderberry Honey

YIELD: 1½ cups of syrup plus ½ cup of elderberry honey

1¾ cups (160 grams) dried elderberries (*Sambucus canadensis*)

1¾ cups honey

¼ cup (16 grams) cinnamon bark chips (*Cinnamomum verum*)

3 tablespoons (17 grams) dried cut and sifted ginger root (*Zingiber officinale*)

1 teaspoon (3 grams) black peppercorns (*Piper nigrum*)

1½ cups water

½ ounce elecampane root tincture (*Inula helenium*), preferably 50 percent alcohol or higher (see page 140 for general instructions for preparing tinctures)

3½ ounces elderberry tincture (*Sambucus nigra*), preferably 50 percent alcohol or higher

Here is a syrup that can be taken throughout the winter months to boost immunity and increase circulation. With its antiviral and immune-stimulating qualities, it can help to weather a cold or flu. The herbs also offer decongestant and anti-inflammatory actions and can help to break a fever by increasing sweating. For children or those who are sensitive to spicy herbs, substitute additional elderberries for the peppercorns and ginger. This recipe uses my syrup triple extraction process, as described on page 151. It also yields a small bonus jar of elderberry honey, because who doesn't need more elderberry honey? Prepare the tinctures four weeks prior to making the syrup by following the directions on page 140 or use store-bought tinctures.

1. Using all of the dried elderberries and the honey, prepare the elderberry-infused honey as described on page 149.

2. Meanwhile, make a concentrated decoction: In a small saucepan with a lid, gently simmer the cinnamon, ginger, and peppercorns in the water, covered, for 20 minutes. Periodically check the water level to make sure it doesn't get too low. Strain and measure your tea. If you have more than ½ cup, return it to the pan and continue to gently simmer the tea, uncovered, until you concentrate the tea to ½ cup.

3. Strain the elderberry honey. Measure ½ cup of the infused elderberry honey for the syrup, and jar the remaining elderberry honey separately.

4. Combine the three preparations: Mix the concentrated ginger decoction, the 4 ounces elderberry honey, and the elecampane and elderberry tinctures. Pour into a bottle, label, and cap.

5. Store in the refrigerator. The syrup should keep for 1 to 2 years if you used 50 percent alcohol or higher tinctures. Do not use if you see signs of spoilage, including bubbling, off-smells, or mold. Dosage for adults: 2 teaspoons up to four times a day. See page 133 to calculate dosage for children.

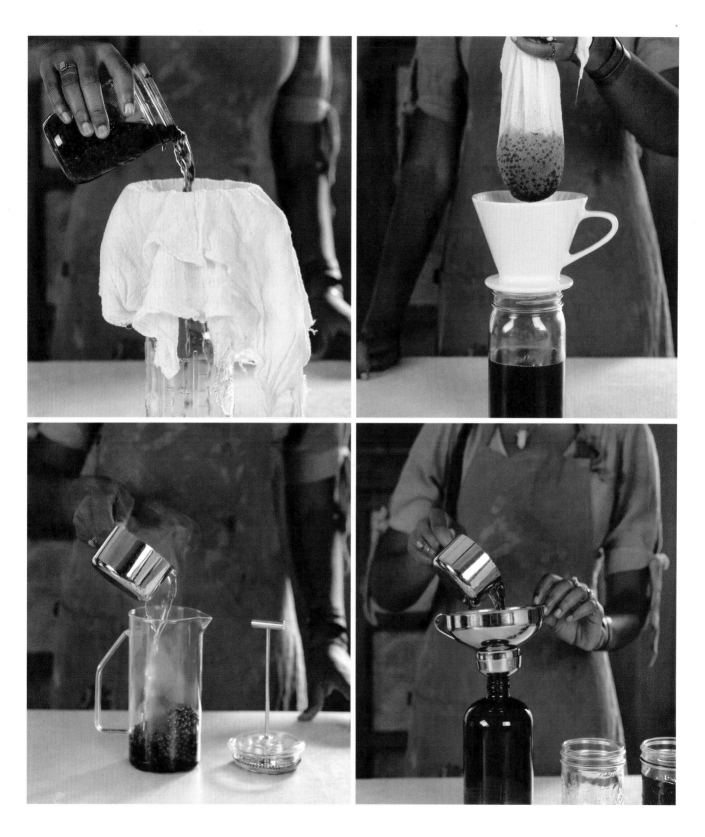

# Quick Cough Syrup for Productive Coughs

YIELD: 4 ounces

2 ounces elderberry honey (page 152)

1 ounce elecampane root tincture (*Inula helenium*)

½ ounce usnea lichen tincture (*Usnea* spp.)

½ ounce echinacea root or seed tincture (*Echinacea purpurea*)

This warming and decongestant syrup is helpful for productive coughs with plenty of mucus. Elder is a faithful ally in colds and flu as it's antiviral, antibacterial, immune-stimulating, and anti-inflammatory. Use store-bought tinctures or prepare your own following the directions on page 140. The tinctures can be made from fresh or dried herbs and should be 50 percent alcohol or higher.

Combine all the ingredients in a half-pint canning jar, seal the lid, and shake until the tinctures are incorporated into the honey. Pour into a 4-ounce bottle. The syrup doesn't need to be refrigerated and will last 2 to 3 years. Dosage for adults: 1 teaspoon up to four times a day. To determine a dosage for a child, follow the directions on page 133.

# Quick Cough Syrup for Dry, Spasmodic Coughs

YIELD: 4 ounces

2 ounces elderberry honey (page 152)

1 ounce wild cherry tincture (*Prunus serotina* or *Prunus virginana*), made from dried bark

½ ounce mullein leaf tincture (*Verbascum thapsus*)

½ ounce spilanthes leaf and flower tincture (*Acmella oleracea*)

This is a soothing syrup that's helpful for dry, hacking coughs—the relentless kind of cough that keeps you up at night or the irritating cough that starts at the back of your throat and is unproductive. Use store-bought tinctures or prepare your own following the directions on page 140. The tinctures should be 50 percent alcohol or higher. Echinacea root can be substituted for the spilanthes.

Combine all the ingredients in a half-pint canning jar, seal the lid, and shake until the tinctures are incorporated into the honey. Pour into a 4-ounce bottle. The syrup doesn't need to be refrigerated and will last 2 to 3 years. Dosage for adults: 1 teaspoon up to four times a day. To determine a dosage for a child, follow the directions on page 133.

# Infused Oils & Salves

Herbal oils for topical use are prepared by infusing botanicals into high-quality skincare oils. They can be used as a stand-alone remedy, such as massage oil, or transformed into salves, lotions, creams, and body butters. Salves and herbal oils soothe skin irritation, dryness, and inflammation and can help with insect bites, rashes, dry lips, scrapes, bruises, sore joints, muscle aches, and dry, chafed skin. Some of my favorite herbs for infusing into oils are chickweed, violet, calendula, plantain, yarrow, comfrey, St. John's wort, and arnica. Salves are easy to transport and to apply; their superpowers are lubrication and staying power. But because herbal oils and salves hold in moisture and heat, they should not be used for weepy skin conditions, infections, and fresh burns. Don't apply infused oils or salves to poison ivy rashes, weepy eczema, pimples, boils, fresh sunburn, deep wounds, or fungal and bacterial skin infections. Instead, use water-based applications such as herbal compresses, soaks, baths, and poultices.

When choosing your oil, look for those with a long shelf life (slower to become rancid) that are unrefined and cold-pressed or expeller-pressed. Extra-virgin olive oil is a reliable option because of its longevity and skin permeability. If you're making a massage oil or body care product, consider sesame, sunflower, coconut, jojoba, or sweet almond oil. Oil isn't the strongest solvent, but it can moderately extract or dissolve certain constituents, including lipids, essential oils, and resins, especially if the oil is heated. Herbal oils are easy to prepare if you mind this fundamental principle: in the presence of water, oil can harbor bacteria or fungi and subsequently ferment or mold. To prevent microbial growth, use dried herbs rather than fresh herbs (which can add moisture, in the form of plant juices), and use dry and clean tools. If you're using homegrown or gathered herbs, make sure your plant material is dried thoroughly. If purchasing dried botanicals, they should be fresh and high quality.

I prefer heating my infused oils because it's a quicker process than cold-infusing, and it results in the most potent remedy. Heat augments the extraction, pulling more medicinal constituents into the oil. This is especially true for resinous botanicals—the heat gently melts and dissolves the resin. Back in the day, I made my herbal oils by infusing fresh plant material in a canning jar of oil for two weeks, but I found that my oils often went bad or they ended up being weak medicine. Today, I make all my oils with dried herbs and heat with one exception: St. John's wort. Heat and blending destroy St. John's wort's medicinal constituents. To prepare St. John's wort oil, I use the freshly wilted whole flowers (picked yesterday) and place them in a jar of oil in a sunny window for four weeks.

## Directions for Infused Herbal Oils

STEP 1: Combine equal parts by volume of your dried herb, or herbal mixture, and your oil in a blender or food processor and blend (see photo A, page 156). For example, if you measure out 1 cup of herbs, use 1 cup of your oil of choice. Note that these are general proportions—an exact weight-to-volume measurement is not necessary with oil preparations to be used topically. As you would imagine, the oil will be more medicinal, or concentrated, if you use a higher proportion of herbs to oil. It's perfectly fine to combine multiple herbs in a single jar or pot for a

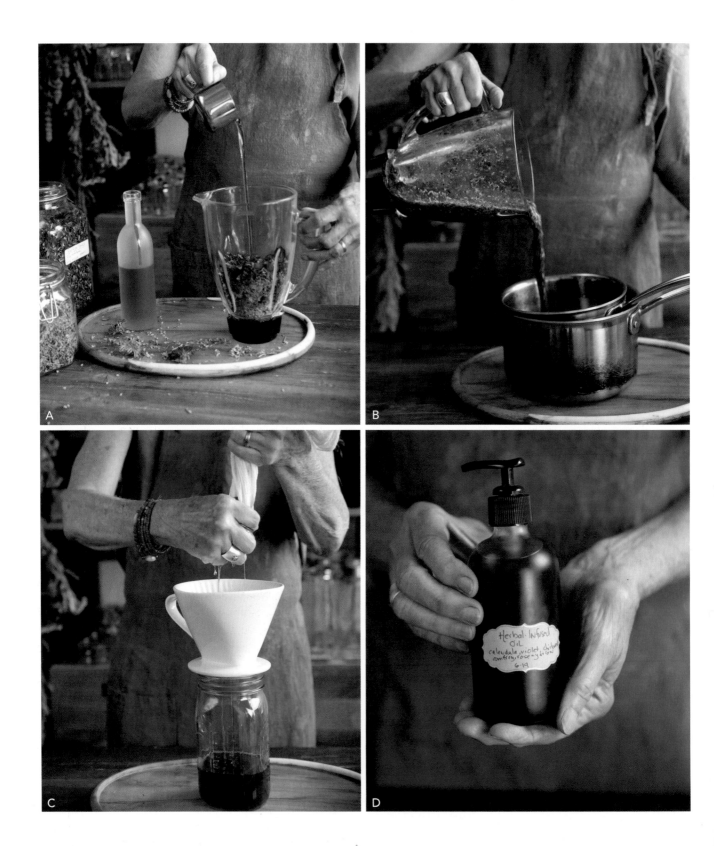

specific formula rather than making separate individual oils. Blend the herbs and oil until you achieve a thick, pesto-like consistency.

STEP 2: In a double boiler, heat the herb-oil mixture on low for 5 hours (B). You can improvise a double boiler by following the directions on page 136. Monitor the oil temperature with a cooking thermometer, and keep the oil temperature around 120°F (a little warmer than bathwater). Take the mixture off the heat periodically if necessary to keep the temperature from getting too high. Add water to the bottom pot as needed. (If you'd like to make infused oils in your slow cooker or oven, conduct a trial run to determine if your setup will work: Heat some water on low heat for a few hours, periodically checking the temperature. If the water temperature remains close to 120°F, you're good to go.)

STEP 3: Strain the oil while it's still warm yet comfortable to touch (C). After your infusion is complete, strain and press it with a fine-weave cloth or cheesecloth, using the instructions on page 137. The oil will be much easier to strain when it is warm.

STEP 4: Label and store (D). Label and cap your oil after it cools to room temperature, to prevent condensation from developing inside the jar. Herbal-infused oils will typically last two to three years when refrigerated or one year unrefrigerated, depending on the stability of the oil used.

Now that you have a lovely herbal-infused oil, you can prepare a healing salve using the instructions below.

## Directions for Herbal Salves

STEP 1: Measure the infused herbal oil, and then heat it slowly to 110°F in a double boiler.

STEP 2: For every ½ cup of herbal oil, add 1 to 1½ ounces (by weight 14 to 21 grams) of grated or beaded beeswax. (Beeswax beads are also sold as beeswax pellets or pastilles.) Start with 1 ounce (14 grams) of beeswax for a salve with a soft consistency. Later you can add more beeswax to make it firmer, if you like. Keep in mind that harder salves are less likely to melt in a hot car or bag but are harder to apply.

STEP 3: Completely dissolve the beeswax into the oil. To test the consistency of your salve, place a spoonful of the oil-beeswax mixture in the freezer for three minutes. Then pull the spoon out and let it come to room temperature to test its hardness. If it's too soft, add more beeswax and let it dissolve. When the salve has reached the desired consistency, turn off the heat. At this point, vitamin E can be added to the salve to prevent rancidity and for its own skin-healing attributes. For every 10 ounces of oil, add 2 capsules vitamin E oil or ½ teaspoon liquid vitamin E oil. This is also when you would add any skin-safe essential oils at the proper dilution rate (consult a trusted aromatherapy book or, for lavender, use one to two drops per 1 ounce of salve) and stir with a chopstick.

STEP 4: Label and store. While your salve is still warm, pour it into jars using a measuring cup for easy pouring, label the contents, and allow it to cool before capping. Salves typically last one to three years unrefrigerated. Refrigeration of your back stock is not necessary but prolongs the shelf life.

Cleanup: I recommend using a rag or paper towel to clean the double boiler and measuring cup while they're still warm. Then proceed with multiple cleanings of very hot water and soap to finish the job.

# Weedy & Wonderful Soothing Salve

YIELD: 10 ounces, or 10 (1-ounce) salve jars

¾ cup (20 grams) dried calendula flower (*Calendula officinalis*)

¼ cup (30 grams) dried comfrey root (*Symphtum officinale*)

¼ cup (14 grams) dried violet leaf (*Viola sororia* or *V. odorata*)

¼ cup (7 grams) dried chickweed leaf (*Stellaria media*)

1½ cups extra-virgin olive oil, or substitute jojoba or almond oil

¼ cup (28 grams) grated or beaded beeswax, plus a little more if a harder salve is desired, or substitute carnauba wax for a vegan salve

2 capsules or ½ teaspoon liquid vitamin E oil (optional)

10 drops lavender essential oil (*Lavandula angustifolia*) (optional)

This salve contains my favorite topical herbs. Use it to soothe and heal dry, chafed hands and feet and chapped lips. These healing weeds ease skin irritation and inflammation and can assuage insect bites, rashes, and bruises.

Infuse the calendula, comfrey, violet leaf, and chickweed into the oil following the instructions on page 155. After straining, measure out 8 ounces of the infused oil. (If you have any extra, save it to use as massage oil.) If you don't quite have 8 ounces, add a tad more olive oil to bring the volume up to 8 ounces. Finish making the salve, adding the beeswax and the vitamin E and essential oil if using, following the instructions on page 157.

Note: Comfrey contains toxic types of pyrrolizidine alkaloids (PAs). Topical use on unbroken skin is not thought to be a problem since PAs are poorly absorbed through the skin. Avoid using on cuts, scrapes, abrasions, or broken skin.

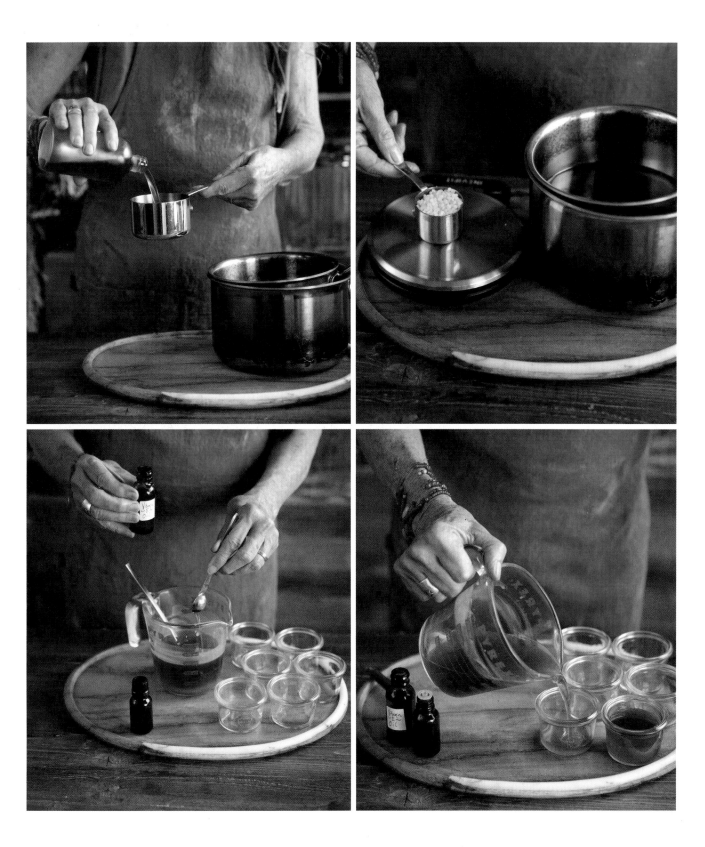

# Herbal Soaks, Compresses, Baths & Poultices

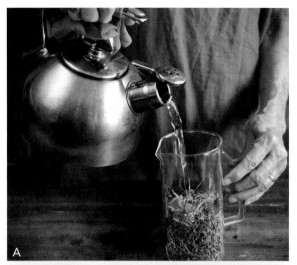

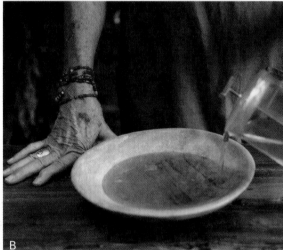

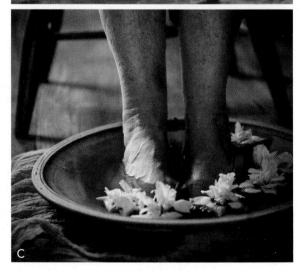

Water-based herbal preparations—poultices, compresses, baths, and soaks—are straightforward yet potent topical remedies. I find them to be more efficacious than infused oils and salves because they're more concentrated and water is a superior solvent for most medicinal constituents. Some of my favorite herbs for water-based preparations include rose, lavender, calendula, comfrey, chickweed, violet, plantain, garden sage, white sage, and witch hazel. Soaks, compresses, and baths ease muscular and joint pain and inflammation. All of the water-based preparations are ideal applications for infections and weepy skin conditions like poison ivy, acne, or weeping eczema. Use them to soothe rashes, hives, insect bites, burns, psoriasis, and sunburn. Adjust the temperature of the preparation depending on the condition you're treating. Teas, compresses, and poultices can all be applied cold, offering relief and vascular constriction for hot, inflamed skin conditions. For muscular tension and cramps, a warm compress, soak, or bath is soothing and relaxing.

## Herbal Soaks, Baths, and Compresses

Herbal soaks are concentrated teas used to immerse specific areas of the body. It's easy enough to rig up a foot or hand soak, or you can submerge a substantial part of the body, such as the bum, in a large shallow basin (this is called a *sitz bath*). An herbal bath is the voluminous version of an herbal soak. Herbal baths are helpful when a wide area of the skin is affected (such as hives, insect bites, or rashes) or there are widespread aches. An herbal compress involves soaking a washcloth in an herbal tea and applying it to the skin. Compresses are handy applications for parts of the body that aren't easily immersed, such as the eyes, neck, or face.

## Directions for Herbal Soaks
*See the photos on page 160.*

STEP 1: Prepare the concentrated tea (A). By volume, add 1 part dried herb, or herbal combination, to 1 part boiled water, and let sit, covered, for 20 minutes. For larger batches, use weaker proportions: 1 part herb(s) to 4 parts water.

STEP 2: Strain with a French press, potato ricer, tea strainer, or through a fine-mesh strainer or a colander lined with a cotton cloth (B).

STEP 3: Soak the part of the body in need of attention for 20 minutes (C); repeat up to three times a day. For a cold soak, cool the tea to the desired temperature before soaking. Refrigerate leftover tea for up to four days, reserving for subsequent applications.

## Directions for Herbal Compresses

Follow Steps 1 and 2 for Herbal Soaks above.

STEP 3: Submerge a compress cloth in the concentrated tea and wring out the excess moisture (A). Apply the compress for 20 minutes and reapply several times throughout the day (B). For a warm compress, dunk a washcloth or clean cotton cloth in the warm tea, wring, and apply. For a cold compress, refrigerate the tea before soaking the cloth.

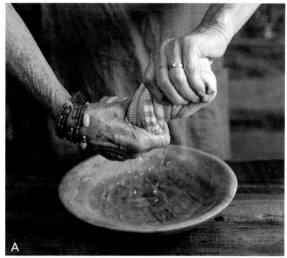

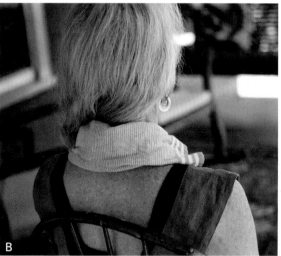

## Directions for Herbal Baths

Follow Steps 1 and 2 for Herbal Soaks above.

STEP 3: Add your strained tea concentrate to a warm bath. Add a few dried petals or fresh flowers for self-indulgent luxury because you are worth it, my friend.

## Herbal Poultices

Poultices are prepared by blending herbs (fresh or dried) into a green slurry or paste and applying the paste to the affected area. (The most primitive version is the aptly named *chew and spit* poultice, which is applied, as you might imagine, solely on one's own body.) Cover the paste with a clean, dry cloth or bandaging material. Poultices are a messy business, but they're formidable remedies. Adding a binder such as clay, marshmallow powder, or calendula oil makes it easier to apply and stay put. Clay is especially helpful for drying weepy skin conditions such as poison ivy. Marshmallow powder is an effective binder and soothing emollient for dry, irritated skin conditions. Calendula oil is a soothing anti-inflammatory, helping to quiet itchy skin conditions. Avoid oil, however, if an infection is present.

## Directions for Herbal Poultices

STEP 1: If using dried herbs, premoisten them: In a saucepan, bring a small amount of water to a boil, turn off the heat, and add a sufficient amount of the dry herbs until the mixture forms a thick paste. Stir and let cool. Then blend completely in a blender. If using fresh herbs, put them in a blender or food processor (A) and slowly add very hot water (not boiling), pouring a little in at a time and blending until the mixture reaches the consistency of a thick slurry.

STEP 2: Transfer the herb mixture to a bowl (B). You can then drizzle in an herbal infused oil, such as calendula, or add clay or marshmallow powder. These additions help bind the mixture and make it easier to apply.

STEP 3: Apply the poultice (C). Spread the preparation on the affected area and cover with a clean, dry cloth or bandaging material (D), depending on the size of the area you're treating. Store any excess poultice in the refrigerator for up to four days.

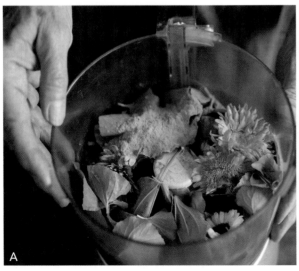

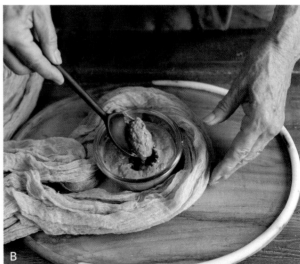

# Soothing Herbal Poultice

YIELD: 2 cups

½ cup very hot water (not boiling), or more as needed

1 heaping handful (about 1 cup) fresh violet leaves (*Viola* spp.), or more as needed

1 heaping handful (about 1 cup) fresh plantain leaves (*Plantago* spp.), or more as needed

1 handful (about ¾ cup) fresh calendula flowers (*Calendula officinalis*), or more as needed

2 tablespoons powdered clay (any cosmetic clay or bentonite clay will do), or more as needed

10 drops lavender essential oil (optional)

This cooling and moistening poultice is helpful for dry, irritated skin conditions such as psoriasis, rashes, chicken pox, and chafed skin. It can also be used for insect bites, mild abrasions, cuts, and scrapes. The combination of herbs provides a soothing blend of healing properties that are demulcent, anti-inflammatory, and vulnerary (wound-healing). If using dried herbs, substitute ¼ cup of the dried herb for one handful of the fresh herb.

Using a food processor or a blender, combine the hot water with the violet leaves, plantain leaves, calendula, clay, and essential oil, if using, and blend until the poultice is smooth, with the consistency of pesto. You may need to add more herbs, clay, or water to achieve the desired consistency. Transfer to an airtight jar and refrigerate for up to three days; apply as needed.

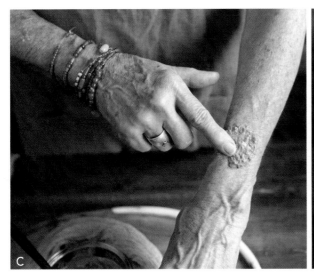

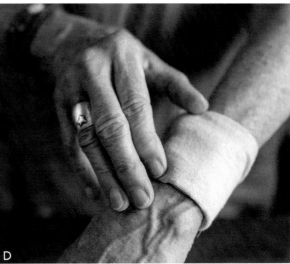

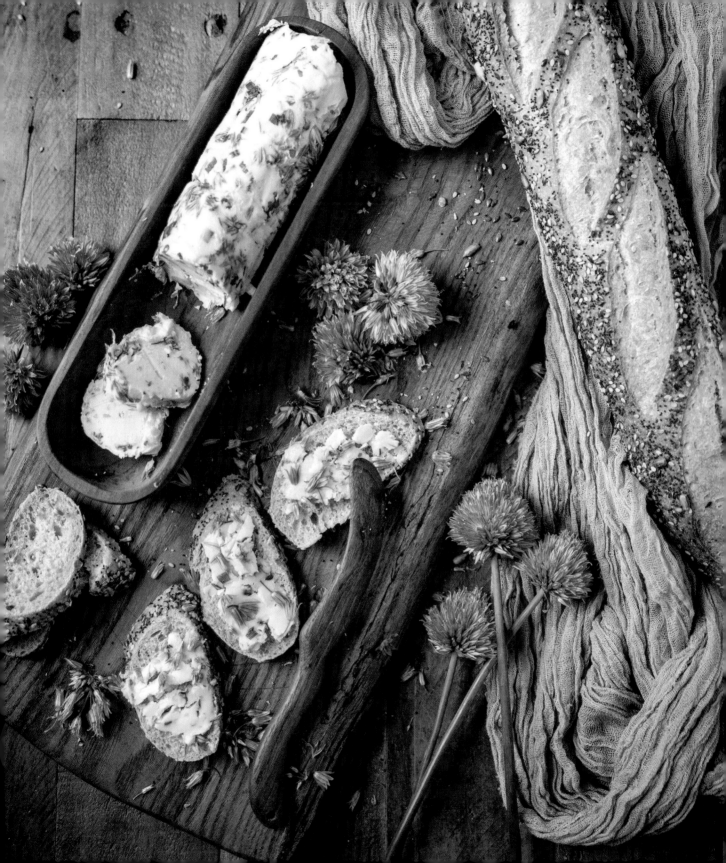

# Herbal Compound Butters

It's hard to imagine anything more alluring or satisfying than butter, but once you slip herbs, spices, and citrus zest into the mix, you'll no longer be questioning how *the best* could get any better. Slather herbal butters on baked roots, toast, and crackers or use them to top grilled veggies or meat. Fruity-sour and sweet butters are delicious with pancakes, muffins, or waffles.

Compound butters can be frozen, giving you an elegant method of preserving fresh culinary herbs, especially those that don't dry well like chives, cilantro, or parsley. I prefer to use organic, grass-fed butter for its increased nutrition, but any salted butter will do. Butter logs are not only pretty; they make it easier to slice off a portion neatly. If you avoid dairy, substitute one of the many nondairy "butters" or, for a sweet butter, try coconut manna. These plant alternatives will have a different consistency from butter. You might not be able to roll them into a log; instead, serve them in a small bowl.

## Directions for Compound Butters

STEP 1: Bring the butter to room temperature. The warmer, the softer, and the easier to stir.

STEP 2: Add the herbs and other flavorings according to the specific recipe (see pages 166 and 167) or your own creativity. Thoroughly mix by hand with a sturdy spoon.

STEP 3: Enjoy your butter right then and there while it's fresh and velvety, or roll it into a log on a piece of waxed paper, twist the ends of the paper closed, and place the log in an airtight container in the refrigerator. It will keep for one to two weeks. To freeze compound butters, place the log, nestled still in waxed paper, in a small ziptop bag, label, and place in the freezer. Use within six months.

Chive-Garlic Butter (recipe, page 166)

# Compound Butters

*For the six recipes that follow (or to create your own), follow the instructions on page 165.*

## Cilantro-Lime-Serrano

Our family loves this butter on wild salmon and black bean dishes. You won't be complaining if you add it to roasted stuffed peppers or grilled fish tacos. Substitute jalapeño pepper for the serrano if you prefer.

YIELD: About 1 cup

- 1 cup (2 sticks) salted butter, at room temperature
- ¼ cup finely chopped cilantro leaves
- 2 teaspoons grated lime zest
- 2 teaspoons finely minced garlic
- ¼ to ¾ teaspoon very finely minced serrano pepper, including seeds, to taste

## Juniper-Sage

Juniper, sage, and black pepper are savory sisters with snappy flavors. Spread this butter on thick slices of sourdough toast, baked potatoes, roasted winter squash, or grilled veggies.

YIELD: About 1 cup

- 1 cup (2 sticks) salted butter, at room temperature
- 2 tablespoons minced fresh garden sage leaves
- 2 tablespoons minced fresh rosemary leaves
- 1½ teaspoons finely minced garlic
- 10 dried juniper berries, crushed with a mortar and pestle
- ⅛ to ¼ teaspoon coarsely ground black pepper, to taste

## Cranberry-Orange

This tart butter is equally at home saddled up to roast turkey or chicken as it is resting against the soft cheek of a pancake or waffle. The butter is marbled with crimson pockets of cranberry juice that won't dissolve into the butter but will readily soak into food.

YIELD: About 1 cup

- 1 cup (2 sticks) salted butter, at room temperature
- ½ cup fresh or thawed frozen cranberries, finely chopped
- 1 tablespoon evaporated cane juice or brown sugar
- 2 teaspoons grated orange zest

## Chive-Garlic

Spread this butter on bread to prepare garlic toast, or spoon it into the gaping mouth of a piping hot sweet potato or potato. The chive blossoms brighten the mix; substitute additional green chive leaves when the flowers aren't in season.

YIELD: About 1 cup

- 1 cup (2 sticks) salted butter, at room temperature
- 3 tablespoons fresh chive flowers (separated from the flower head by hand)
- 2 tablespoons finely minced fresh chives
- 1 tablespoon finely minced garlic

## Spiced Rose

If your mother's cinnamon toast took a trip to Turkey, you'd receive a postcard three months later with this recipe written on the back (alongside greasy, rose-stained fingerprints). Cinnamon and cardamom add depth to the silkiness of butter; rose petals seal the deal with a kiss. If you can get your hands on maple sugar (crystallized maple syrup), use it in place of the brown sugar.

YIELD: About 1½ cups

- 1 cup (2 sticks) salted butter, at room temperature
- 2 cups (35 grams) loosely packed fresh rose petals (organic, non-sprayed)
- ¼ cup dark brown sugar
- 1 tablespoon ground cinnamon
- ½ teaspoon ground cardamom
- ½ teaspoon vanilla extract

## Hibiscus-Raspberry-Orange

Scarlet and sour, this festive confection easily lends its fruity luster to biscuits, scones, waffles, cupcakes, pancakes, and thick slabs of rustic seeded bread toasted to crunchy perfection. If you don't care for sweets, add less sugar.

YIELD: About 1 cup

- 1 cup (2 sticks) salted butter, at room temperature
- ¼ cup dark brown sugar, or to taste
- 3 tablespoons (10 grams) finely crumbled freeze-dried raspberries
- 1 tablespoon hibiscus powder
- 2 teaspoons grated orange zest

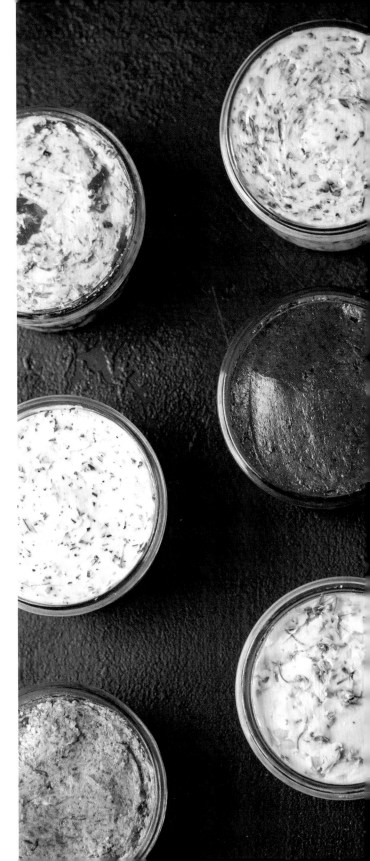

# Herbal Finishing Salts

Herb-infused finishing salts are a delightful alchemy between earth and sea, plant and mineral. Herbal salts are surprisingly easy to conjure up and make a nice alternative for preserving fresh culinary herbs. In the early fall, I prepare big batches of salts from the herbs we harvest before the first frost. If your love language involves homemade gifts, as mine does, you'll appreciate having a pantry full of finishing salts in pretty little jars ready for birthdays and holiday gift-giving.

Finishing salts get their name from the fact that they are traditionally added to a dish after it's prepared. But you needn't be held back by this convention as long as you understand how salt behaves. Coarser salts, with a larger flake, add a gust of crunch and saltiness, but if you add them earlier in the cooking process, the salt dissolves and loses its texture. Sometimes you don't want splashes of saltiness and instead prefer a finer grain for even distribution. Experiment with salt textures, and you'll be a more dexterous cook. Add herbal salts to marinades and dressings or rub them onto meats and seafood before roasting, grilling, or pan-frying. I enjoy my finishing salts daily on popcorn, eggs, and beans. When I need a quick party trick, I add herbal salts to goat cheese and drizzle in olive oil, resulting in a salty, creamy dip. Herbal salts are so central to the life of my kitchen that they live next to the stove, coming out to play at nearly every mealtime. It's all too easy to overdo it with these salt blends if you treat them like herbal seasoning and add liberal amounts to food. They are genuinely salty, so go easy at first!

We live in extraordinary times, with a dazzling array of salts. We have salts that are smoky, volcanic, or kissed by the subtle flavors of seaweed or minerals. Himalayan pink salt and Real Salt (from Utah) are mined from ancient marine fossil deposits; their rosy hue is derived from their high content of minerals and trace elements. If you're concerned about microplastics in your sea salt (yes, sadly, that is a thing), these mountain-mined salts are a good bet. Substitute Himalayan pink salt for Real Salt in the recipes below, if needed. Use the weight measurements in these recipes instead of volume because salt density varies depending on its crystal size. Also, pay special attention to the texture of the salt when purchasing—these recipes call for coarse salt (they may not be labeled as "coarse," but they should look coarser than table salt).

## Directions for Herbal Finishing Salts

STEP 1: Destem and finely mince your fresh herbs. If you are following the recipes beginning on page 170, use the weight measurements given for the salt for greater accuracy, since I call for salts with a variety of crystal sizes. You can also create your own blend, using equal parts fresh herb(s) to salt by volume. For instance, if you are making a rosemary/thyme salt, add 1 cup total of combined fresh rosemary and thyme leaves to 1 cup of coarse sea salt. If you don't have fresh herbs on hand, you can use high-quality dried herbs; simply cut the quantity of herbs called for in half.

STEP 2: Blend the ingredients in a food processor or spice blender until the consistency is even. Don't go overboard. I like my finishing salts the texture of beach sand rather than table salt. If you don't have a food processor or spice blender, finely mince your fresh herbs and then combine with the salt.

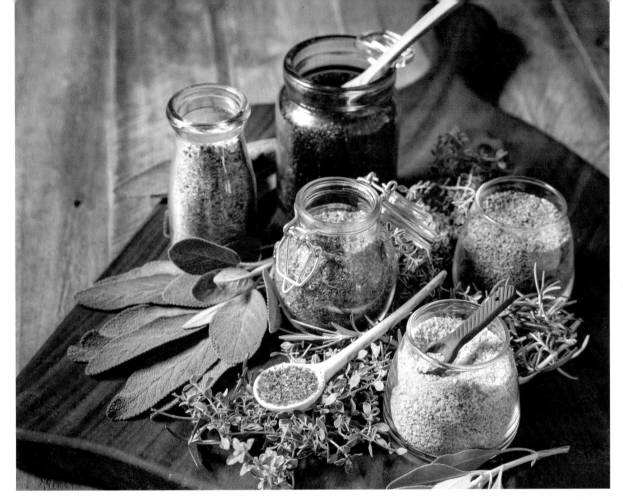

*Clockwise from top left:* Smoky BBQ Salt Rub; Midnight Nettles Gomasio; Dusky Desert Finishing Salt; Lemon–White Sage Finishing Salt; Crimson Cajun Salt (recipes, pages 170 to 171)

STEP 3: Dry the finishing salts (if you used dried herbs, skip this step). Spread the mixture on a serving tray or rimmed baking sheet and place it in an area with good airflow. I dry my salts on a table or counter underneath a ceiling fan. Depending on the humidity, it may take two to four days for the salt to dry. If your blend is heavy on fresh herbs and light on salt, it will take longer to dry. Periodically stir and break apart any clumps. If you need your finishing salts right away or you live in a humid climate, you can dry herbal salts in a dehydrator. Or dry them in an oven: Place the mixture on a rimmed baking sheet. Use the lowest heat setting and leave the oven door slightly ajar. Stir every half hour and break up any clumps. Depending on the recipe, it may take a few hours for the mixture to dry. Let the salt cool before storing. The heat from the oven evaporates some of the herbs' essential oils, diminishing the salt's aroma and flavor. Therefore, if you have the time, the slow drying (open-air) method is preferred.

STEP 4: After your blend is thoroughly dry, store in airtight glass containers.

# Finishing Salts

*For the five recipes that follow (or to create your own), follow the instructions on page 168.*

## Lemon–White Sage Finishing Salt

This is one of my favorite herb-infused finishing salts, and its uplifting aroma makes it delightful to prepare. If you haven't tried white sage (*Salvia apiana*) as a culinary herb, you're in for a real treat. White sage is similar to its kissing cousin, garden sage, but with a more intense flavor. Like garden sage, white sage's pungent, resinous flavor complements fatty foods. Indeed, our taste buds may be speaking for our stomachs in this department, as sage is one of the best culinary herbs for enhancing fat digestion. Try this finishing salt in stuffing, along with black pepper and anise seeds, or add the blend to meatloaf, poultry, and roasted roots. (White sage is overharvested in the wild. Grow your own white sage or purchase from an organic farmer. Substitute garden sage if needed. Do not gather from the wild or buy wildcrafted white sage.)

YIELD: 1½ cups

1½ cups (420 grams) coarse Real Salt

1 handful (21 grams) whole fresh white sage leaves (*Salvia apiana*)

3 tablespoons grated lemon zest (from 3 lemons)

## Dusky Desert Finishing Salt

This pungent blend is especially tasty on poultry and adds variety to goat cheese, baked potatoes, and stuffing. Combine it with olive oil and vinegar to create a flavorful salad dressing, or sprinkle on sweet potato and black bean casseroles and burritos. Try it as a garnish on squash bisque or sliced and roasted squash—its smokiness slow dances with the sweetness of winter squash.

YIELD: 1¼ cups

⅓ cup (90 grams) coarse Real Salt

⅓ cup (80 grams) coarse wood-smoked sea salt

⅓ cup (75 grams) coarse Hawaiian, or black, lava sea salt

⅓ cup (23 grams) tightly packed fresh rosemary leaves

¼ cup (7 grams) tightly packed whole fresh garden sage leaves

2 teaspoons minced fresh garlic

15 dried juniper berries (mashed with a mortar and pestle or the back of a knife)

1 teaspoon grated orange zest

¼ teaspoon coarsely ground black pepper

## Midnight Nettles Gomasio

Gomasio, or sesame salt, is a traditional Japanese seasoning. This herbal version adds a splash of ebony to salads, dressings, and stir-fries along with a hearty dose of antioxidant anthocyanins. It's also rich in minerals from both the sesame seeds and the nettles. Try it sprinkled on salad, soup, roasted roots, and grilled fish. Look for black sesame seeds in the Asian food section of your supermarket or order them online. Don't confuse black cumin seeds for black sesame seeds—they look similar but are not interchangeable. If you can't find black sesame seeds, substitute unhulled sesame seeds.

YIELD: About 2 cups

1¾ cups black sesame seeds

½ cup (120 grams) coarse Hawaiian, or black lava, sea salt

¼ cup (6 grams) dried nettles leaves (*Urtica dioica*)

Heat a dry skillet over medium heat. When the skillet is warm, add the sesame seeds and toast, stirring frequently, for a few minutes until their aroma fills the room. It's easy to burn the seeds, so don't walk away! Turn off the heat, pour the seeds onto a plate, and let cool. Combine the seeds with the salt and nettles in a food processor and blend. Gomasio doesn't need to dry; it's best eaten fresh. Keep refrigerated and use within three to four months.

## Smoky BBQ Salt Rub

This salt is delicious on veggie scrambles, home fries, or French fries, or as an ingredient in hamburgers or veggie burgers. As you can imagine, it's also a righteous rub for grilling meat or veggies.

YIELD: 1¼ cups

1 cup (280 grams) coarse Real Salt

3 tablespoons (47 grams) coarse wood-smoked sea salt

3 tablespoons (8 grams) fresh rosemary leaves

2 tablespoons (4 grams) fresh thyme leaves

2 tablespoons paprika

1 tablespoon red pepper flakes

1 tablespoon garlic powder

1 tablespoon yellow mustard seeds

## Crimson Cajun Salt

Hands down, this is my favorite of the salt blends. Its zesty heat matches its fiery hue. I sprinkle it on scrambled or fried eggs most mornings. It's also my go-to popcorn condiment along with nutritional yeast. And if you like Mexican food as much as I do, you'll find the salt blend perfectly complements black bean burritos, quesadillas, and tortilla soup.

YIELD: 1¼ cups

1 cup (260 grams) coarse red Alaea Hawaiian sea salt

2 tablespoons (4 grams) fresh thyme leaves

2 tablespoons grated orange zest

2 tablespoons chipotle powder

1 tablespoon paprika

# Herbal Pestos

You already know pesto is delicious. But it's also medicinal. Nuts are a high-quality source of healthy fats and protein. Garlic is antimicrobial and supports the cardiovascular system and protects against cancer. Add healing herbs into the mix, and suddenly you've concocted a dish of superhero proportions. Not only is pesto tasty, nutritious, and healing, it also allows you to preserve culinary herbs and wild edibles. Freeze pesto in ice cube trays; once frozen, pop out the green cubes into ziptop freezer bags for use throughout the winter. The day before I host a party, I'll thaw out a cube, stir it into goat cheese, and top with coarsely ground black pepper. A jar of pesto in the refrigerator serves as a handy condiment to smear on wraps, sandwiches, and toast.

Pesto invites adventure and creativity into the kitchen as few other dishes will. Throw pungent greens, salty cheese, and earthy nuts into the food processor and the flavors effortlessly meld. Once you move beyond the familiar combination of basil and pine nuts, there is a vast world of pesto possibilities. Be free with your nuts: fool around with the sweetness of cashews and pecans, the bitterness of walnuts, and the rooted familiarity of peanuts. Dry-toasting nuts elevates their nuttiness, allowing them to fully come into their own. For the greens, you can go with medicinal and aromatic herbs, such as tulsi, lemon balm, bergamot, or bee balm, or nutrient-dense and mild-mannered herbs like chickweed and violet. Wild greens such as amaranth, stinging nettles, and lamb's-quarters need to be steamed before adding them to pesto to soften them and to disarm the sting of nettles. Add a touch of sour in the form of lemon or lime juice to balance the richness of the nuts and oil. A pinch of curry powder adds a mysterious depth and complexity without overtaking the pesto's flavor. If you avoid dairy, try substituting nutritional yeast, olives, or nut-based "cheeses" for the cheese.

You'll find my recipe for Lemon Balm Pesto on page 173, Chickweed Pesto on page 254, Basilicious Benediction Pesto on page 391, and Nettles Pâté (pesto's denser cousin) on page 384. The following proportions are merely guidelines; modify them to your whim, season, and harvest.

### GENERAL PROPORTIONS FOR HERBAL OR WILD FOODS PESTO:

- 3 cups fresh herbs, firmly packed (for example, tulsi, lemon balm, basil, chickweed, violet, or bee balm) or 2 cups steamed greens (such as nettles, lamb's-quarters, kale, chard, spinach, or wild amaranth)

- 1 to 1½ cups nuts or seeds (almonds, pistachios, walnuts, hazelnuts, cashews, pecans, peanuts, sunflower seeds, or pine nuts), preferably dry toasted

- 1 cup oil (extra-virgin olive oil, avocado oil, pumpkin seed oil, grapeseed oil, or sunflower oil), plus more if needed

- ¾ cup freshly grated Parmesan cheese (optional)

- 3 to 6 garlic cloves, to taste

- 1 to 2 tablespoons lemon or lime juice, to taste (optional)

- Sea salt, to taste

Put all the ingredients in a food processor and blend until the pesto reaches a uniform consistency. Some folks like a chunky pesto, while others blend until creamy. You may need to add more oil if the food processor sputters. Taste before seasoning with salt; the amount will vary depending on your taste, the quantity and type of cheese you use, and whether your nuts are salted.

# Lemon Balm Pesto

**YIELD:** 2 cups

- 3 cups (115 grams) packed fresh and tender lemon balm leaves (*Melissa officinalis*)
- 1 cup shelled roasted and salted pistachios
- 1 cup extra-virgin olive oil
- ¾ cup (60 grams) freshly grated Parmesan cheese
- 2 tablespoons fresh lemon juice
- 3 to 5 garlic cloves, to taste
- A few pinches sea salt, to taste

Back in the day, when I ran an in-person herbal school, my students would pick one herb and give a presentation on its medicinal qualities along with a sample: a spot of tea, a taste of tincture, or sometimes a nibble of the plant. When a student told me she'd be preparing lemon balm pesto, I gave an encouraging smile, belying my apprehension. I am a decidedly adventurous eater, but this pesto felt wrong.

Never have I been so happy to eat crow. On the day of her presentation, I politely held myself back from seconds to let others have a go. When my team recipe-tested this book, this pesto emerged as one of the recipe testers' all-time favorites. You'll know just what to do with this pesto when you taste it. But to offer some starting points, may I suggest smothering it on broiled fish or rotisserie chicken. It holds its own snuggled up with pasta or even slathered on sourdough toast. If you avoid cheese, substitute ½ cup nutritional yeast for the Parmesan. Lemon balm leaves are more tender earlier in the growing season. Later in the summer, use only the tender top leaves for pesto. Be sure to remove the leaves from the fibrous stem before adding them to the food processor.

Add all ingredients except the salt to a food processor and blend until uniform. Taste and add salt to your preference. Refrigerate in an airtight container for up to one week or freeze for up to six months.

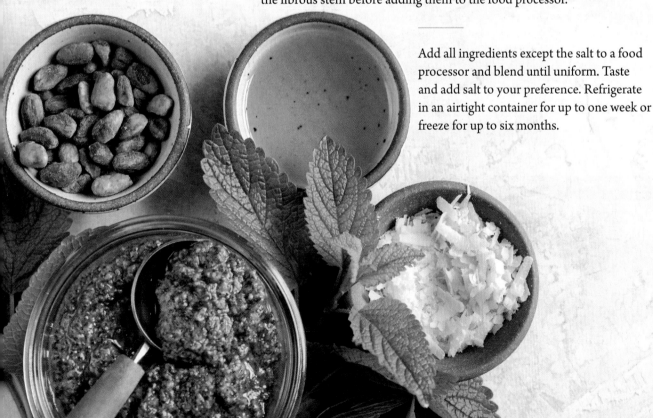

# Herbal Immunity Broth Concentrate

YIELD: 4 quarts

Carcass from a 4-pound chicken (use a rotisserie chicken or bake your own, using your favorite recipe)

1½ gallons water

½ cup apple cider vinegar

2 cups (40 grams) tightly packed dried whole maitake mushrooms (*Grifola frondosa*)

2 cups (40 grams) dried whole shiitake mushrooms (*Lentinula edodes*)

1 cup (30 grams) dried astragalus root slices (*Astragalus propinquus*), or substitute 30 grams of cut and sifted astragalus root

1 cup (20 grams) tightly packed dried nettle leaves (*Urtica dioica*)

1 cup (15 grams) packed dried whole calendula flowers (*Calendula officinalis*)

½ cup (30 grams) dried wakame seaweed (*Alaria esculenta*), broken into 2- to 3-inch pieces before measuring (see Tip)

1 whole leek including fibrous portions, sliced lengthwise and washed well, coarsely chopped

1 large onion, including skin, coarsely chopped

4 celery stalks, coarsely chopped

4 carrots, coarsely chopped

Herbal broths, stocks, and soups are ancient medicinal preparations that have seen a comeback with the resurgent interest in bone broth. Here is my recipe for an herbal broth that's ideal for supporting immunity and for recovering from surgery or prolonged illness. In our home, we eat this broth throughout the winter months—along with copious amounts of raw garlic—and we rarely catch a cold or come down with the flu, even with a child in school.

Making this broth concentrate is an all-day affair; start early in the morning on a day when you plan on staying home for the entire day or, alternatively, prepare it in a slow cooker. Slow cooking in water optimally extracts the minerals from the nettles and seaweed. It also extracts the long-chain polysaccharides—which support immunity—found in the astragalus root and maitake and shiitake mushrooms. If you're familiar with preparing bone broth, feel free to modify this recipe with your choice of bones. Vegetarians can omit the chicken bones and simmer the broth for one hour. I give specific proportions for the vegetables, but you can certainly use what you have on hand. In our home, we save our vegetable scraps—celery tops, onion skins, shiitake stems, leafy green stems, and the like—in a ziptop bag in the freezer for our stock material. On broth-making day, it's a cinch to add the entire bag of frozen veggies to the pot.

Technically, this is more of a stock than a broth, as it's highly concentrated and doesn't contain herbs and spices. For the most part, people (including picky little ones) won't detect this broth in their food, which means you've got a stealthy way to sneak minerals and immune support into dishes like chili, stew, marinara sauce, and soups. Its culinary anonymity allows it to slip into any cuisine; its potency means it can be compactly frozen and stored for future meals. As a general guideline for how to dilute the concentrate and deliver the correct amount of medicine from the herbs and mushrooms, add the concentrate to dishes with about ½ cup of the broth for each serving of food.

This broth concentrate is a lovely contribution to the Thai Calendula Chicken Soup on page 239—you can use the broth, along with the chicken meat left over from preparing this recipe, in the soup recipe.

The herbs in this recipe are appropriate for children and when breast-feeding. When pregnant, omit the calendula.

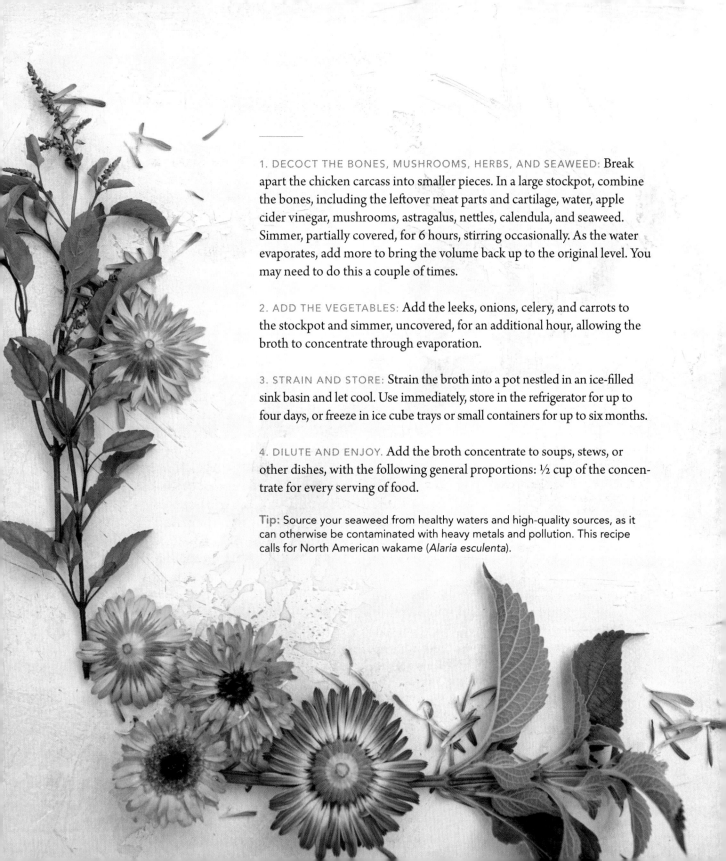

1. **DECOCT THE BONES, MUSHROOMS, HERBS, AND SEAWEED:** Break apart the chicken carcass into smaller pieces. In a large stockpot, combine the bones, including the leftover meat parts and cartilage, water, apple cider vinegar, mushrooms, astragalus, nettles, calendula, and seaweed. Simmer, partially covered, for 6 hours, stirring occasionally. As the water evaporates, add more to bring the volume back up to the original level. You may need to do this a couple of times.

2. **ADD THE VEGETABLES:** Add the leeks, onions, celery, and carrots to the stockpot and simmer, uncovered, for an additional hour, allowing the broth to concentrate through evaporation.

3. **STRAIN AND STORE:** Strain the broth into a pot nestled in an ice-filled sink basin and let cool. Use immediately, store in the refrigerator for up to four days, or freeze in ice cube trays or small containers for up to six months.

4. **DILUTE AND ENJOY.** Add the broth concentrate to soups, stews, or other dishes, with the following general proportions: ½ cup of the concentrate for every serving of food.

**Tip:** Source your seaweed from healthy waters and high-quality sources, as it can otherwise be contaminated with heavy metals and pollution. This recipe calls for North American wakame (*Alaria esculenta*).

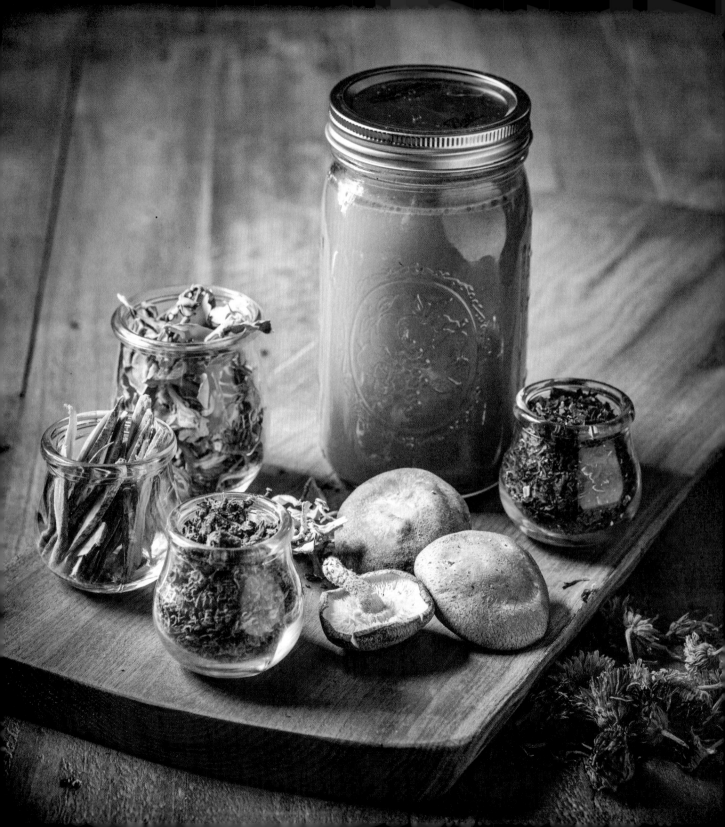

# Edible Flowers

I am an unabashed *fleuravore*. When I have a special dinner guest during the growing season, I search the garden for edible blossoms, dreaming up all the ways I might translate those precious splashes of color into evocative delicacies. In addition to the sensory pleasures of eating flowers, there are medicinal and nutritional perks. You're probably familiar with the high micronutrient content of berries, but did you know that edible flowers are also good sources of dietary flavonoids and related antioxidant compounds? It might seem challenging to ingest enough petals to supply a significant quantity of flavonoids in your diet, but some edible flowers are quite large: daylily, rose of Sharon, Chinese hibiscus, and Roselle hibiscus are a few examples.

## Guidelines to Fleuravory

**DON'T EAT FLOWERS THAT HAVE BEEN SPRAYED WITH CHEMICALS.** Roses and other cut flowers from florists have been sprayed with toxic fungicides and pesticides, and bedding plants, like pansies, are typically grown with chemicals that persist even after you plant them. Instead, grow your own flowers or purchase them from organic growers.

**EAT A SMALL AMOUNT AT FIRST.** Some flowers, such as daylily and yucca, can cause uncomfortable throat irritation or gastric upset in sensitive individuals.

**REMOVE THE INNER REPRODUCTIVE PARTS (THE STAMENS AND PISTILS) OF LARGER FLOWERS.** These floral parts can taste bitter or acrid. Daylily, Chinese hibiscus, squash, and rose of Sharon are a few of the flowers that are best neutered before nibbling.

**PULL SMALLER FLOWERS AND FLORETS FROM THE LARGER FLOWER HEADS OR FLOWERING STALKS.** Remove the tiny yellow florets from calendula, sunflower, and dandelion flower heads as the green base from which they grow is bitter and chewy. The individual blossoms of bee balm, wild bergamot, and anise hyssop should also be plucked from their tough flowering stalks.

**KNOW WHAT YOU ARE EATING.** Be sure of your identification, and don't rely on common names alone, which can be misleading. Instead, use scientific names and identifying characteristics. Some flowers are deadly poisonous or will make you very sick.

**TASTE YOUR FLOWERS FIRST.** Some blooms taste sweet or mild—these can easily slip into savory or sweet dishes. Others, such as nasturtium, wild bergamot, and chives, possess a bolder flavor; their spiciness is best featured in creamy dips or as a piquant splash in salads or salsas. Culinary herbs such as rosemary, fennel, and sage have flowers that taste similar to the leaves.

Herbal Immunity Broth Concentrate (recipe, page 174)

### Edible Flowers

- Anise hyssop (*Agastache foeniculum*)
- Apple blossom and crabapple (*Malus*, several species)
- Bee balm (*Monarda didyma* and other *Monarda* spp.)
- Bergamot, wild and lemon (*Monarda fistulosa* and *Monarda citriodora*)
- Black locust (*Robinia pseudoacacia*)
- Calendula (*Calendula officinalis*)
- Carnation (*Dianthus caryophyllus*)
- Cherry, flowering (*Prunus*, various spp.), in moderation
- Chives (*Allium schoenoprasum*)
- Dandelion (*Taraxacum officinale*)
- Daylily (*Hemerocallis fulva*)
- Dill (*Anethum graveolens*)
- Fennel (*Foeniculum vulgare*)
- Garlic chives, or Chinese chives (*Allium tuberosum*)
- Hibiscus, Chinese (*Hibiscus rosa-sinensis*)
- Hibiscus, roselle (*Hibiscus sabdariffa*)
- Hollyhock (*Alcea rosea*)
- Honesty, or money plant (*Lunaria annua*)
- Johnny jump-ups, or heart's-ease (*Viola tricolor*)
- Lavender (*Lavandula angustifolia* and other species)
- Lilac (*Syringa vulgaris*)
- Mustard (*Brassica* spp.)
- Nasturtium (*Tropaeolum*, several species)
- Pansy (*Viola*, various species and hybrids)
- Pineapple guava (*Acca sellowiana*)
- Pineapple sage (*Salvia elegans*)
- Purple dead nettle (*Lamium purpureum*)
- Quince (*Cydonia oblonga*)
- Redbud (*Cercis canadensis*)
- Red clover (*Trifolium pratense*), in moderation
- Rose (*Rosa* spp.)
- Rose of Sharon (*Hibiscus syriacus*)
- Rosemary (*Salvia rosmarinus*)
- Sage, garden (*Salvia officinalis*)
- Snapdragon (*Antirrhinum majus*)
- Squash (*Cucurbita pepo*)
- Stock, hoary (*Matthiola incana*)
- Sunflower (*Helianthus annuus*)
- Thyme (*Thymus* spp.)
- Violet (*Viola sororia* and *Viola odorata*)

Edible flowers of spring, *clockwise starting at one o'clock*: Cherry blossom, pansies, dandelion, redbud, quince, purple dead nettle, mustard, crab apple, pansies, and honesty; common blue violet flowers in the center.

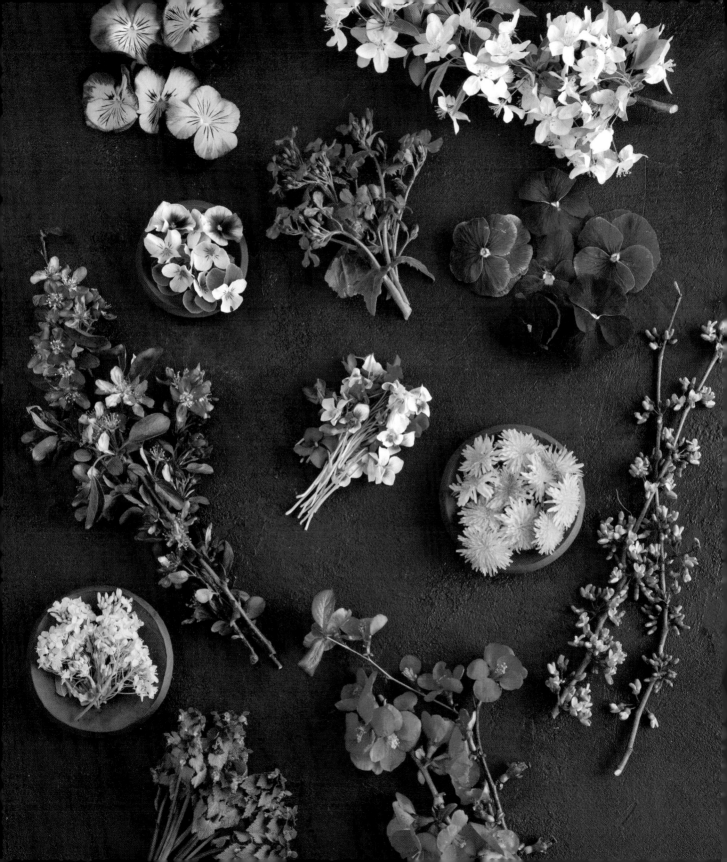

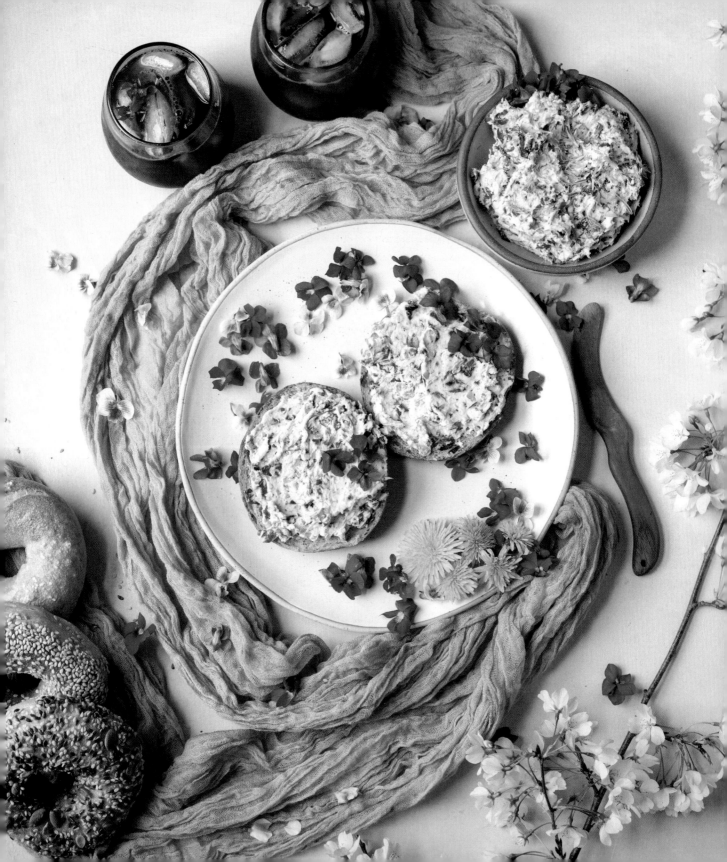

# Fairy-Floral Springtime Spread

YIELD: 2 cups

1 cup (100 grams) pecan halves

¼ cup (36 grams) dried cranberries, sweetened or unsweetened

15 dandelion flower heads (*Taraxacum officinale*)

1 cup fresh violet flowers (*Viola sororia* or *V. odorata*)

10 ounces soft goat cheese, at room temperature

Sea salt, to taste

2 to 4 tablespoons maple syrup, to desired sweetness

When my daughter was little, she would spend afternoons in the yard, picking dandelions and violets. She would then serve the springtime blooms, dished up in miniature seashells, to her fairy dolls in an elaborate tea party of pocket-sized proportions. This fairy-floral spread is an homage to the preciousness of childhood and the magic of springtime. Here, we have a slightly sweet spread that can be served with crackers, bagels, croissants, crepes, or bread. If you avoid dairy, try a neutral, soft nut cheese in place of the goat cheese. Throughout the growing season, you can make this spread by substituting mild-tasting edible flowers such as rose, calendula, and rose of Sharon. Be confident of your identification (see the dandelion and violet profiles on pages 257 and 401) and be sure your flowers aren't sprayed.

1. Toast the pecans in a dry skillet over medium heat, stirring frequently, for 1 to 2 minutes, until brown and aromatic. Do not leave unattended, as the nuts can burn quickly. Place toasted pecans immediately on a cutting board to cool, and then chop finely.

2. Coarsely chop the dried cranberries. Pull the yellow florets ("petals") from the dandelion flower heads, composting the bitter green base. Leave the violet flowers whole.

3. Combine the goat cheese, pecans, cranberries, flowers, salt, and maple syrup in a bowl and taste. Add more sea salt and maple syrup, if needed. Serve at room temperature. The spread will store in the refrigerator for a few days; however, this is a dish that is best prepared soon before eating.

# Herbal Culinary Oils

When I open my spice cabinet and see my assorted jars of herbal oils and vinegars nestled among my spices and herbal salts, I feel inspired to cook. Herbal culinary oils are delectable in salad dressings, marinades, and sauces. They lend flavor to sautés and stir-fries. And nothing is handier after a busy day of work when I don't have the energy to add fresh herbs to dinner. You might have seen recipes for herbal oils made with fresh (not dried) herbs, but I strongly recommend against this—the combination of oil and fresh herbal juices creates a hospitable environment for the growth of bacteria and fungi. In a few instances, botulism bacteria have grown in unrefrigerated garlic oil. While this is rare, the stakes are high, as botulism toxin can be fatal. Prepare culinary herbal oils with dried herbs and spices to avoid this risk. I also recommend sterilizing jars to reduce the likelihood of microbial contamination.

### Directions for Herbal Culinary Oils

STEP 1: Sterilize a quart jar and let it dry completely. (Moistness in the jar could cause your oil to spoil.) See page 136 for instructions on sterilizing jars.

STEP 2: Add your ingredients and oils to the jar, and cap. Label with the date and ingredients, and place in a dark cabinet for two weeks. Mark your calendar to remind you when to strain.

STEP 3: Strain the oil infusion through a straining cloth, following the steps outlined on page 137.

STEP 4: Pour the strained oil into a sterilized and dry bottle or jar, then label. Keep refrigerated to prolong shelf life. Use within 6 months, checking for signs of spoilage.

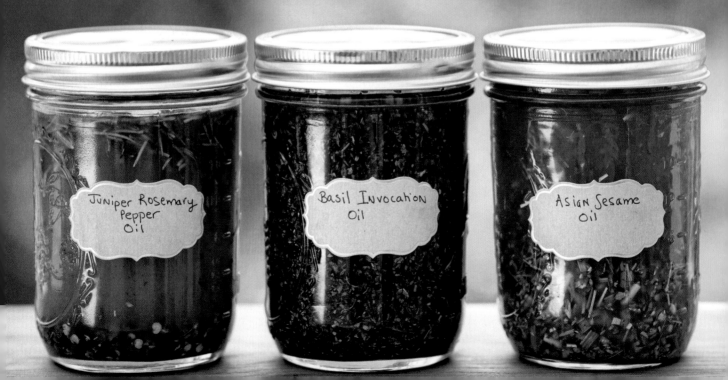

# Herbal Culinary Oils

*For these three recipes or to create your own, follow the instructions on page 182.*

## Basil Invocation Oil

I like to use this green oil, dripping with aromatics, as a homemade pasta sauce or when reheating pasta dishes. Add red pepper flakes, fresh garlic, and coarsely ground black pepper to the basil oil for a delectable dipping oil.

YIELD: 1¼ cups

- 1¾ cups extra-virgin olive oil
- ¾ cup (15 grams) dried Genovese basil leaf (*Ocimum basilicum*)
- ½ cup (12 grams) dried tulsi leaf (*Ocimum tenuiflorum*)

## Ginger-Lemongrass Sesame Oil

This spicy sesame oil can be used to sauté greens or tofu or as an addition to Thai-inspired marinades. Combine it with rice vinegar to make a dressing for seaweed salads and Napa cabbage salads.

YIELD: 1½ cups

- 1¼ cups unrefined expeller-pressed sesame oil
- ½ cup toasted expeller-pressed sesame oil
- ¼ cup (8 grams) dried lemongrass leaf (*Cymbopogon citratus*)
- 3 tablespoons (21 grams) dried ginger, cut and sifted root (*Zingiber officinale*)
- 2 tablespoons garlic powder
- ¼ to ½ teaspoon cayenne powder, to taste

## Juniper-Rosemary-Pepper Oil

Juniper, garlic, and black pepper lend a pungent flair to this effervescent oil. Try it with poultry, stuffing, and wintertime squash soups. Combine the oil with freshly grated Parmesan cheese, finely chopped sundried tomatoes, and Kalamata olives for a flavorful dip or pasta topping.

YIELD: 1¼ cups

- ¼ cup (6 grams) dried sliced shiitake mushrooms
- 14 (2 grams) dried juniper berries (*Juniperus communis*), bruised with a pestle
- 2 tablespoons garlic powder
- 1 teaspoon black peppercorns, bruised with a pestle
- 1 teaspoon red pepper flakes
- 1½ cups extra-virgin olive oil
- 3 tablespoons (6 grams) dried rosemary leaf

# Herbal Vinegars

Herbal vinegars hold the enchantment of a bygone era when household pantries were lined with homemade conserves, ferments, and jarred medicine. Culinary vinegars allow you to enjoy the flavors and medicinal qualities of your favorite kitchen herbs year-round. Spicy herbs readily chum up with vinegar, which explains why vinegar is often the base for enlivening botanicals, including the ever-popular fire cider (recipe on page 187).

Vinegar is produced by bacterial fermentation of alcohol into acetic acid and water. The acidity varies, depending on the type of vinegar and the manufacturer. Apple cider vinegar is the most popular for medicinal preparations, but you can use any type of vinegar that strikes your fancy. I prefer balsamic vinegar as the base of my culinary herbal vinegars because my family enjoys its flavor in salad dressings.

In general, water and alcohol are stronger solvents than vinegar for most medicinal constituents. That said, there are several reasons you might use vinegar to extract an herb's medicinal qualities. For starters, medicinal vinegars are a reasonable option for people who avoid alcohol-based tinctures. Vinegar draws out minerals more effectively than alcohol and thus makes an excellent solvent for mineral-rich herbs such as nettles, dandelion, chickweed, and violet; these vinegars are an excellent option for sneaking extra nutrition into your diet. When you add vinegar to foods that are high in minerals, such as dark leafy greens, the acidity helps the body assimilate those minerals. Drizzle mineral-rich herbal vinegars on cooked greens for a double dose of minerals. Finally, vinegars provide an easy—and sometimes undetectable—method for ingesting medicine.

Culinary vinegars can be used as a base in salad dressings and marinades and added to cooked kale, spinach, or chard. Add equal parts infused honey to medicinal vinegars to make an oxymel, a sour-sweet medicinal preparation that can make vinegars more palatable. You might likewise combine your herbal vinegar with a little sugar or fruity honey to make a vinegary sipping beverage known as a *shrub*.

## Fresh versus Dried Herbs in Herbal Vinegars

Most herbalists prefer to make culinary vinegars, including spicy versions like fire cider, from fresh herbs rather than dried. If you go this route, check the percentage of acid on the label of your vinegar: look for 5 to 6 percent or higher to minimize the chance of spoilage. The water content of fresh herbs dilutes the vinegar—thus lowering its acidity—rendering the vinegar less shelf-stable (the acidity of the vinegar is what keeps microbial growth at bay). Vinegars made from fresh herbs should be refrigerated to prolong their shelf life. For medicinal and mineral-rich vinegars, I recommend using dried herbs, as your finished product will have a longer shelf life.

Vinegar-based extracts have a shorter shelf life than alcohol-based tinctures. Herbal vinegars made from fresh herbs should generally be used within six months to one year. Vinegars made from dried herbs will last one to three years. Watch for signs of bubbles, off-smells, or visible mold to let you know the vinegar has spoiled.

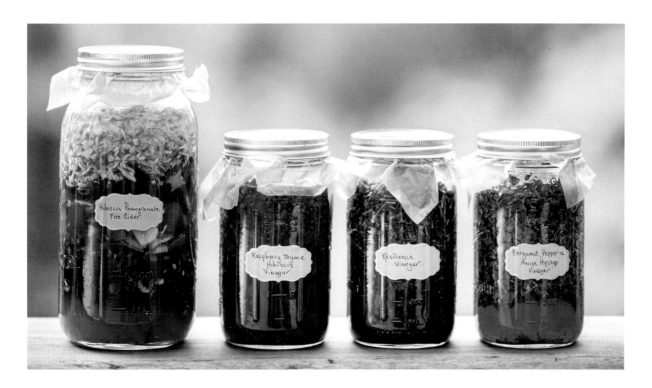

## Dosing Herbal Vinegars or Vinegar-Based Tinctures

Vinegar preparations of herbs aren't as potent as alcohol-based tinctures, so the dosage of a vinegar-based preparation will be higher. The following are general guidelines for adults. Calculate doses for children by following the directions on page 133. If you're taking herbal vinegars by the spoonful, take during meals, rinsing it down with water, as the vinegar will be better assimilated and the acid will be less likely to aggravate digestion or damage tooth enamel. Those prone to acid reflux may find the vinegar irritating to their digestive system.

- Herbal vinegars made from tonic food herbs, such as nettles, chickweed, dandelion, cleavers, and violet, can be taken liberally: 1 tablespoon (15 ml) one to two times a day. (These are plants we can eat large quantities of as food, so you can see why it's safe to ingest larger amounts in vinegars.)
- The general adult dosage for vinegars made from stronger medicinal herbs like passionflower, skullcap, milky oats, and valerian is 1 teaspoon (5 ml) one to three times a day. There are exceptions, though, such as black cohosh, gentian, and lobelia, which traditionally have a lower dose. You'll find the dosage for the herbs covered in this book in the Herbal Profiles beginning on page 136.

### Directions for Herbal Vinegars

STEP 1: Wash and sterilize an appropriately sized canning jar, using the directions found on page 136.

STEP 2: Add the vinegar and herbs to the canning jar.

IF USING FRESH HERBS: Wash your desired fresh herb(s) and chop coarsely. Loosely fill the jar to the top with the herbs, and fill the jar with your vinegar of choice. Note that the proportions are not exact: the tighter you pack the herbs, the stronger the vinegar will be flavored, and it will be a more concentrated medicine. If you're preparing a culinary vinegar with a strong-tasting herb or spice, use less, perhaps filling the jar only one-quarter full.

IF USING DRIED HERBS: Fill the jar halfway with dried herbal material and top the jar off with vinegar. The dried herbs should be in fine pieces and not powdered, which would make straining a challenge. If you're using home-dried herbs, you'll want to crumble the plant material into smaller pieces.

STEP 3: Label and seal the jar with a plastic lid or a canning jar lid lined with natural waxed paper (vinegar will corrode metal canning jar lids).

STEP 4: Place the jar in a dark cabinet for four weeks to infuse. You can sneak a little after a few days if needed.

STEP 5: Strain following the directions on page 137. Store the vinegar in a sterilized jar or vinegar bottle with a lid that won't readily corrode, and label with the ingredients and date.

STEP 6: Store and enjoy. If the vinegar is prepared from fresh herbs, store in the refrigerator and use within six months to one year. If it's prepared from dried herbs, store in a dark cabinet and use within one to three years.

# Herbal Vinegars

*For these four recipes or to create your own, follow the instructions beginning on page 184.*

## Bergamot, Pepper & Anise Hyssop Vinegar

This is one of my favorite herbal culinary preparations. The sweetness of anise hyssop tempers the pungency of black pepper and bee balm, or wild bergamot. With a lovely red hue (amplified by adding more bee balm flowers to the mix), this vinegar makes a beautiful gift. If you don't have homegrown bee balm or anise hyssop, they can be a bit hard to find. If necessary, substitute oregano and tarragon, respectively.

YIELD: About 3 cups

½ cup (11 grams) dried anise hyssop leaf and flower (*Agastache foeniculum*), or substitute ½ cup dried French or Mexican tarragon leaves

½ cup (8 grams) dried bee balm leaf and flower (*Monarda* spp.), about half leaves and half flowers (or substitute 3 tablespoons dried oregano)

1 heaping teaspoon (3 grams) whole black peppercorns

## Hibiscus-Pomegranate Fire Cider

Fire cider is vinegar infused with spices and herbs and sweetened with honey. Many cultures throughout the world prepare a version of this rousing concoction. Fire cider clears out the sinuses—thanks to the onions, horseradish, hot peppers, and ginger—and wakes up the immune and circulatory systems. People take it to ward off colds and respiratory infections. If a virus does take hold, fire cider lessens sinus congestion by thinning mucus and stimulating its excretion.

Rosemary Gladstar, treasured herbal grandmother, popularized fire cider a few decades ago. This rendition strays from tradition with the addition of pomegranate and hibiscus. These fiery-colored botanicals add a fruity contrast to the spices along with a splash of antioxidant flavonoids. Fire cider, with all its spicy ingredients, can aggravate heartburn, peptic ulcers, and gastrointestinal inflammation, and it will be too heating on a long-term basis for those with fiery constitutions. Mix the ingredients in a bowl and transfer to a half-gallon canning jar or two 1-quart jars to infuse. The dosage is 1 teaspoon (5 ml) as needed.

YIELD: 5 cups

- 4 cups apple cider vinegar
- 1 cup (20 grams) dried hibiscus flower (*Hibiscus sabdariffa*)
- 1 cup pomegranate arils (about 1 pomegranate)
- ¾ cup (65 grams) grated fresh horseradish root
- ½ cup (55 grams) grated fresh ginger root
- 1 medium red onion, diced
- 1 medium garlic bulb, cloves separated, peeled, and finely chopped
- ¼ to ⅔ cup honey, to taste
- 3 to 5 medium jalapeños, including seeds, diced, to taste

## Resilience Vinegar for Strong Bones & Teeth

Add this mineral-rich vinegar to salad dressing or pour it over cooked greens. It doesn't have an unpleasant "medicinal taste," allowing it to travel through many types of cuisines anonymously. The plants in this vinegar are some of the highest mineral-containing herbs around. Nettles, chickweed, and dandelion are all traditional "blood cleansers," helpful for addressing skin conditions like acne, eczema, and psoriasis. The daily dosage is 1 tablespoon (15 ml) once or twice a day with food.

YIELD: 2½ cups

- 2¾ cups balsamic or apple cider vinegar
- ¾ cup (15 grams) dried chickweed leaf (*Stellaria media*)
- ¾ cup (12 grams) dried nettles leaf (*Urtica dioica*)
- ½ cup (18 grams) dried oatstraw leaf and stem (*Avena sativa*)
- ¼ cup (5 grams) dried dandelion leaf (*Taraxacum officinale*)

## Raspberry-Thyme-Hibiscus Vinegar

This sweet scarlet vinegar is my idea of a fun time. Even those who are not herbally inclined will gladly pour it all over their salad and ask for seconds.

YIELD: 3 cups with honey, 2½ cups without

- 2½ cups red wine vinegar
- 1½ cups (37 grams) freeze-dried raspberries
- ½ cup (11 grams) dried hibiscus flower (*Hibiscus sabdariffa*)
- ½ cup honey (optional)
- A small handful (8 grams) fresh thyme sprigs or 2 tablespoons (4 grams) dried thyme

# Herbal-Infused Rich Syrups

Herbal cocktails are all the rage in my trendy mountain town, and I'm not complaining. I'll suffer a hibiscus rose margarita when I'm out with my girlfriends. Herbal syrups can flavor and sweeten boozy libations and alcohol-free mocktails alike. Whenever I throw a party, I set up a self-serve bar with sparkling water, bitters, and an assortment of simple syrups alongside fancy glasses. The kids are the first to mix up their own swanky (nonalcoholic) drinks, and the grownups soon follow suit, reaching for the gin, vodka, and tequila. The following recipes are based on a rich simple syrup; possessing twice as much sugar as plain simple syrup, the extra sugar allows them to stay fresh far longer. Because they're extra sweet, a little goes a long way. Once you understand the basic preparation of herbal simple syrups, you can experiment with your favorite herbs, using similar proportions, and concoct your own variations. Unlike herbal syrups intended for their medicinal actions, herbal-infused rich syrups simply enliven beverages with their aroma and flavor.

## Directions for Herbal-Infused Syrups

(Follow these general directions for the herbal variations on page 189. See page 406 for the Violet Simple Syrup recipe.)

STEP 1: Heat the sugar and water over medium-low heat, stirring until the sugar dissolves. Heat for a few more minutes until the sugar water is steaming but not yet boiling.

STEP 2: Remove from heat and stir in your herb(s). Cover and let steep for 20 minutes.

STEP 3: Strain, as outlined on page 137, label, and refrigerate.

STEP 4: Store and enjoy. Rich simple syrup will keep, refrigerated, up to six months. Check for any signs of spoilage, including bubbling, mold, or off-smells.

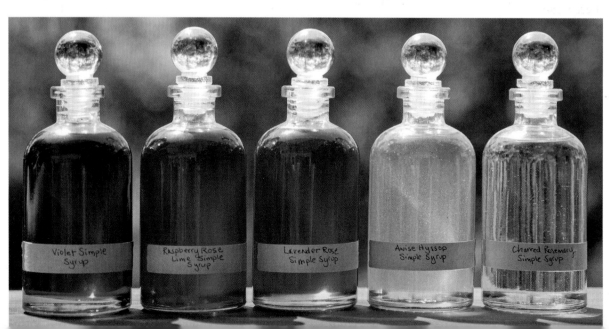

# Herbal-Infused Syrups

## Anise Hyssop Simple Syrup

Try this root beer–flavored syrup in sparkling water for a nonalcoholic sparkler, or add it to rum- or vodka-based drinks.

YIELD: 2 cups

- 2 cups organic white sugar
- 1 cup water
- 1½ cups (20 grams) dried anise hyssop leaf and flower (*Agastache foeniculum*)

## Charred Rosemary Simple Syrup

Toasting the rosemary releases its essential oils and adds a smoky flavor. This syrup pairs just as well with lemonade as it does with gin and sparkling water.

YIELD: 2 cups

- 2 cups organic white sugar
- 1 cup water
- 6 (13 grams) fresh rosemary sprigs (*Salvia rosmarinuss*)

Heat the sugar and water as described in Step 1 on page 188. Meanwhile, toast the rosemary: Heat a dry skillet, preferably cast iron, on medium-high. When the skillet is hot, place the rosemary sprigs on the skillet, pressing down with the back of a spatula to crush the leaves. Toast-smoosh on both sides until the tips of the leaves begin to turn brown and the kitchen smells of rosemary. Don't abandon the stove, as the rosemary could ignite. After the rosemary is gently charred, add it to the sugar water and proceed to steep and finish as described on page 188.

## Lavender-Rose Simple Syrup

This syrup adds a floral twist to iced herbal tea or green tea.

YIELD: 2 cups

- 2 cups organic white sugar
- 1 cup water
- 1 cup (28 grams) dried lavender flowers (*Lavandula angustifolia*)
- ½ cup (10 grams) dried rose buds or petals (*Rosa* spp.; organic; not sprayed)

## Raspberry-Rose-Lime Simple Syrup

With its crimson hue and fruity flavors, this festive syrup makes the rounds with me to wintertime gatherings. Try it in margaritas or with sparkling water (see page 365).

YIELD: 2½ cups

- 1 cup (140 grams) frozen or fresh raspberries
- 2¾ cups organic white sugar
- 1 cup water
- ½ cup (10 grams) dried rose petals or buds (*Rosa* spp.; organic; not sprayed)
- 1 tablespoon grated lime zest

Heat the raspberries, sugar, and water in a pot on low heat until the sugar is completely dissolved. Turn off the heat, add the rose petals and lime zest, and let steep for 20 minutes. Strain, label, and store as described on page 137.

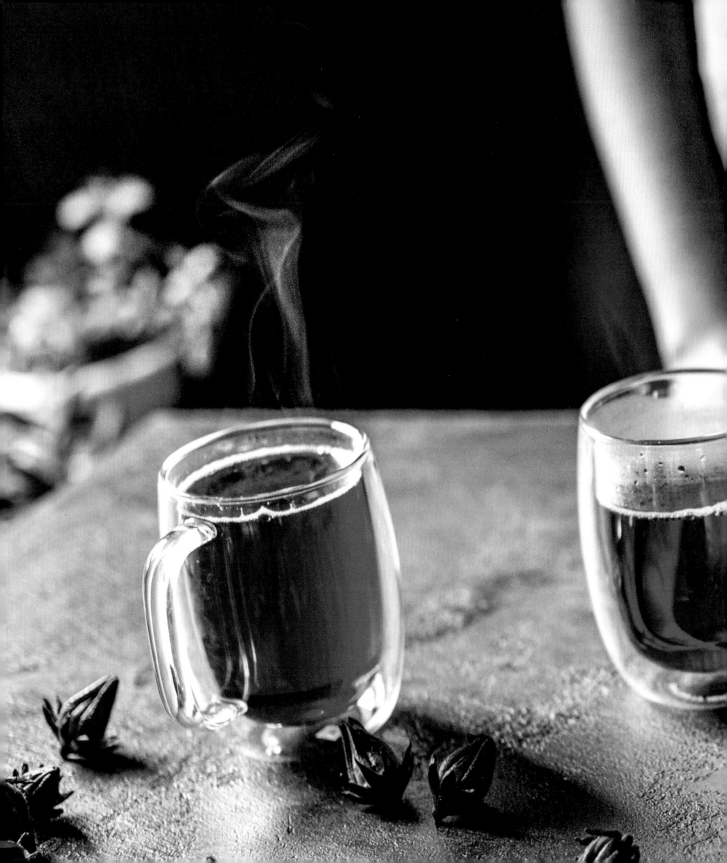

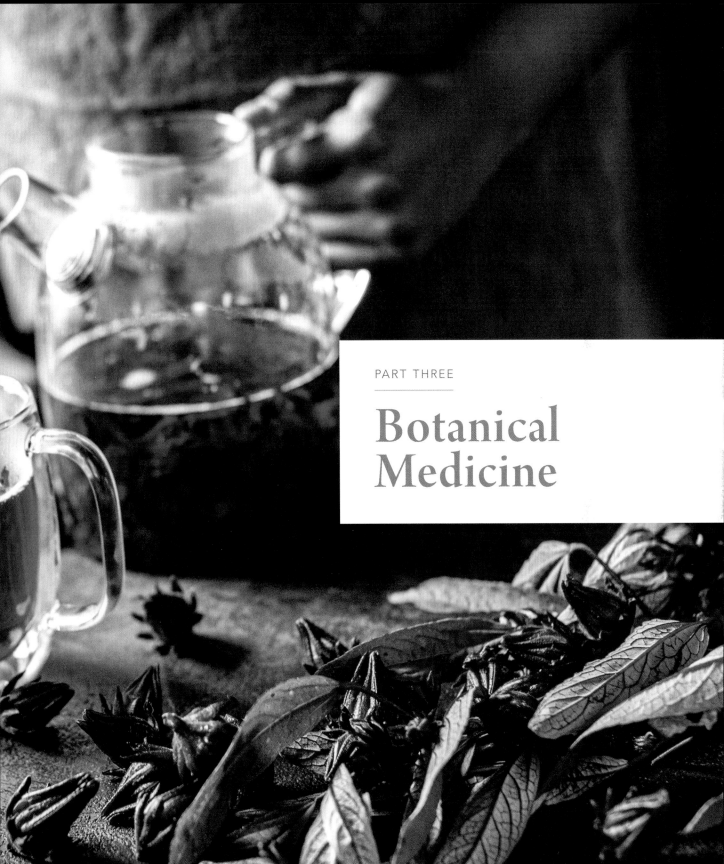

PART THREE

# Botanical Medicine

CHAPTER EIGHT

# Foundations in Herbalism: Herbal Action Terms, Energetics & Safety

> Good people,
> Most royal greening verdancy,
> Rooted in the sun,
> You shine with radiant light.
> In this circle of earthly existence
> You shine so finely,
> It surpasses understanding.
>
> ~ Hildegard of Bingen

In this chapter you'll find essential botanical medicine principles: herbal action terms and energetics, which give you a framework for understanding how herbs work in the human body. If you're new to herbal medicine, don't skip these sections, as they are the roots of holistic herbalism. You'll also find important safety information. My favorite mushroom identification books start with the poisonous mushrooms you're likely to encounter. It's a sobering reminder that one wrong move could be your last! In this same fashion, I'm starting out the Botanical Medicine section of this book with an introduction to herbal safety and poisonous plants.

This book covers growing herbs and making medicine and introduces you to 30 botanicals. Once you've gotten the lay of the land, you'll want to build on the information here by learning more about the ancient craft of botanical medicine. For more on specific disorders and their herbal treatment, I encourage you to consult a comprehensive herbal book. See our list of Recommended Reading in the HealingGardenGateway.com.

# Herbal Action Terms

Herbal terminology provides a shorthand way to communicate about how herbs affect the body. Some actions will be familiar as they are standard medical terms. For example, you've likely come across the term *diuretic* in relation to coffee, tea, or alcohol—substances that increase urinary output. On the other hand, if you're new to herbalism, some terms might sound a bit foreign. For instance, *galactagogue* isn't what you might imagine (an herb that stimulates alien lactation in a galaxy far, far away). The term actually describes an herb that stimulates breast milk production in *humans*! (*Galactagogue*'s Latin root, *lact,* is also found in the words *lactation* and *lactate,* all relating to breastfeeding.)

Why bother with these seemingly archaic medical action terms? For starters, they're widely used in the herbal world; you'll hear them in lectures and read them in books and magazines. Learning herbal action terms also helps you understand how herbs work on a deeper level, including how they affect a person's constitution, and gives you a framework for learning about new remedies.

Let's take the term *diuretic* and explore its full spectrum of effects—or actions—on the human body. Diuretic herbs' ability to increase urinary output helps address urinary tract infections by flushing out the bacteria and reduces the incidence of kidney stones. Increasing urination also has the effect of reducing water retention in the body, such as premenstrual bloating or fluid buildup in the extremities. (Note that bloating, or edema, in the extremities can be a sign of a serious medical condition, including congestive heart failure or kidney disease.) Now, let's look at how a diuretic herb might intersect with a person's energetics, or constitutional leanings. People who run dry (with dry skin, hair, and nasal passages or frequent thirst) don't typically need to remove extra fluid from their body, so diuretics can aggravate their dry constitution. Examples of some diuretic remedies are dandelion leaf, corn silk, goldenrod, and stinging nettles.

As another example, consider the term *astringent.* Astringent herbs contain tannins or gallotannins that create a puckering sensation and tightening of tissues. If you've ever eaten an unripe persimmon or steeped black tea for too long, you've tasted tannins and experienced astringency. We use astringent remedies to assuage a wide variety of maladies, both topically and internally. Herbalists use astringent botanicals to reduce gastrointestinal inflammation, alleviating the symptoms of diarrhea, peptic ulcers, leaky gut syndrome, ulcerative colitis, and irritable bowel syndrome. These high-tannin remedies are classic herbal gargles for sore throats. Topically, astringents possess antimicrobial and anti-inflammatory properties. They are applied to the skin as poultices, washes, and compresses to treat rashes, mild burns, and wounds, and they are used in mouthwashes for dental infections, periodontal disease, and loose, bleeding gums.

Concentrated astringents shouldn't be ingested for an extended time (up to four days to a couple of weeks, depending on the astringency) because of the tannin's ability to bind to digestive enzymes and consequently impair digestion. Moreover, astringents, being drying in nature, are too drying as a daily tonic for people with a dry constitution. Examples of some astringent herbs include tea (black and green), meadowsweet, yarrow, uva-ursi, rose, blackberry, and raspberry.

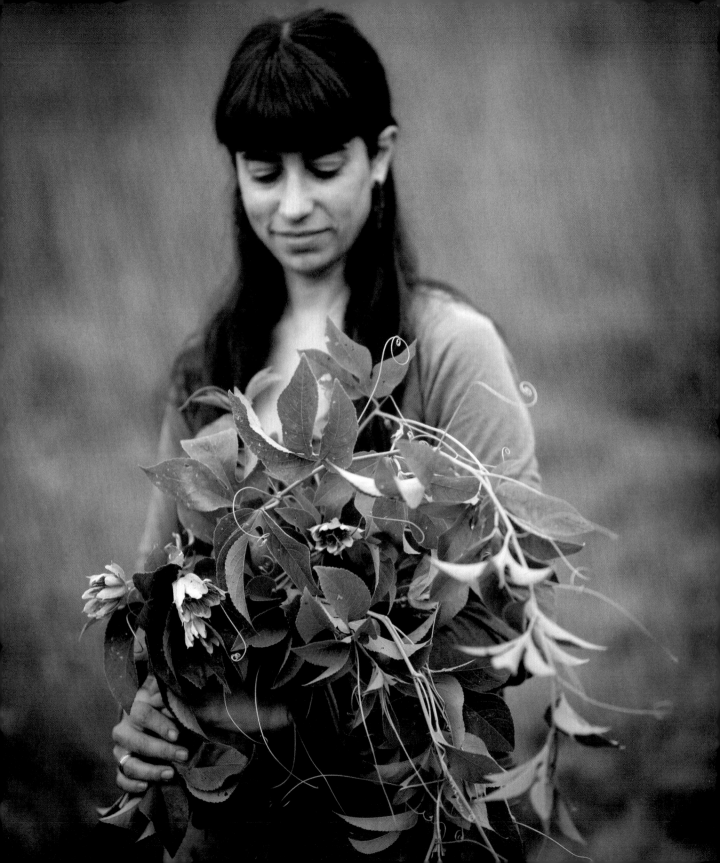

## HERBAL ACTION TERMS

Adaptogen: A tonic herb, nontoxic in nature, that supports balance in many bodily systems (homeostasis) and promotes resilience, helping the body to deal with physical, mental, and emotional stress

Alterative: Supports healthy cellular metabolism and the body's natural processes of detoxification, cleansing, and elimination; also known as blood cleanser

Analgesic/anodyne: Provides pain relief (either topically or internally)

Antianxiety: Helps lessen anxiety; also known as anxiolytic

Antibacterial: Inhibits bacterial infections

Anticatarrhal: Dissolves, removes, or prevents excess mucus in the respiratory passages

Antidepressant: Lessens the frequency or intensity of depressive states

Anti-inflammatory: Alleviates inflammation; can be a topical or internal remedy

Antimicrobial: Inhibits a broad spectrum of microbial pathogens, including bacteria, fungi, viruses, and protozoans

Antirheumatic: Relieves the discomfort of musculoskeletal inflammation

Antispasmodic: Eases cramps or spasms in skeletal or smooth muscle tissue

Antiviral: Inhibits viral infections

Aphrodisiac: Elevates or sustains sexual or sensual desire and arousal

Astringent: Tightens or constricts the mucous membranes and skin, effectively relieving inflammation

Bitter: Stimulates digestive, liver, and gallbladder function

Cardiotonic: A tonic herb that has a beneficial effect on the heart and blood vessels

Carminative: Aids the release or decreased production of intestinal gas

Cholagogue: Stimulates the flow of bile from the liver via the gallbladder

Decongestant: Relieves nasal congestion and inflammation

Demulcent: A mucilaginous (slimy) herb that soothes and protects irritated mucous membranes and the skin

Diaphoretic: Stimulates perspiration

Diuretic: Increases urination

Emetic: Induces vomiting

Emmenagogue: Stimulates menstruation

Expectorant: Aids in the removal of mucus (along with trapped debris and pathogens) from the lungs

Galactagogue: Encourages breast milk production

Hemostatic: Helps reduce or stop bleeding

Hepatic: Supports general liver function

Hypnotic: Promotes sleep

Hypoglycemic: Lowers blood sugar levels

Hypotensive: Lowers blood pressure

Immune tonic: A tonic, daily herb that supports and bolsters the immune system

Immunomodulator: A tonic, daily herb that regulates and balances the immune system

Immunostimulant: A short-term herb that stimulates the immune system in fighting off infection

Laxative: Stimulates bowel movements and fecal elimination

Lymphagogue: Promotes the flow of lymph (lymphatic fluid) through the lymphatic system, relieving stagnation and swelling in the lymph nodes and supporting immune function

Nervine: An herb that supports the nervous system

Parturient: Supports childbirth

Partus preparator: Helps prepare the body for childbirth

Phytoestrogen: Compounds produced by plants that can bind to estrogen receptor sites in the body and subsequently cause an estrogen-like effect

Sialagogue: Promotes salivation

Styptic: Helps to reduce bleeding

Vasodilator: Dilates the blood vessels

Vermifuge: Expels parasites from the body; also known as anthelmintic

Vulnerary: Promotes tissue repair; can be a topical and/or internal remedy

# Herbal Energetics

Have you ever noticed how iced lemon water or lemonade is particularly refreshing when you're overheated? Or how cucumber salad hits the spot when you're sweating through a July picnic? Lemons and cucumbers have a cooling quality. Conversely, during the cold of winter, spicy hot soup and herbal chai warm the bones. Spices like cinnamon, cayenne, and black pepper have a warming quality. Each herb has an energetic effect on the body—warming or cooling, drying or moistening.

Traditional systems of herbalism are built around the energetics of healing plants and the constitutions (energetic leanings) of people. You've probably noticed how some folks are proverbially warm while others are always cold and pile on the layers. Or how some folks have dry skin, hair, and mucous membranes, whereas others have oily hair and skin and excess mucus in their sinuses and lungs. It's beyond the scope of this book to cover herbal energetics in detail. To learn more about plant–human matchmaking, I highly recommend herbalist Rosalee de la Forêt's book *Alchemy of Herbs*. You'll find each herb's energetics listed in the Medicinal Properties section in the individual herbal profiles starting on page 210.

Although this is a simplified approach, you can start with matching an herb's energetics to a person's constitution by following these general principles. People who run cold benefit from warming herbs;

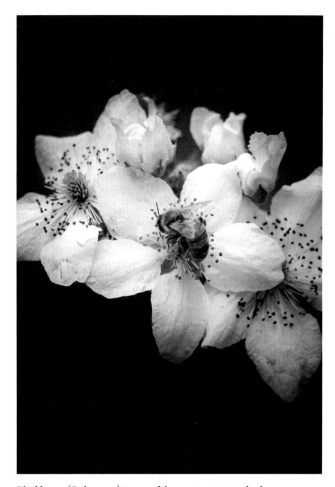

Blackberry (*Rubus* spp.) is one of the most astringent herbs

those who run hot benefit from cooling herbs. If you have dry skin and sinuses, moistening herbs will be your allies. If you tend to have excess mucus in your sinuses and lungs and you have oily skin, look to drying herbs.

# Herbal Safety

Even though herbs are generally quite safe, there are still crucial safety considerations. Herbs can have harmful interactions with pharmaceuticals, or they can be unsafe in pregnancy or while nursing. Herbal products can be mislabeled (contain a different herb from what the label lists), or they can be adulterated with other herbs or even pharmaceutical agents. This is why, if you aren't growing and making your own, it's imperative you purchase herbal products from reputable manufacturers who test their products and have safety protocols in place. The field of herbal safety is expanding as we learn more about the potential for adverse reactions and drug–herb interactions. Even so, surprisingly little is known about most herbs and their interaction with medication, with the exception of the most popular medicinal herbs. Unfortunately, there is also a lot of misinformation online, based on conjecture and tenuous evidence.

When taking a new herb, consult with your health care providers about possible interactions with any prescribed medicines. That said, most health care providers are not educated on herb–drug interactions, compounded by the fact that patients do not always let them know the herbs or supplements they are taking. You'll likely need to do additional research. I highly recommend the *American Herbal Products Association's Botanical Safety Handbook* (Second Edition), as it is the most comprehensive book on herbal safety. You can also join the American Botanical Council—they have an extensive online herbal library available for members. For the herbs covered in depth in this book, I've listed each herb's contraindications (side effects and potential drug–herb interactions) in the "Precautions" sections at the end of the herbal profiles.

## Compounding Actions

Herbs can compound the effect of pharmaceuticals with the same action. For example, if an herb is a diuretic, it's likely to amplify the impact of pharmaceutical diuretics. The same goes for herbs that are hypotensive, hypoglycemic, or anticoagulant.

## Herbs in Pregnancy and Breastfeeding

When considering the ingestion of any herb in pregnancy, begin with assuming that the herb *isn't* safe. Then you can look for evidence that the herb is, in fact, appropriate and safe. In other words, fewer botanical remedies are appropriate in pregnancy than the long list of herbs that are contraindicated in pregnancy. Use herbal remedies only when they are known to be safe, and be especially careful about where you source your herbs—adulterated and mislabeled herbs have harmed developing babies. The first trimester is especially tenuous. The developing baby is highly susceptible to substances, including herbs, pharmaceuticals, and environmental chemicals, that can disturb its proper development. So, it's better to err on the side of caution and avoid herbs unless they are completely safe and absolutely necessary.

When it comes to herbs and breastfeeding, most herbal constituents pass through the mammary glands into breast milk and accordingly can affect breastfeeding babies, which is why drinking herbal teas and then breastfeeding can be an effective delivery method for gentle, baby-safe herbs like mint, fennel, chamomile, and catnip. But toxic herbs and stimulating laxatives should be avoided while breastfeeding. Plants that contain pyrrolizidine alkaloids (outlined on page 200) should be completely avoided, as they can damage the baby's liver.

## When to Seek Medical Care

It's important to realize that herbs aren't always an appropriate solution for treating injuries, addressing serious health conditions, and combating infections, especially in the case of life-threatening or virulent infections. Seek conventional medical care when needed, and don't let herbal idealism get in the way of healing.

## Poisonous Plants

Poisonous plants grow throughout the world. We're not just talking about wild plants here—people grow poisonous ornamentals in their yards and gardens and inside their homes, often unknowingly. There are no generalizations when it comes to toxic plants—some are deadly after a single nibble, and others are poisonous only if they are used incorrectly. Factors such as dosage, part ingested, time of year, and individual human and plant biochemistry will establish the fine line between medicine and poison. Poisonous plants most commonly elicit obvious symptoms such as nausea, vomiting, tremors, stupor, and salivation. But sometimes illness or even death can take days, weeks, or months to manifest, such as with pyrrolizidine alkaloids, discussed below. All gardeners and herbalists should have accidental poisoning from plants on their radar. With some plants, all it takes is one mistake to have fatal consequences.

Children should be taught the seriousness of poisoning through plants from an early age. It is imperative to keep an eye on young children, who are tempted to put most anything in their mouths. For adults, carelessness is frequently the cause of poisoning. Plants can look surprisingly similar, and if you aren't aware of the poisonous plants in your midst, you might not be as naturally prudent. For example, gardeners have poisoned themselves by mistaking foxglove (*Digitalis purpurea*) for comfrey (*Symphytum officinale*). If you're new to the plant world, it's easy to forget which herbs you planted where and to become confused. Therefore, label your plants, and stay vigilant when harvesting!

### Proper Identification

When it comes to properly identifying species, you'll want to carefully read written descriptions, preferably ones that use technical terms and exact measurements, and look at multiple photographs, and then make sure that your plant-at-hand matches *all* traits. Use several sources to help with identification, and double-check your handiwork with experts to verify identification. If you have any doubt whatsoever, do not harvest. When the stakes are high, there's no reason to be casual or cavalier.

### Common Poisonous Plants

I recommend familiarizing yourself with the poisonous plants in your area—look for free resources produced by governmental agencies. Be especially cautious with these plant families: carrot (Apiaceae), buttercup (Ranunculaceae), pea (Fabaceae), spurge (Euphorbiaceae), nightshade (Solanaceae), and lily (Liliaceae), but remember there are poisonous plants in dozens of plant families. It's beyond the scope of this book to cover poisonous plants in depth, but here are a few deadly plants that you'll want to know; start by researching if they grow wild or are cultivated in your area.

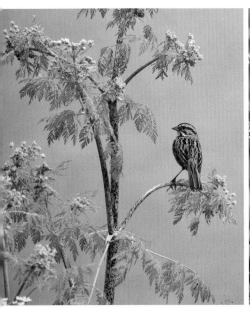
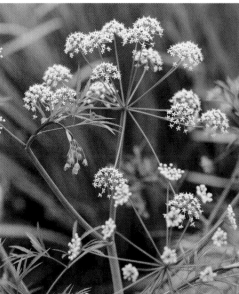
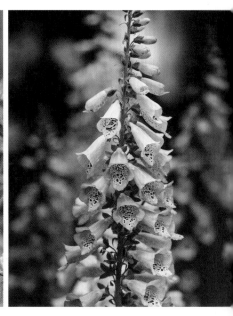

FOXGLOVE (*Digitalis purpurea*, and other *Digitalis* species, Plantaginaceae) is deadly poisonous and can be confused with several medicinal plants, including comfrey, elecampane, mullein, and borage.

POISON HEMLOCK (*Conium maculatum*, Apiaceae) is deadly poisonous and can be confused for several wild medicinals, including yarrow, Queen Anne's lace (also called wild carrot), and some species of angelica.

GROUNDSELS, RAGWORTS, STAGGERWEED, AND LIFE ROOT. This is a large group of flowering plants (in the genera *Senecio, Packera, Jacobaea, Ligularia,* Asteraceae) that contains some deadly poisonous members. They can be confused with other wild plants you may want to gather, particularly goldenrod or arnica.

WATER HEMLOCK (*Cicuta* spp., Apiaceae) is a small genus with four species of deadly poisonous plants in the carrot family. The plant can be confused with several wild edible and medicinal herbs that grow in a similar habitat, including elderberry, angelica, and spikenard.

## Pyrrolizidine Alkaloid–Containing Plants

Pyrrolizidine alkaloids (commonly referred to as *PAs*) are a large class of compounds that can be harmful or benign, depending on their molecular structure. Harmful PAs can cause veno-occlusive disease of the liver—a serious condition that is often deadly. Symptoms typically don't appear until the damage is irreparable. Common plants that contain harmful PAs include comfrey, borage, ragwort, boneset, and the various species of coltsfoots and butterburs. The damage from harmful PAs relates to the concentration of the compound in the plant, the part of the plant that is used, the dosage of the medicine, the person who is ingesting the medicine, and the duration of ingestion. Damage can happen quickly—within a few weeks—if consumption and concentration are high enough, especially in susceptible individuals. We are still learning about the types of PAs and the potential for harm—it is an evolving

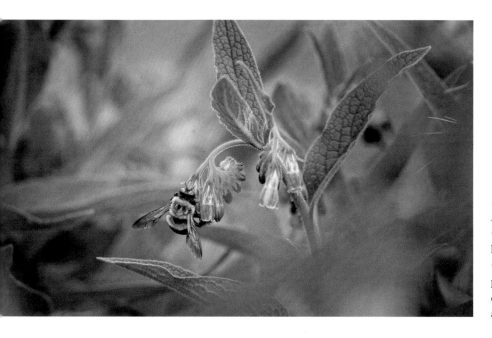

*From left to right:* Poison hemlock (*Conium maculatum*), water hemlock (*Cicuta* sp.), and foxglove (*Digitalis purpurea*), all deadly poisonous; comfrey (*Symphtum officinale*) contains pyrrolizidine alkaloids

field, and new information may come to light after the publication of this book.

Children and developing fetuses are the most susceptible to damage from PAs. It is my recommendation that children, pregnant and nursing folks, and those with compromised liver health should not ingest PA-containing plants. Others should seek expert advice before ingesting them and limit their use by decreasing the dosage and duration of treatment. Topical use of PA-containing preparations on unbroken skin is generally considered safe because absorption of these compounds through intact skin is extremely minimal, but limit topical use to two weeks to be on the safe side.

When in doubt, err on the side of caution—there are other suitable herbs that can be substituted for PA-containing botanicals or PA-free preparations may be commercially available. For example, gotu kola and calendula can be used internally in lieu of comfrey for stimulating tissue repair, and PA-free butterbur and borage oil preparations are available at health food stores and select pharmacies. Note that you may read different advice from other herbalists regarding these plants. I tend to be more conservative after reading the science and case reports: the stakes are high—death and permanent liver damage—even if they are rare. Bottom line, since there are plenty of other viable solutions, why risk it?

A special consideration for gardeners is the natural transfer of PAs to nearby plants. Apparently, plants that produce PAs can pass on the compounds to neighboring plants that don't naturally possess PAs. In one study, plants that were mulched with *Senecio* leaves (containing high levels of PAs) demonstrated uptake of the compounds. In light of these recent studies, I recommend planting comfrey away from other medicinal plants and not using it in homemade herbal fertilizers or as a mulching ingredient. At the time of this writing, I couldn't find any research on the effects of fermentation on PAs. Composting PA-containing plants likely reduces or destroys the compounds, but you may want to keep comfrey leaves out of the compost to err on the side of caution.

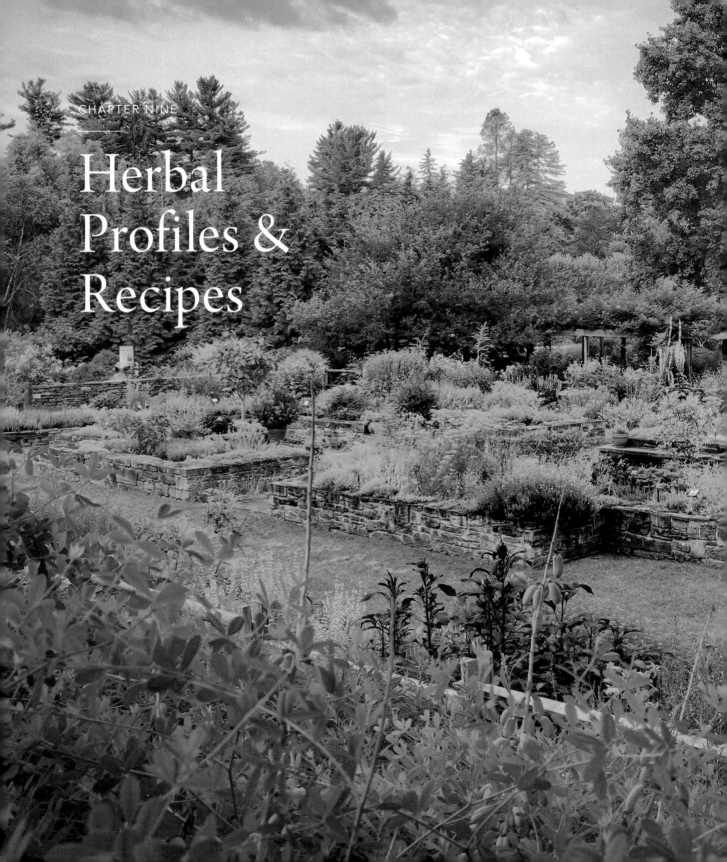

CHAPTER NINE

# Herbal Profiles & Recipes

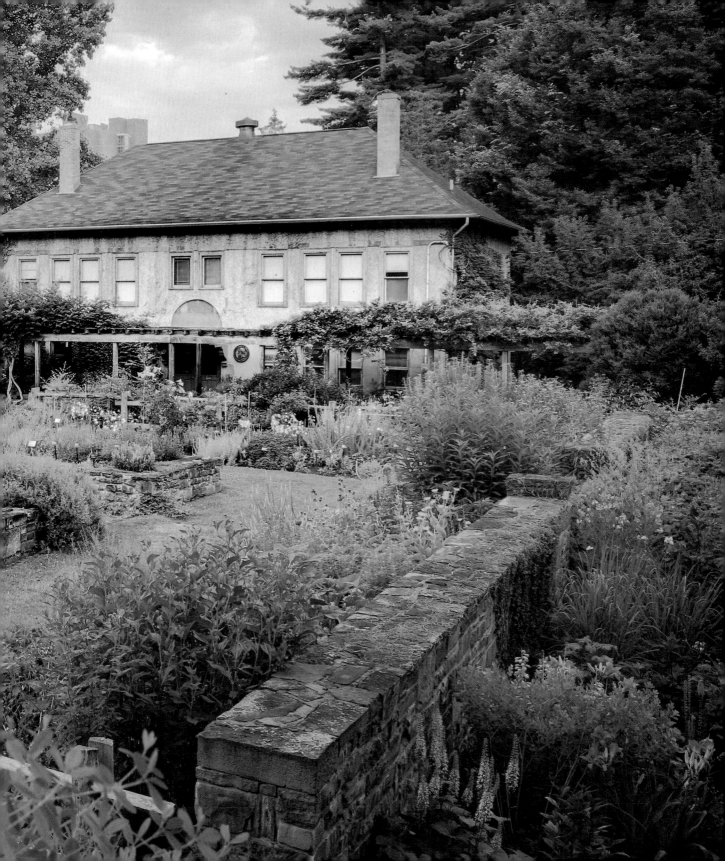

I chose the herbs featured in this chapter based on their ease of cultivation in a wide variety of climates and their medicinal versatility. I hope you'll turn to these pages year after year, growing closer to each plant and forging a lifelong friendship through learning its growth patterns, likes and dislikes, and medicinal qualities. Read this section carefully as it will help you use the herbal profiles and understand each category.

# How to Use the Herbal Profiles

### Key Botanical Terms and Scientific Names

Cultures around the globe have long had ways of categorizing and communicating about plants based on medicinal and edible uses and physical traits. Our modern scientific system of naming plants originated in 1735 when Swedish botanist Carl Linnaeus developed a system of classifying life based on biological similarities, appearances that related to genetic relationship. This branch of science—*taxonomy* (biological classification)—set out to categorize all life into distinct groupings within a rank-based form of classification. We still use this basic system today, with a few modifications. Since our understanding of botany and plant relationships is ever evolving, this fluid system is in constant refinement. Recent advances in genetics have resulted in massive reclassifications and scientific disagreement in the last two decades, which is why some scientific names and plant families listed in this book are different from those in older references.

So, why bother with scientific names? It boils down to this simple fact: plants can have several common names but only one scientific name. Here's a prime example: there's a tree in eastern North America that goes by four different names, including blue beech, ironwood, hornbeam, and musclewood. That same tree species has only one scientific name: *Carpinus caroliniana*. Another example involves the hemlock tree and poison hemlock. The hemlock tree (*Tsuga* spp.) is a medicinal member of the pine family; it is unrelated to poison hemlock (*Conium maculatum*), an herbaceous perennial in the carrot family. The only thing they have in common is the name hemlock! See the Common to Scientific Name Index on page 428.

Every living organism known to science has one scientific name, which is also called a binomial name ("two names": genus + species). For example, dandelion's scientific name is *Taraxacum officinale. Taraxacum* is the genus and *officinale* is the species. A genus is a group of related species. A species is defined as a group of living organisms capable of breeding, or exchanging DNA. Species names are also called the *specific epithet,* or *epithet,* but most of the time, people use the term *species.* The specific epithet often describes something unique about that species. For example, red maple's (*Acer rubrum*) species name—*rubrum*—describes the red flowers and immature fruits; the genus *Acer* is used for all maple species. Sugar maple's (*Acer saccharum*) species name—*saccharum*—means "sweet," for the sugary sap that gives us maple syrup. Sometimes the epithet commemorates a botanist instead of the culture or peoples originally interacting with the plant. These early human–plant relationships, especially with medicinal or edible plants, are worthy of honor; especially considering early botanical explorations were often part of the overarching milieu of colonization, replete with rampant genocide, land stealing, and appropriation.

A genus name is used only for that genus of plants, never repeated for another genus. But a species name can be used more than once in different genera to describe unrelated plants. For example, many botanically unrelated plants have the species name *officinale,* because they all are or were the "official" medicinal species in the genus. (These were listed as the official medicinal species in the old pharmacopeias, or medicinal herb books.) As with our red maple, many species of plants have the species name *rubrum* or *rubra,* but this doesn't necessarily mean they are related to each other; instead, they happen to have red flowers or fruits.

Occasionally, you will see two possible abbreviations following the genus name. The abbreviation *spp.* is an umbrella term that signifies all the species in a given genus. For example, if you read "willow (*Salix* spp.)," it signifies every species in the *Salix* genus. The abbreviation *sp.* signifies that the species is unknown. For example, if you read "*Arnica* sp." as a caption on a photograph, it means the genus was identified to *Arnica,* but the exact species was unknown.

Botanical families are groups of related genera. All scientific plant families end in the suffix *–aceae* (pronounced ay-see-ee). For example dandelion is in the Asteraceae, or sunflower, family. There are many common names for the Asteraceae, including the sunflower, aster, or daisy family. But there's only one scientific name for the family.

## Identification and Poisonous Plants

In this book, I don't cover the identification of garden medicinals, on the supposition that you are growing the herbs from seed or acquiring them from herbal nurseries that have correctly identified them. In contrast, I do give identifying traits for the herbs that might already be weeds in your garden or landscape—dandelion, chickweed, violet, and nettles. Please be aware that it's beyond the scope of this book to outline all the possible look-alikes you may encounter, as each location has its unique flora. See a regional field guide to learn more.

Be absolutely sure of your identification before harvesting any plant, whether cultivated or weedy. There are many plants and mushrooms that can make you sick or that are deadly poisonous. People can become confused about unlabeled garden medicinals, and sometimes nurseries incorrectly label plants. Double-check the identity of any plant

---

*Page 202–203:* Robison Herb Gardens at Cornell Botanic Gardens in Ithaca, New York

in question. Sometimes a new herb—even one that has been correctly identified—can cause an unusual reaction, ranging from gastric intolerance to a full-blown allergy. Please see the sections "Herbal Safety" on page 198 and "Poisonous Plants" on page 199.

## Cultivation

ZONES: These are based on the USDA Plant Hardiness Zones. If you live outside the United States, match the lowest possible temperature in the zone with the lowest possible temperature in your climate. Sun requirements for herbs vary depending on where you live. If you live in the warmer reaches of a plant's range, it will likely tolerate more shade. Conversely, if you live in a colder climate, the herb will take more sun.

SOIL: Whenever possible, I've listed the optimal pH range for the herb, but keep in mind that most plants will tolerate a broader range of pH levels than their ideal.

SIZE: A plant's size varies by its age and the soil fertility, climate, and amount of sun it receives.

LIFESTYLE: This describes the plant's life cycle.

*Annual* plants complete their life cycle in one year or one growing season. (Flowering, fruiting, and dying in one year or less.)

*Biennial* plants are purely vegetative (nonreproductive) their first year of life and flower, set seed, and die during their second year of life. Examples are burdock and mullein.

*Perennial* plants live more than two years. Can be an herb, shrub, or tree.

*Herbaceous perennial* plants regrow from dormant roots every year and don't put on any woody growth above ground. Examples of herbaceous perennial herbs include echinacea, bee balm, and elecampane.

*Woody perennial* plants grow leaves from buds on woody growth (hard brown twigs or branches) every year. Can be vines, shrubs, or trees.

PROPAGATION: See Chapter Five for plant propagation specifics.

PROBLEM INSECTS AND DISEASES: Here you'll find the most common problems encountered with particular plants, but the list is by no means comprehensive. If you can't figure out the problem with your plant, consult with your local extension office or public agricultural department. Consult Chapter Three, Holistic Solutions for Plant Diseases and Problematic Insects, to learn about addressing these garden issues.

HARVESTING: See Chapter Six, Harvesting and Drying Herbs, for more information.

# Medicinal Properties

PART USED: I list the primary part(s) of the plant used medicinally. It's important not to stray from this traditional knowledge because other parts of the plant aren't necessarily medicinal or may even be toxic.

MEDICINAL PREPARATIONS: For an explanation on weight-to-volume tinctures, please see page 142. For instructions on how to prepare infusions and decoctions, please see pages 146 and 147. To learn more about calculating dosage, including children's dosages, see page 133.

ACTIONS: Herbal action terms provide a shorthand way to communicate about how herbs affect the body. For a glossary of terms and explanation of why these terms are useful, see page 196.

ENERGETICS: Each herb has an energetic effect on the body—in general terms, they can warm or cool the body, or they can be drying or moistening. Traditional systems of herbalism are built around the energetics of healing plants and the constitutions (energetic leanings) of people. See page 197 to learn more.

PRECAUTIONS: These are my best interpretations of the scientific literature and traditional texts of possible adverse events, drug–herb interactions, and side effects. Remember, this field is continually being refined as we learn more about drug–herb interactions and increase the reporting of adverse events. To learn more about herbal safety, see page 198.

## Recipes and Measurements

Some of the recipes in this book have weight measurements (in grams), along with the volume measurements (in milliliters, fluid ounces, teaspoons, tablespoons, cups, and quarts). You'll have greater success with these recipes if you weigh the ingredients with a kitchen scale. If a weight measurement isn't given, the ingredient isn't variable or the recipe needn't be followed exactly, and a volume measurement will be fine. Tea recipes assume you are using dried, cut, and sifted dried herbs (store-bought bulk herbs; not powders) unless otherwise specified. Use twice or three times the volume for homegrown herbs unless you've broken the material down finely. For more on recipes and measurements, including calculating tea recipes for homegrown herbs, please see page 147.

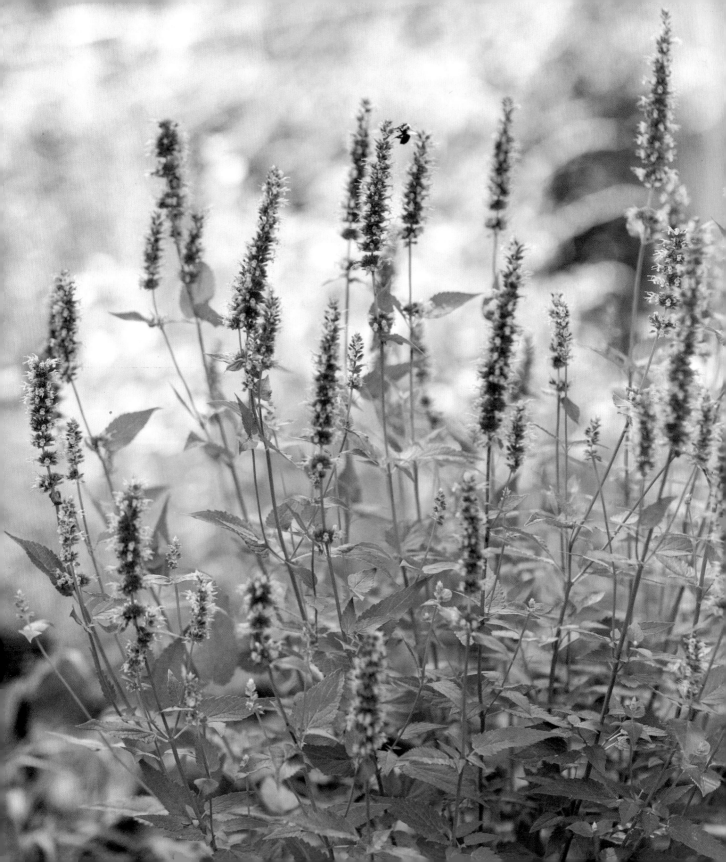

# ANISE HYSSOP
## LICORICE MINT

SCIENTIFIC NAME: *Agastache foeniculum*
LAMIACEAE, mint family
AKA: lavender giant hyssop

Few herbs are as foxy as anise hyssop, and even fewer are such magnetic pollinator attractors—butterflies, bees, and hummingbirds visit the plants daily throughout the long flowering season. It's a fashionable garden herb, and for good reason: it's relatively unfussy with a high curb appeal. Despite its acclaim among herb and native plant enthusiasts, the dried herb isn't readily available in stores. Yet another reason to grow your own! Anise hyssop's alias—licorice mint—aptly describes its aromatic flavor, a blend of licorice, mint, and anise.

Anise hyssop is native to upland woods and dry prairies of North America. It spreads locally by seed, so the plant grows semi-wild in scattered locales elsewhere. Native peoples of the North American prairie have long used anise hyssop as a beverage tea and a culinary and medicinal herb for digestive and respiratory complaints. Korean licorice mint (*Agastache rugosa*), or *Tu huo xiang*, looks similar to anise hyssop and is used in Chinese medicine to assuage digestive upsets and allay the symptoms of cold and flu. It has the same growing requirements as anise hyssop. The two plants are challenging to distinguish and possess a similar aroma and flavor. I feel they are interchangeable, medicinally, and their traditional medicinal uses are overlapping. Contemporary herbal and culinary use of anise hyssop comes from both the traditional Asian use of Korean licorice mint and the Native American use of anise hyssop. A recent garden introduction, agastache, 'Blue Fortune', is a hybrid of the two species with longer floral spikes and an extended flowering season.

If there were a contest for the herb with the most confusing common names, anise hyssop would win the gold medal. Anise hyssop isn't related to true anise (*Pimpinella anisum*), a lacy herb in the carrot family, but the two herbs share a similar flavor and aroma, and both are digestive aids. True hyssop (*Hyssopus officinalis*) is also in the mint family and bears purple floral spikes, but the similarities end there. True hyssop is quite bitter and antimicrobial; it is a strong medicinal that you wouldn't sip as a beverage tea. Finally, licorice mint is botanically unrelated to licorice (*Glycyrrhiza glabra*), an herb in the bean family, which is also a digestive and respiratory remedy.

A cultivar of licorice mint (*Agastache* sp.) growing at Longwood Gardens

## Cultivation

**ZONES:** 3–9; sun to partial sun

**SOIL:** pH 6–7; moist to dry soil

**SIZE:** 2 to 4 feet tall; 1 to 2 feet wide

**LIFESTYLE:** Short-lived herbaceous perennial

**PROPAGATION:** Sow the seeds directly on the surface of the soil and lightly tamp in. Germination occurs in one to two weeks. Roots can be divided into three or four divisions in the early spring or fall. Space the plants 9 to 12 inches apart.

**SITING AND GARDEN CARE:** Anise hyssop is a short-lived perennial with a lifespan of a few years. Thankfully for its fans, it prances about the garden, self-sowing freely. In some climates it can be a bit disorderly; you'll need to mulch, or you'll find yourself with a gaggle of baby hyssops. You'll also want to deadhead the spent flowers before they go to seed. In the warmer reaches of licorice mint's range, grow the plant in light shade with moister soils. In cooler regions, plant anise hyssop in average to drier soil and full sun. The herb is known for its deer and rabbit resistance.

If you want lush licorice mint (and who doesn't?), pinch back the growing tips every week in the spring to flesh out the plant. If you don't encourage bushiness, the plant tends to be somewhat spindly and produces fewer blooms later in the season. Interplant the herb with other crops as a beneficial companion plant. It provides shelter for lacewings, a beneficial garden insect whose prey includes aphids, spider mites, scales, and many other problem insects.

You might have seen pretty perennials labeled "Agastache" or hummingbird mints in the nursery, with showy crimson, coral, and peach spikes, and billed for their ability to attract hummingbirds and withstand drought. It's important to note that while some species of *Agastache* have been used as botanical remedies, they aren't necessarily medicinal and should not be considered interchangeable with the licorice mints (*Agastache foeniculum* and *Agastache rugosa*). In other words, not all agastache species are medicinal.

**PROBLEM INSECTS AND DISEASES:** Anise hyssop is favored by gastropods—see the general measures for controlling slugs and snails on page 73. Some growers have problems with spider mites, powdery mildew, and rusts.

**HARVESTING:** After you pinch back the tips, use the tender young "pinchings" in herb-infused waters, or add them, finely sliced, to salads and marinades. But the biggest harvest comes later in the season. When the flowers are a few weeks old, harvest the flowering stems, leaving about 9 inches of growth at the base of the plant. In most climates, the plants will send out another flush of growth and enjoy a second season of flowering. Leave half the flowering stalks intact for their charm and for the pollinators, and let them go to seed if you want more plants in the garden. Dry the flowering stems in hanging bunches. After drying, strip the leaves and the flowers off the stem and combine them, yielding one of the prettiest dried herbs that any apothecary jar will ever see.

## Medicinal Properties

**PART USED:** Flowering herb—leaves and flower spikes

**MEDICINAL PREPARATIONS:** Tea, tincture, infused honey, syrup, mead, herbal steam, elixir, homemade soda, ice cream, infused vinegar, and herbal butter

**TINCTURE RATIOS AND DOSAGE:** Fresh (1:2 95%) or dry (1:4 60%); either preparation 2–4 ml up to three times a day

**TEA RATIOS AND DOSAGE:** Infusion of 2 teaspoons dried leaves and flowers per 1 cup water up to three times a day

**ACTIONS:** Nervine, expectorant, carminative, antiemetic, and diaphoretic

**ENERGETICS:** Slightly warming and drying

## Medicinal Uses

Anise hyssop makes a tasty beverage tea and is used as a sweetener in cooking by Native peoples of the prairie states, including the Cheyenne, Dakota, Omaha, Pawnee, and Winnebago tribes. Children have an affinity for the sweet flavor of this herb; in formulas, it can mask the more unpleasant flavors of other medicinals. Anise hyssop has a long tradition of use by Native peoples as a respiratory herb, both as a steam and an herbal infusion. It is a gentle medicinal in the same league as chamomile, linden, or mint and is safe for most people, including children and elders.

### RESPIRATORY SYSTEM

Combine licorice mint with catnip and lemon balm in a tea or syrup, serving as a gentle remedy for coughs, fever, and colds. The herb can break up respiratory congestion as a steam inhalation along with thyme and bee balm. Anise hyssop is a gentle sedative, safe for children, and can be used to encourage sleep and ease headaches associated with sinus congestion. Korean licorice mint is also a traditional fever and cold remedy.

### DIGESTIVE SYSTEM

Korean licorice mint is a traditional remedy for nausea, vomiting, and bloating. Anise hyssop has similar therapeutic qualities.

## Minty Dreams of Kitties & Butterflies Tea

This tasty tea blend is helpful for insomnia, mild anxiety, and digestive upset, especially gassiness. All of these herbs are traditional beverage teas and remedies for children, two guideposts for their gentle nature. If you're breastfeeding, you can sip on the tea, which will pass through the breast milk, to soothe fussy or colicky babies.

4 cups water

2 tablespoons dried lemon balm leaf (*Melissa officinalis*)

1½ tablespoons dried anise hyssop leaf and flower (*Agastache foeniculum*)

1 tablespoon dried passionflower leaf and flower (*Passiflora incarnata*)

2 teaspoons dried catnip leaf and flower (*Nepeta cataria*)

1 teaspoon dried chamomile flower (*Matricaria recutita*)

In a small pot, bring the water to boil. Add the herbs, turn off the heat, and infuse, covered, for 20 minutes. Strain. Adults, drink one to three cups daily as needed. See page 133 for calculating dosage for children.

## Culinary Uses

If you're not a fan of the flavor of licorice or its sidekick anise, you might still enjoy anise hyssop. Finely chop the leaves and add them to salad, herbed goat cheese, and fruit salad for an anisey flair. Licorice mint companionably flavors all manner of confections, including ice cream, sorbet, granitas, icing, cake, cookies, cordials, and smoothies. To infuse the flavor, prepare a concentrated tea and use it in place of the water in a recipe, or infuse the herb into milk or butter. (Gently heat the herb and milk or butter for 20 minutes and strain. Be sure the butter or milk returns to the right temperature before proceeding with the recipe.) Strip the fresh flowers from the dense floral spike and use them like herbal confetti.

Iced tea prepared from anise hyssop, mint, and lemon balm is divinely refreshing. Licorice mint infused vinegar makes a tasty base for fruity salad dressings, such as raspberry balsamic vinaigrette. The infused honey slips charmingly into herbal teas, masking unpleasant flavors. Add licorice mint honey to herbal cough syrups or use it as a stand-alone respiratory remedy. The infused simple syrup is a tasty base for herbal libations and fancy botanical cocktails; see the recipe on page 189.

PRECAUTIONS: **None known or recorded.**

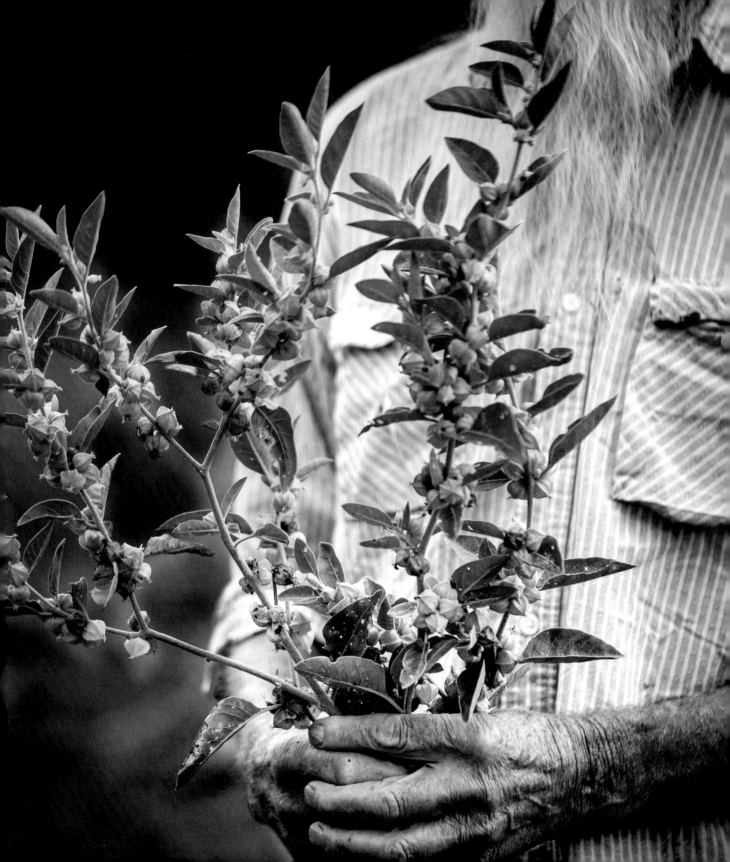

# ASHWAGANDHA

SCIENTIFIC NAME: *Withania somnifera*
SOLANACEAE, nightshade family
AKA: Indian ginseng, winter cherry

Nothing approximates the bracing scent of freshly dug ashwagandha root. To those in the know, the musky aroma is reminiscent of horse sweat or horse urine, earning the herb its name, which translates to "scent of a horse." In Ayurvedic medicine—an ancient system of constitutional medicine hailing from India—ashwagandha root is one of the most important tonic herbs for vitality and virility and is consequently called "Indian ginseng" by Westerners.

Native to India, the Middle East, and northern Africa, ashwagandha has now spread throughout southern Eurasia and much of Africa. It's easy to grow in average garden soil, and the root can reach sizable proportions in one growing season, making it a worthwhile crop for temperate herb gardeners.

Despite its medicinal merits, the odor of the root may not be your cup of tea!

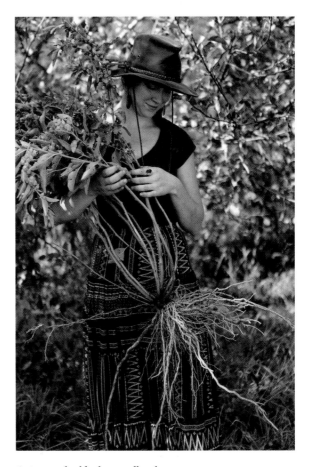

A six-month-old ashwagandha plant

## Cultivation

ZONES: In zones 3–7 can be grown as an annual; in zones 8–13 grows as a small shrub; full sun

SOIL: pH 6–8 (ideal 7.5–8); well-drained soil; will tolerate drought

SIZE: As an annual in temperate gardens: 2–4 feet tall, 1–2 feet wide; in the tropics: 3–5 feet tall, 3–4 feet wide

LIFESTYLE: Grown as an annual in areas with hard frosts; woody shrub in warmer climates

PROPAGATION: Sow the seeds on the surface of the soil as they are light-dependent germinators, and keep the soil temperature warm (77°F is optimal). Germination occurs in one to two weeks. If you live in a climate with hard freezes well into spring, plant the seeds indoors or in a greenhouse at the same time you plant tomatoes. Plant outdoors after the danger of frost has passed. Space the plants 2 feet apart.

SITING AND GARDEN CARE: Ashwagandha prefers dryer soils but will tolerate fertile, moist garden soil and even clayey soils. Although it grows better in slightly alkaline soils, it can be grown in acidic to neutral conditions. As with humans, adversity fosters a complexity of character in this herb. Ashwagandha grown without regular watering and fertilizing is more potent.

If you live in an area where the temperatures stay above 20°F, the herb may overwinter, especially if you mulch heavily. Depending on how warm your area is, it may be a woody evergreen or it may be an herbaceous perennial (dying back to the ground and re-emerging with warmer temperatures). In areas with hard frosts, it's grown as an annual—the roots are still potent but will be smaller than tropical-grown plants. If you live in a colder climate, you may want to cover the plants with plastic or floating row cover to provide a little extra warmth during both ends of the growing season.

The bright-red inedible fruit—sometimes called winter cherry—is cloaked in a papery husk, much like a mouse-sized tomatillo or ground cherry. To save seeds, ferment the fruits for a few days in water; the bacteria "eat" off the pulp, leaving you with cleaned seeds after repetitive rinsing and fermentation. (See page 106 for more.) Dry the seeds on a plate and store for spring.

PROBLEM INSECTS AND DISEASES: Aphids can be a problem. If flea beetles are a problem in your garden, they will also plague ashwagandha. Use row covers and ground cloth to keep them from the plants. I've had success with waiting until the starts are larger before planting them in the garden—the more mature plants seem to have bolstered defenses.

HARVESTING: Harvest the roots in the fall before the first frost. Wash and chop the roots when fresh; the roots get tougher as they dry. The roots can be woody, so you may need to use pruners and a butcher's knife to process them. Dry on screens or in loose-weave baskets (see page 124).

## Medicinal Properties

PART USED: Root

MEDICINAL PREPARATIONS: Powder, tincture, capsules, tea, and ghee

TINCTURE RATIOS AND DOSAGE: Dry (1:4 60%) 2–4 ml up to three times a day (fresh tincture not recommended)

TEA RATIOS AND DOSAGE: Decoct 1–2 teaspoons dried root per 1 cup water up to three times a day

POWDER: In Ayurvedic medicine, a typical dosage is 1 gram per day of the powder mixed in a bit of warm milk

ACTIONS: Adaptogen, antianxiety, nervine, immunomodulator, anti-inflammatory, neuroprotective, antioxidant, antitumor, and aphrodisiac

ENERGETICS: Warming

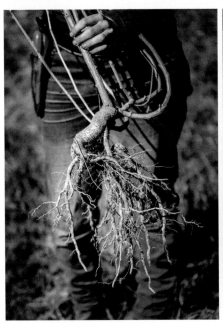 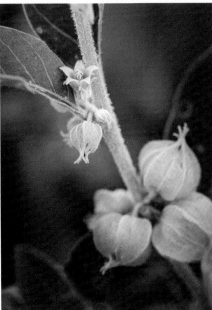 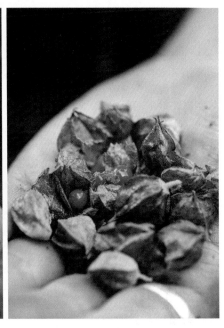

A seven-month-old ashwagandha root; close-up of ashwagandha flowers and developing fruit; ashwagandha fruit for seed-saving

## Medicinal Uses

Ashwagandha is one of India's premier tonic medicinal herbs used for a wide variety of conditions, including anxiety, insomnia, fatigue, infertility, sexual debility, stress, memory loss, arthritis, and asthma. It is revered as a grounding, rejuvenative tonic, safe for elders and children alike.

### NERVOUS SYSTEM

Ashwagandha's species name, *somnifera*, refers to its traditional use in treating trouble sleeping. The root addresses the underlying causes of insomnia, especially if it stems from stress or anxiety. If you suffer from chronic insomnia, you might take a daily tonic formula consisting of milky oats, tulsi, and ashwagandha, along with a separate nighttime formula of passionflower, skullcap, and hops. In Ayurvedic medicine, the herb is highly prized for restoring emotional equanimity in the case of chronic anxiety, overwork, or burnout. It is simultaneously calming, restorative, and nourishing, which gives a person energy.

### REPRODUCTIVE SYSTEM

Ashwagandha is a traditional tonic for increasing sexual appetite and fertility in males. Ashwagandha also helps ease menopausal symptoms and is a traditional remedy for female infertility and low libido.

### IMMUNE SYSTEM

The immune balancing qualities help bolster weakened immune systems, as well as dampen the overzealousness of the immune system in autoimmune conditions and allergies. Contemporary herbalists use ashwagandha for hypothyroidism and as an adjunct treatment for radiation therapy in cancer.

> PRECAUTIONS: Avoid ashwagandha in pregnancy. If you are sensitive to plants in the nightshade family, you may react to this plant similarly. The root appears to potentiate the effects of barbiturates; concurrent use should be avoided or closely monitored. Diabetics taking ashwagandha should monitor glucose levels closely with the guidance of a physician. It is traditionally avoided during colds and flu. Do not consume the fruit.

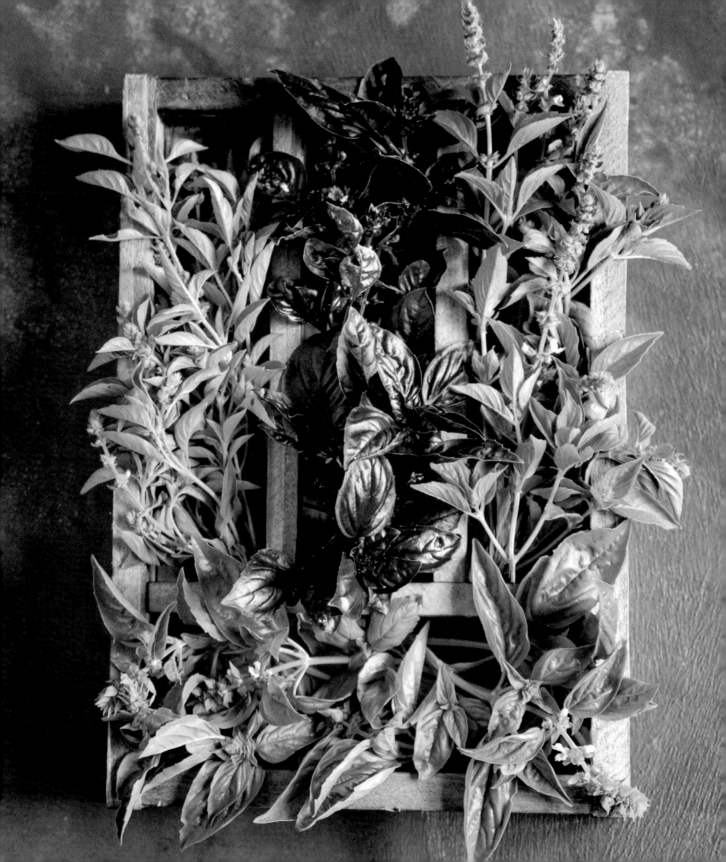

# BASIL

SCIENTIFIC NAME: *Ocimum basilicum*
LAMIACEAE, mint family
AKA: a plethora of varietal names

Basil is the crown jewel of the vegetable and herb garden, with endless culinary possibilities and myriad forms. This mint family herb is a well-known companion plant, helping to repel pesky insects and attract bees. Equally at home in a container and in the soil, potted basil happily grows on patios or porches with ample sunshine. Basil has been cultivated for thousands of years and is native to the tropics of Africa to Southeast Asia. There are numerous varieties—one could have an entire garden dedicated to housing every type of basil known.

The purple cultivars dress up the garden and can be added to dried flower arrangements and infused into vinegar, lending a radiant fuchsia color. I love the twist of citrus found in lime basil and lemon basil. Genovese basil is one of the most popular sweet basil varieties; its large leaves are well suited for preparing pesto.

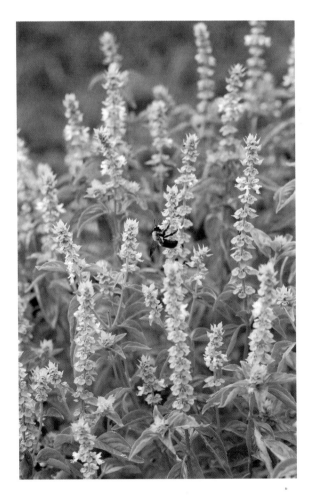

Basil varieties, ***top left to right***, Mrs. Burns' lemon basil, amethyst improved basil, lime basil, and on the bottom Genovese basil 'Prospera'; Genovese basil

## Cultivation

ZONES: Can be grown in all climates during the frost-free months; full sun

SOIL: pH 5–8 (6.4 is ideal); well-drained but fertile soil

SIZE: 1–2 feet tall; 1 foot wide on average (size depends on variety)

LIFESTYLE: Annual to short-lived, frost-tender perennial (only some varieties)

PROPAGATION: Sow seeds directly in the garden after the danger of frost has passed, or start seeds indoors five weeks before the last frost and transplant outside after the frost-free date. Germination occurs in 6 to 10 days at 70–80°F. Don't overwater the seedlings; they are prone to damping-off. Basil takes readily from stem cuttings. Space plants 1 foot apart.

SITING AND GARDEN CARE: Basil thrives in full sun and warm soils—the plants take off when the days are hot and the nights are balmy. Soil should be fertile but not too rich. The plant likes to be well watered, but note that watering from above can increase the risk of soil-borne diseases. Pinch the tips every week to encourage bushiness and deter flowering.

Basil thrives as a potted herb. The purple varieties are especially fetching in mixed herbal containers, particularly complementing gray-hued botanicals such as lavender, 'Vana' tulsi, and silver-leafed thyme. Containers give some protection against slugs, but the herb is a beacon for gastropods, and they'll likely find their way to the plants despite your best measures. Check the plants at night and look under the pot during the day. Basil's elongated flowering stalks are abuzz with bees and other pollinators in the late summer.

PROBLEM INSECTS AND DISEASES: Even though it's relatively hassle-free in the garden, basil is affected by slugs (described above) and a few serious diseases, such as fusarium wilt, bacterial leaf spot, gray mold, damping-off, and root rot. Basil downy mildew (*Peronospora belbahrii*) is especially destructive—it initially causes the leaves to turn yellow, and then the underside of the leaves turns purplish-gray and fuzzy. Certain varieties, such as 'Lemon', 'Thai', and various purple basil types, are less susceptible to the above diseases. Varieties of *Ocimum americanum* are the least susceptible to basil downy mildew.

HARVESTING: To ensure a long and bountiful harvest, pinch back fresh growth each week. These "pinchings" can be prepared into medicine or food or dried in open baskets or on screens. After the plants are mature, harvest longer stems and dry in hanging bunches. If you leave 6 inches of the plant intact, it will regrow, giving you another harvest. I like to leave a few plants intact so the pollinators, especially the bees, can visit their flowers. Take care not to bruise the leaves when gathering as they easily oxidize and turn black.

## Medicinal Properties

PART USED: Leaves and flowers

MEDICINAL PREPARATIONS: Tea, tincture, pesto, infused oil, infused vinegar, herbal butter, and herbal finishing salts

TINCTURE RATIOS AND DOSAGE: Fresh (1:2 95%) or dry (1:4: 60%); either preparation 2–4 ml up to three times a day

TEA RATIOS AND DOSAGE: Infusion of 1 to 2 teaspoons dried leaves and flowers per 1 cup water up to three times a day

ACTIONS: Nervine, antispasmodic, carminative, antimicrobial, diaphoretic, antioxidant

ENERGETICS: Slightly warming and drying

## Medicinal Uses

Basil is best known for its culinary uses but is also a versatile medicinal. This garden gem possesses some of the same qualities as its cousin, tulsi (holy basil; *Ocimum tenuiflorum*). Both herbs are used to lift the spirits, impart vitality, brighten the mind, and alleviate anxiety.

### NERVOUS SYSTEM

Sweet basil is enlivening, helping to allay fatigue and mental dullness. It's a gentle circulatory stimulant and a traditional remedy for improving memory and concentration. It pairs well with rosemary and gotu kola in this capacity. Ayurvedic herbalist Vasant Lad says that basil "gives the seed-power of pure awareness." For an overworked mind, a massage with basil-infused oil can ease mental tension, tightness, and headache.

### DIGESTIVE SYSTEM

Its pungent flavor and warming quality make basil an excellent aid to digestion, helping reduce gas and nausea. Warm tea, prepared from ginger, catnip, and basil, with a touch of added lemon juice, makes an excellent remedy for steadying queasiness due to motion sickness, illness, or the side effects of chemotherapy.

### RESPIRATORY SYSTEM

The spicier varieties of basil, with clove undertones, are more antimicrobial, heating, and helpful for reducing respiratory congestion. A warm basil infusion is valuable for treating the sinus congestion associated with colds and flu.

## Culinary Uses

Basil's snappy, minty flavor can be folded into diverse cuisines. Mince the fresh leaves into ribbons, and sprinkle on raw tomato and mozzarella salads and cold pasta salads. Thai basil is an essential flavoring in Thai soups and curries. Add basil at the very end of cooking; prolonged heating can ruin its flavor.

Basil can be muddled into lemonade and fancy cocktails, such as cucumber-basil mojitos, lemon-basil martinis, and strawberry-basil margaritas. The

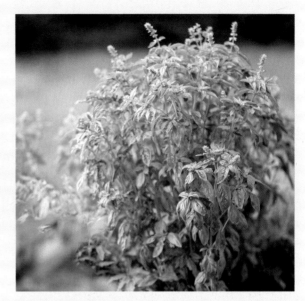

Genovese basil 'Prospera' is resistant to downy mildew, with some resistance to fusarium

tangy-sweet herb perks up water with its aromatics; see my recipe for Basil-Cucumber-Lemon Water on page 220. And then there is pesto, a sauce originating from Genoa, in northern Italy. Traditional ingredients include olive oil, pine nuts, Parmesan cheese, raw garlic, and, of course, Genovese basil. I combine sweet basil with holy basil (tulsi) into an extra medicinal version of pesto—see my recipe for Basilicious Benediction Pesto on page 391.

> **PRECAUTIONS:** Basil is contraindicated in higher doses (medicinal strength) during pregnancy because of its ability to stimulate the menses and its traditional role as an aid in childbirth. That said, most people do not avoid small doses of culinary basil or even pesto (which certainly is a high dose) in pregnancy and there are no reports of basil's actions in this regard. To be on the safe side, if you have a history of miscarriage or signs of threatening miscarriage, you might consider avoiding higher doses of basil in pregnancy.

# Basil-Cucumber-Lemon Water

YIELD: 4 cups (32 ounces)

1 small cucumber

1 lemon

4 basil sprigs (about 5 inches), such as Genovese, lime, lemon, or other variety

4 cups room-temperature water

Ice, to serve

Have you noticed some people seem to be missing the "thirst gene" and need an enticement to drink even one glass of water? In this glass, cucumber and lemon, two of the earth's finest thirst-quenchers, are the lure. This famous duo is as cooling as they come, and basil adds an aromatic sparkle. Any basil variety will do, but if you haven't tried lime basil, a citrusy basil cultivar, it's high time you become acquainted.

1. Slice the cucumber and lemon into thin slices. Bruise the basil with the back of a knife or with a mortar and pestle.

2. Combine all ingredients in a half-gallon jar or pitcher and shake or stir briskly for 1 minute. Infuse for 1 hour at room temperature.

3. Strain into ice-filled cups, and garnish with slices of cucumber and lemon (from the infusion jar) and a sprig of the crushed basil. For a cocktail version, add 1 ounce gin to every glass.

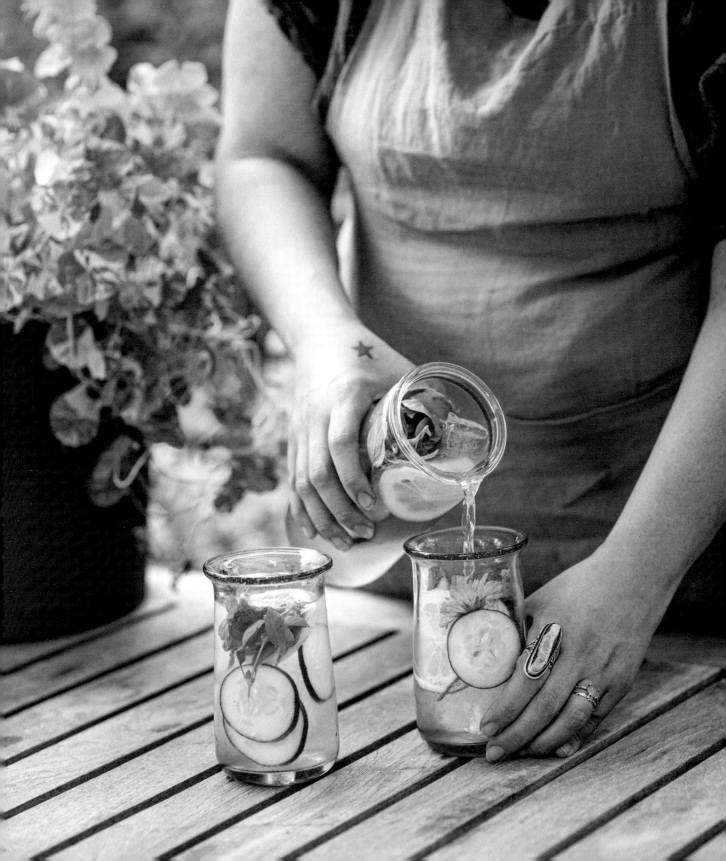

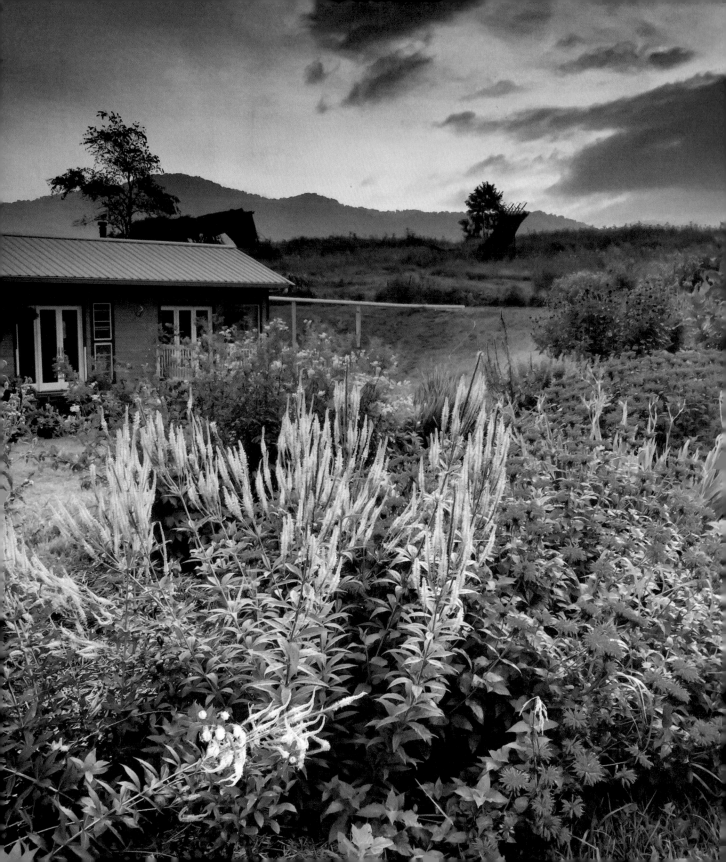

# BEE BALM
## WILD BERGAMOT

SCIENTIFIC NAME: *Monarda* spp.
LAMIACEAE, mint family
AKA: Oswego tea, horsemint, wild oregano, sweet leaf, baby-saver plant

Bergamots and bee balms are some of the showiest medicinals for the garden, with their tousled tops of crimson and lavender. The flowers are edible, adding a vivid zest to any meal. The aromatic leaves are an important traditional spice and medicine for Native American peoples across the continent. Like its minty brethren basil, the tender shoots are delectable prepared as a pesto. If that's not enticing enough, the bergamots lure throngs of butterflies, bees, and hummingbirds to the garden. You won't easily find the dried herb or tincture for sale, which means to experience them as a food or medicine, you'll need to grow your own.

There are over 20 species in the *Monarda* genus, all of which are native to North America. It is important to use scientific names with this group, as common names are many and often used interchangeably. The plants might be called wild bergamot, bee balm, Oswego tea, or horsemint, depending on where you live and with whom you are talking. The name wild bergamot is especially confusing, as bergamot is also applied to the essential oil from the similarly scented *Citrus bergamia*. It is the citrus oil, and not *Monarda,* that flavors Earl Grey tea.

This group of herbs is beloved to gardeners—there are countless cultivars to pick from, with variously colored blooms and statures. Some of the strains are less likely to spread throughout the garden, while others show resistance to powdery mildew (a common fungal issue with the genus). Most *Monarda* species are herbaceous perennials that spread via stolons or clumping, but *M. citriodora* is an annual and *M. punctata* is a short-lived perennial.

The species of *Monarda* have overlapping medicinal uses. They aren't necessarily interchangeable because their essential oil profiles vary, but we can make some generalizations about their therapeutics.

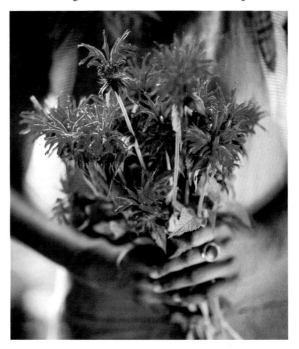

Bee balm (*Monarda didyma*) growing with culver's root (*Veronicastrum virginicum*) in my North Carolina garden

## Cultivation

### MONARDA FISTULOSA
(Wild Bergamot, or Sweet Leaf, or Bee Balm)

ZONES: 3–9; full sun to light shade

SOIL: pH 5–8; average to well-drained soil

SIZE: 3–4 feet tall; indefinitely wide

LIFESTYLE: Running herbaceous perennial

### MONARDA DIDYMA
(Bee Balm, or Oswego Tea, or Bergamot)

ZONES: 4–9; sun to part shade

SOIL: pH 5.5–7; fertile garden soil to rich, moist soil

SIZE: 3–4 feet tall; indefinitely wide

LIFESTYLE: Running herbaceous perennial

### MONARDA CITRIODORA
(Lemon Bergamot or Lemon Bee Balm)

ZONES: 3–10; sun to light shade

SOIL: pH 5.5–8; average to well-drained soil

SIZE: 2–3 feet tall; 1–2 feet wide

LIFESTYLE: Annual

### MONARDA PUNCTATA
(Horsemint or Spotted Bee Balm)

ZONES: 3–10; sun to light shade

SOIL: pH 5.5–7.2; average to well-drained soil; thrives in sandy and coastal soils

SIZE: 2–3 feet tall; 1–2 feet wide

LIFESTYLE: Clumping, biennial to short-lived perennial

PROPAGATION: The seeds of all *Monarda* species are Lilliputian-tiny and must be planted on the surface of the soil and misted or bottom watered to avoid burying them too deeply in the soil. Germination typically takes place in 6 to 21 days at 65–70°F. In the case of the running bee balms (*M. didyma* and *M. fistulosa*), it's easier to propagate the plant through root division. This is also the only way to propagate cultivars and have the plants retain the distinctive characteristics of their parents. Space *Monarda* plants 1 foot apart except for *M. citriodora,* which can be spaced 9 inches apart.

SITING AND GARDEN CARE: Wild bergamot (*M. fistulosa*) and bee balm (*M. didyma*) spread vigorously by runners, similar to how mint spreads. Plant them where they can go hog wild, or contain their exuberance with a rhizome barrier, as you would for mint or bamboo. The bergamots will attract pollinators to the garden, including hummingbirds, butterflies, bees, and the mystical clearwing hummingbird moth (*Hemaris thysbe*), which resembles a fantastical cross between a lobster, hummingbird, and bumblebee. *M. fistulosa* is a favorite nectary for many species of native bumblebees and butterflies, including the eastern tiger swallowtail, monarch, and great spangled fritillary. Soldier beetles—beneficial garden predators that eat aphids, grasshopper eggs, and other garden pests—are attracted to bee balm species.

Bee balm (*Monarda didyma*) prefers fertile, moist soil (imagine a floodplain). If you live in a hot climate, try planting it in dappled shade or in an area that receives morning sun and afternoon shade. It will flower in part shade, although less lavishly. There are red, purple, and lavender named varieties of this species, with varying heights.

Wild bergamot (*Monarda fistulosa*) thrives in hotter and drier conditions as compared to bee balm. This species has such a wide range (most of North America), with diverse genetics and subspecies, so consider sourcing plants from local native nurseries to ensure you will have plants suited to your specific climate.

---

*Clockwise, from top left:* Horsemint (*Monarda punctata*); lemon bergamot (*Monarda citriodora*); red bee balm (*Monarda didyma*); wild bergamot (*Monarda fistulosa*)

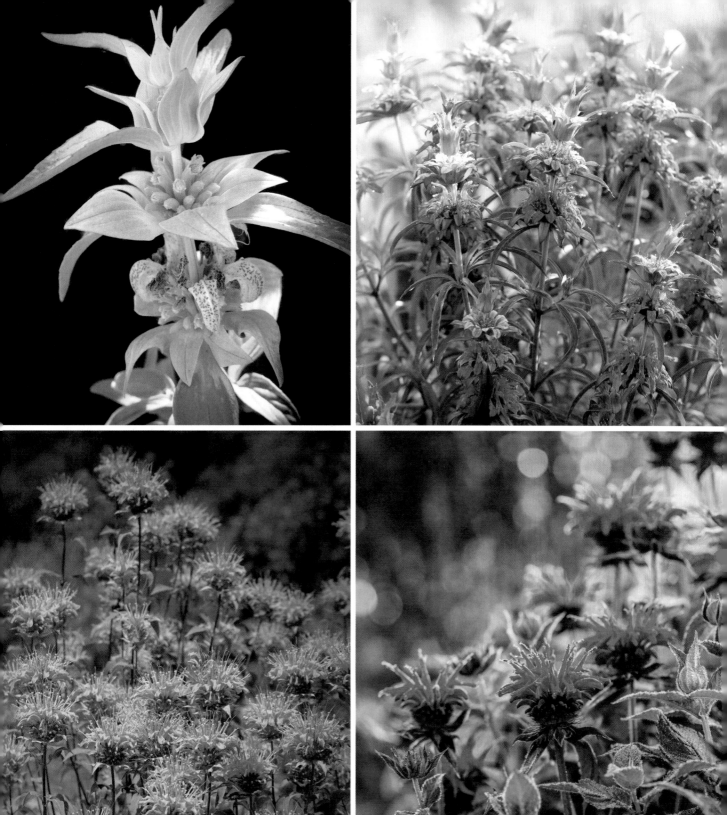

Lemon bergamot, or lemon bee balm (*Monarda citriodora*), is one of the showiest members of this group and something of an anomaly, as it is an annual. Its bloom season is incredibly long. Lemon bergamot leaves have a lemony and spicy aroma. The plant thrives in average to dry garden soils. Pinch it back in the spring to encourage bushiness and more bodacious blooms.

Horsemint (*Monarda punctata*) is one of the first medicinals I ever wildcrafted as a young herbalist in Florida, and it remains dear to my heart. It is perhaps one of the most pungent of the *Monarda* clan, with very high levels of thymol (a monoterpene phenol, which is highly antifungal and antibacterial and found in many other mint family members, including thyme and oregano). Horsemint shines as an antimicrobial and is especially useful as a steam inhalation for respiratory congestion owing to its high essential oil content. Horsemint thrives in sandy soils and tolerates saltiness, making it uniquely suited to the coastal plains of the Southeast, maritime soils, lowland deserts, and the well-drained soils of the Great Lakes.

PROBLEM INSECTS AND DISEASES: All the *Monarda* species are highly susceptible to powdery mildew, a fungal disease that appears as a white powder on the leaves midsummer and that is especially prevalent in sultry climates. Some *M. didyma* cultivars that have demonstrated resistance to powdery mildew are 'Violet Queen', 'Marshall's Delight', 'Mrs. Perry', 'Raspberry Wine', 'Rose Queen', and 'Purple Mildew Resistant'. The white-flowered *M. fistulosa* varietal 'Albescens' is also resistant. After the plants are done flowering and powdery mildew has swept through, the plants are generally peaked and unsavory. I cut them back at this time, and the vegetation regrows and fills in the bare area in a few weeks.

HARVESTING: Harvest the flowering stems when they are in bloom, leaving some for the pollinators, and hang in bundles. If you live in an area where powdery mildew is a serious issue, you may want to harvest your *Monarda* in early summer, before the fungus gets hold of the leaves. The plants will still flower, although the blooms will be lower down on the stem. You can harvest the flowers separately from the leaves at this time and combine them with the leaves that you dried earlier in the season. If you're harvesting the greens for culinary use, such as pesto, pinch back the tender upper growth.

## Medicinal Properties

PART USED: Leaves and flowers

MEDICINAL PREPARATIONS: Tea, tincture, douche, honey, syrup, oxymel, steam inhalation, infused oil, herbed butter, infused vinegar, pesto, dressing, poultice, and compress

TINCTURE RATIOS AND DOSAGE: Fresh (1:2 95%) or dry (1:4 60%); either preparation 2–4 ml up to three times a day

TEA RATIOS AND DOSAGE: Infusion of 1 to 2 teaspoons dried leaf and flower per 1 cup water up to three times a day

ACTIONS: Diaphoretic, antibacterial, antifungal, emmenagogue, anticatarrhal, expectorant, carminative, nervine, antirheumatic, and diuretic

ENERGETICS: Warming and drying

## Medicinal Uses

The bee balms and bergamots are some of the most important medicines of Native American peoples, both historically and currently. All of our Western herbal understanding of the plant comes from the ancient knowledge of Indigenous peoples who use various *Monarda* species to treat fevers, colds, coughs, flu, and respiratory congestion of the lungs and sinuses. Bergamot has a rich tradition of being used to scent the hair, body, or clothing and is placed on the hot rocks inside the sweathouse for its aromatic benefits. Even though all the *Monarda* species can be used medicinally in a similar fashion, each species has its own essential oil profile and energetic signature. Some of the *Monarda* species are more "sweet" and more palatable as a tea or culinary herb (*M. didyma,* for example), while others are quite hot and less enjoyable as a beverage tea or spice (*M. punctata,* for example). Even within each species, there is aromatic variability. Play around with the group—employing your taste buds and sniffer—until you unlock their nuances and impress their aroma upon your heart.

## DIGESTIVE SYSTEM

Wild bergamot is used medicinally to reduce gas and bloating and improve digestion. The leaves and flowers can be added to food as a culinary herb for this purpose or ingested as a tea or infused honey. Anishinaabe herbalist and ethnobotanist Keewaydinoquay taught her students that *M. fistulosa*'s name, the baby-saver plant, comes from its tradition for calming colic in infants, thus saving the babies from their parents' madness over caring for an inconsolable child. Drinking the tea while breastfeeding allows the herb to pass into the breast milk, thus soothing digestive colic. Older children can drink the tea sweetened with honey for digestive upset.

## RESPIRATORY SYSTEM

I like to use the dried leaves and flowers in a bath, sauna, or steam inhalation to help break up phlegm in respiratory congestion. Wild bergamot's essential oils are antimicrobial and anti-inflammatory. Wild bergamot is useful in colds and flu, as it is anticatarrhal and diaphoretic (brings on a sweat to break a fever). Make sure you drink the tea or the tincture (add it to hot tea or water) piping hot if you're attempting to break a fever.

## NERVOUS SYSTEM

Bee balm is a gentle nervine sedative—on par with chamomile and mint—although most folks prefer the flavor of mint or chamomile to bee balm. But individual reactions to herbs can vary. I had a student who found bee balm to be exceptionally hypnotic—just one cup of tea would quickly lure her into dreamland.

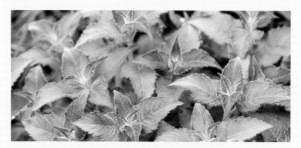

Bee balm at the perfect harvesting stage for culinary use

## TOPICAL USES

I commonly include wild bergamot, along with yarrow and Japanese honeysuckle, in my herbal soaks and compresses to address bacterial and fungal infections. The Lakota use wild bergamot as a compress for sore eyes, and Cherokee healers apply the herb topically to cuts and boils. The flowers contain antioxidant and anti-inflammatory flavonoids and related compounds, including rutin and quercetin.

# Culinary Uses

All *Monarda* species have edible flowers, which add a bright, spicy pungency to savory dishes. Pull the individual flowers from their fibrous flower heads and use as a garnish, or toss in salads for an extra splash of color. The flowers are especially fetching when suspended in ice cubes. The leaves of *Monarda* species can be combined with basil to create a twist on the classic pesto. I find that wild bergamot (*M. fistulosa*) has the best flavor for pesto and makes a lovely pesto on its own, but bee balm (*M. didyma*) is a close runner-up. Horsemint (*M. punctata*) is too intense for pesto. The spicier species can best be enjoyed sparingly in a blend with milder herbs. The leaves of *M. fistulosa* are a traditional culinary herb used to flavor meat, soups, and stews.

> PRECAUTIONS: Do not use in pregnancy, as it is a traditional menstrual stimulant. Like other spicy herbs, bee balm may aggravate heartburn.

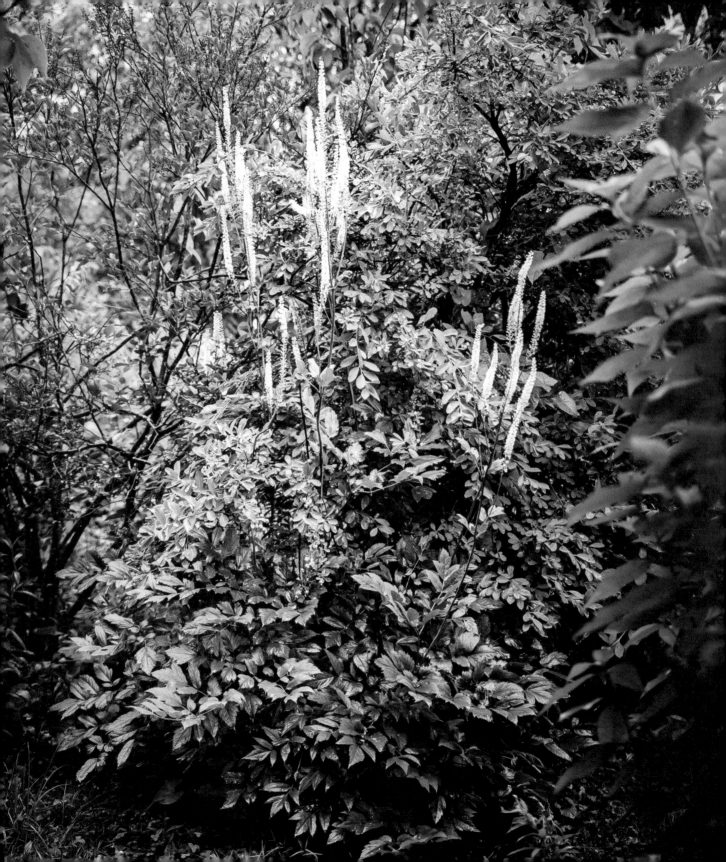

# BLACK COHOSH

SCIENTIFIC NAME: *Actaea racemosa*; formerly *Cimicifuga racemosa*
RANUNCULACEAE, buttercup family
AKA: black snakeroot, bugbane, rattletop, papoose root

Black cohosh is a dashing woodland herb. Its lacy leaves and ivory wands of tasseled blooms climb forested slopes in a midsummer floral procession fit for a dryad kingdom. Black cohosh is more than visually mesmerizing; its flowers and leaves possess a bracing scent, and its gnarled roots are acrid. The herb has been thrust into the herbal limelight in the past few decades as a menopausal remedy, but it's been a treasured ally for childbirth, menstrual cramps, and delayed menstruation for centuries. Native peoples have long used the herb for arthritic pain, coughs, and colds.

Black cohosh is one of the easiest woodland medicinals to grow, thriving in a variety of habitats and soils, including in pots, backyard gardens, clayey soils, and sandy soils. Considering its charisma and medicinal versatility, it is well worth bringing into the landscape. In the wild it has been overharvested and has suffered from habitat loss, which is even more reason to propagate it and expand its populations. Black cohosh is native to central and eastern North America and is especially prevalent in the Appalachian Mountains and New England.

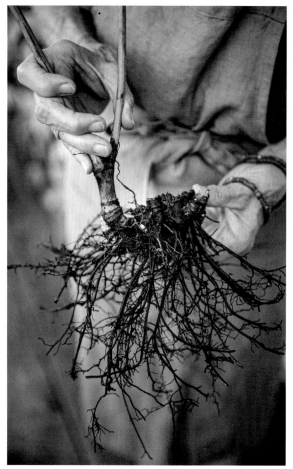

Black cohosh flowering in partial shade at 7Song's garden in Ithaca, NY; a teenage black cohosh root

## Cultivation

**ZONES:** 3–8; full shade to part shade (morning sun and afternoon shade)

**SOIL:** pH 5–6; rich, moist, well-drained soil high in organic matter

**SIZE:** 5–8 feet tall (in flower); 2–4 feet wide

**LIFESTYLE:** Herbaceous perennial

**PROPAGATION:** Black cohosh is most easily grown from division. If you're increasing a wild stand of black cohosh, dig up mature plants in the fall, after they have set seed. Each division should have at least one bud, along with 1 to 2 inches of rhizome and its associated rootlets. (The thick underground part of cohosh is technically a rhizome but is often called a root; I use the two terms interchangeably.) One plant can yield three to eight divisions, depending on its age and root mass. Plant divisions 2 feet apart with the bud pointing upward, covered with 2 inches of soil and additional forest duff.

Planting the herb from seed is a lengthy affair but will yield a population with greater genetic diversity. Germination takes six months to two years (sometimes three!), and the germination rate is lower than other herbs. Use the freshest seeds available and sow heavily, as the seeds are prone to fungal diseases and subsequent rot. Sow the seeds in the late summer in forest garden beds or in large outdoor flats or garden boxes. The seeds can also be stratified in sand with the plastic bag method, starting with one month of warm, moist stratification at approximately 70°F, followed by three months of cold (35–40°F), moist stratification. (See page 88.) Because young seedlings can't tolerate full sun, be sure trays are placed in the shade or under a shade cloth (a 66 percent shade cloth or stronger) until their second year. Keep seed trays around another season, as you may have a second flush of germinating seeds the following spring. Space plants 2 to 3 feet apart.

**SITING AND GARDEN CARE:** Black cohosh tolerates a variety of soil types, but it favors fertile, moist yet well-drained, and slightly acidic soils. If planting in the forest, amend the soil with composted leaves, aged pine bark fines, or composted hardwood bark. Breaking up compact ground and digging in one of the above amendments into the native soil will help increase drainage while adding fertility and organic matter. If all you have to work with is the acidic soil of coniferous forests, amend the earth with a touch of lime to reduce the acidity, and add copious organic matter to increase soil fertility and water retention. Keep plants watered during the heat of summer if it doesn't rain.

In colder climates, the herb can tolerate more sun than you might imagine. The more light, the faster the plants will mature, and the greater the harvest. If your summers aren't too hot, plant black cohosh where it will receive full sun in the morning and shade in the afternoon. In climates that have cloudy and mild summers, it can even be grown in full sun. Check with local growers to see where they've planted black cohosh and how it's faring in that location. The plant is less particular than other forest medicinals about where it will grow, but in general, it prefers to grow under hardwood trees in open woodlands. It naturally grows on slopes or in the lower, flatter reaches of coves, but it doesn't favor waterlogged soils. In central or eastern North America, look for black cohosh's forest-floor cronies: blue cohosh, doll's eye, trillium, and bloodroot. Trees to look for include tulip poplar, basswood, red maple, Fraser magnolia, and sugar maple. To locate good planting sites in the western United States, look for oaks and maples.

**PROBLEM INSECTS AND DISEASES:** Black cohosh is relatively disease-free, especially when interplanted with other herbs; however, it is affected by leaf spots and various root rots. If you're growing black cohosh in the field, inoculate with a bit of woodland soil (preferably from spots where black cohosh grows) scattered throughout the bed to introduce beneficial bacteria and fungi. Consider using an all-purpose mycorrhizal inoculant as well. Cutworms, deer, slugs, rodents, and a leaf-eating beetle can be problems as well.

HARVESTING: Plants grown in amended garden beds will be ready for harvest in the fall of the third year, when they have multiple stems and have reached reproductive maturity. Forest-grown plants will be ready for harvest after three to five years. If the plants are grown from seed rather than root division, add on another year or two. Dig the rhizomes in the fall, and, if possible, replant a division to ensure subsequent regenerative harvests. Wash the rhizomes immediately, taking care to get into the tight nooks and crannies with a bristle brush. Chop when fresh and prepare as medicine or dry on screens. Black cohosh has several look-alikes and is overharvested—do not harvest from the wild.

## Medicinal Properties

PART USED: Rhizome (sold as the "root")

MEDICINAL PREPARATIONS: Tincture, decoction, syrup, and capsules (Use caution with dosing; larger doses can be nauseating or emetic.)

TINCTURE RATIOS AND DOSAGE: Fresh (1:2 95%) or dry (1:5 60%); either preparation ½–1 ml up to three times a day

TEA RATIOS AND DOSAGE: Decoction of ½ teaspoon dried rhizome per 1 cup water up to two times a day. Bitter and acrid!

ACTIONS: Antirheumatic, hormone balancer, parturient, phytoestrogen, nervine, emmenagogue, uterine antispasmodic, anodyne, hypotensive, pulmonary antispasmodic, and emetic (in high doses)

ENERGETICS: Heating and drying

## Medicinal Uses

Black cohosh has a potent flavor—it is bitter, soapy, and acrid. Its aroma and flavor hint at its complex biochemistry—black cohosh straddles the worlds of medicine and toxin. It can cause nausea or vomiting, especially with higher doses, and it has other possible side effects such as indigestion and headaches. I tend to use smaller doses of the plant—on the order of ½ to 1 dropperful of tincture. It's easier to deliver smaller doses in tincture form; plus, the tea is acrid. Some herbalists use larger doses, but smaller doses are plenty effective and less likely to cause side effects. Most of the studies demonstrating black cohosh's efficacy in alleviating menopause symptoms were conducted with minimal doses of the root. The equivalent dosage of a 1:2 95% tincture would be 3 to 9 drops (not droppersful!) of tincture a day!

All contemporary understanding of the herb originates with the traditions and wisdom of North American Indigenous peoples. The Cherokee use black cohosh to stimulate menstruation, ease joint pain, and alleviate colds, coughs, and constipation. The Iroquois use it externally as a soak or steam bath for rheumatic pain. European settlers adopted the plant into their repertoire early on—it became quite popular as a remedy for arthritic pain and hacking, spasmodic coughs, notably for tuberculosis and whooping cough.

### REPRODUCTIVE SYSTEM

Black cohosh is a hormone balancer, specifically balancing the hormonal interplay of the hypothalamus, pituitary, and ovaries. For this purpose, it should be taken regularly—compared to most herbal treatments, consistent daily dosing is crucial, ideally with two doses, morning and night. The root can be used to balance hormones in a number of scenarios, including menopause, menstrual cramps, ovarian cysts, uterine fibroids, infertility, amenorrhea, and irregular cycles. Studies have demonstrated its efficacy in relieving menopausal symptoms such as hot flashes, insomnia, irritability, depression, and vaginal dryness. Black cohosh can give immediate ease to menstrual cramps when combined with other uterine antispasmodics and nervines, such as blue cohosh, motherwort, skullcap, black haw, and passionflower. It also helps stimulate delayed menstruation or a scanty flow. The herb is especially helpful for dull muscular pain in the back, pelvic region, and thighs, with a sense of dragging pain in the uterus.

## MUSCULOSKELETAL SYSTEM

Many herbalists use the root to lessen the pain and inflammation of arthritic conditions, including osteoarthritis, rheumatoid arthritis, fibromyalgia, and tendinitis. It is also used to relieve the inflammation and pain of pulled muscles. I often combine it with meadowsweet, willow, black haw, and valerian for this purpose. Herbalist Michael Moore described black cohosh as being useful to assuage "purple pain"—cold, congestive, and dull aches with the person feeling cold, clammy, and feeble.

## Hormone-Balancing Formula

This blend is helpful for balancing hormones and can be used tonically to address endometriosis, painful menstrual cramps, irregular cycles, PMS, ovarian cysts, infertility, acne, premenstrual headaches, and menopausal symptoms. It's imperative to commit to regular dosages. It may take three months before the full benefit is seen. During this time, the menstrual cycle may be modified, including changes in menstrual flow and length of cycle (longer or shorter). After a few months, the cycle should begin to stabilize. In six months, if the condition has improved, the formula can be discontinued. If it becomes worse again, the formula can be recommenced. At this point, it may be possible to lower the dose to find the smallest, most effective dosage.

**MAKES 6 OUNCES**

3 ounces vitex or chaste tree berry tincture (*Vitex agnus-castus*)

1 ounce black cohosh root tincture (*Actaea racemosa*)

1 ounce dandelion root tincture (*Taraxacum officinale*)

1 ounce vervain leaf and flower tincture (*Verbena officinalis* or *V. hastata*)

Use fresh herb or dry herb tinctures. Combine all tinctures and store in a glass dispensing bottle. Dosage is 3 ml two times a day, morning and night.

---

Black cohosh's flowering stalks are a striking addtion to the woodland herb garden

## Musculoskeletal Anti-inflammatory Formula

This blend contains medicinals that are traditional anodynes, skeletal-muscle relaxants, and anti-inflammatory remedies. It can be used to ease arthritic pain in arthritis, fibromyalgia, and tendinitis and provide relief for muscle strains or "pulled muscles." For chronic inflammation, consider supplementing with fish oil and turmeric and eating one cup of berries daily.

**MAKES 5 OUNCES**

1½ ounces black haw or cramp bark root bark or bark tincture (*Viburnum prunifolium* or *V. opulus*)

1 ounce meadowsweet leaf and flower tincture (*Filipendula ulmaria*)

1 ounce black cohosh root tincture (*Actaea racemosa*)

½ ounce skullcap leaf and flower tincture (*Scutellaria lateriflora*)

½ ounce valerian root tincture (*Valeriana officinalis*)

½ ounce willow bark tincture (*Salix* spp.)

Use fresh herb or dry herb tinctures. Combine all tinctures and store in a glass dispensing bottle. For acute injury or pain, the dosage is 2–4 ml every few hours up to five times a day. (This is a higher dose, suitable for two to three days maximum.) For ongoing daily use, an appropriate dose is 2–4 ml up to three times a day.

> **PRECAUTIONS:** Large doses can be emetic or nauseating. Possible side effects include headache and gastric upset. Black cohosh can alter the length of the reproductive cycle when taken regularly. Do not use in pregnancy (except as a birth aid under the care of a medical practitioner) or breastfeeding due to its emmenagogue qualities, hormonal influence, and potent bioactivity. The herb has been implicated in a handful of cases involving hepatotoxicity (liver damage), which may be attributed to possible adulteration of other *Actaea* species in commerce or may be a rare idiosyncratic reaction. Consult with your health care provider to address any concerns about the herb's effect on the liver.

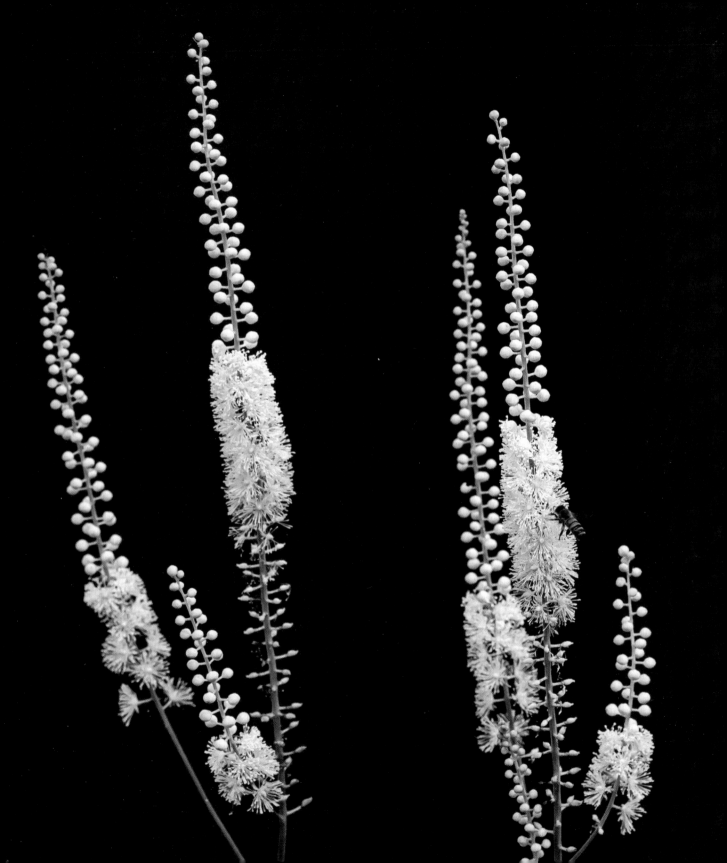

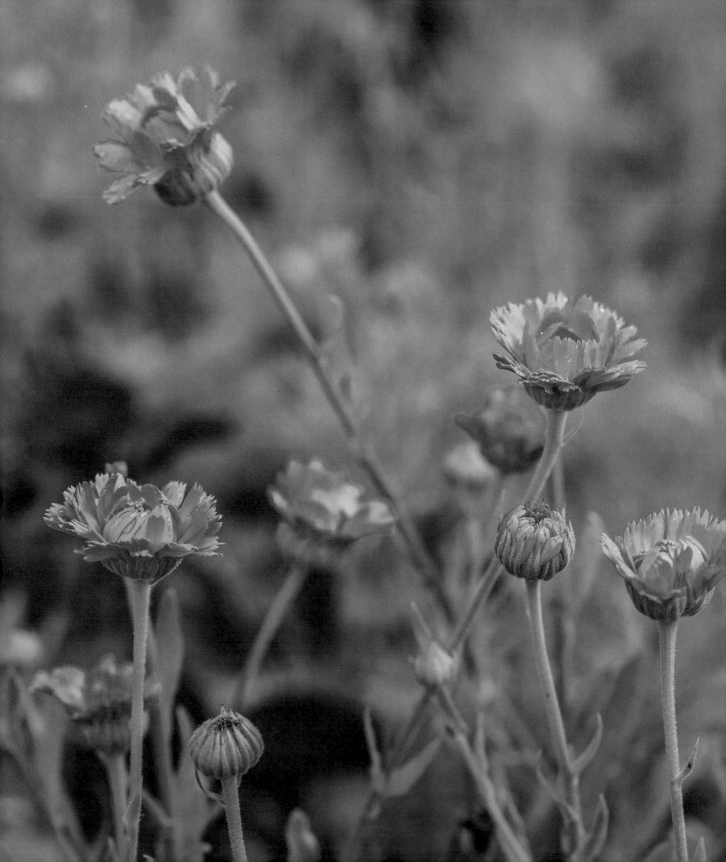

# CALENDULA

SCIENTIFIC NAME: *Calendula officinalis*
ASTERACEAE, aster, or sunflower family
AKA: pot marigold, garden marigold

One of the easiest herbs to grow, calendula is the perfect gateway herb for burgeoning gardeners. The sunshiny blooms are a joy to harvest and prepare as medicine. For centuries, the herb has been a popular remedy for healing wounds, burns, and rashes. The edible blooms—bursting with antioxidant compounds—are infused into immune-supporting teas and nourishing and fortifying soup stocks. Calendula is also called pot marigold, a name that's rightly confusing, as there are other plants in the sunflower family called marigolds.

(Marigolds in the *Tagetes* genus are common garden ornamentals; they are not interchangeable with calendula, medicinally.) Calendula's name originates from the Latin *calendae*, referring to its long blooming season; in certain locales, it is said to bloom every month of the calendar year. The species name, *officinalis*, refers to its historical use in apothecaries as the official medicinal species of its genus. The plant is native to southern Europe and is now widely cultivated throughout the Americas and Europe.

Calendula's medicine is found in the entire flower head, including its sticky, green bottom. (Botanically speaking, the overlapping green structures are bracts, and together, they make up the green base, or involucre, of the flower head.) The resin found in the flower base is antimicrobial and wound healing—its presence is a good indicator of a given variety's medicinal strength. What we call "petals" are actually ray florets, miniature flowers unto themselves (see the photo, *right*). I'll refer to the ray florets as petals for the sake of easy reading. When purchasing dried calendula, look for intact flowers with green undersides along with brightly colored petals, another barometer of freshness and medicinal strength.

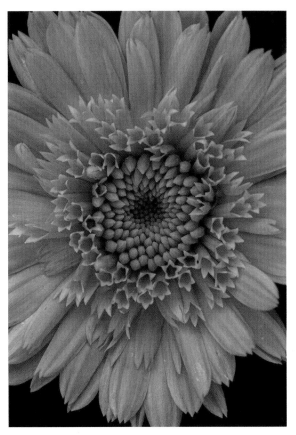

Note calendula's individual flowers, called florets, arranged in a ring around the center of the flower head

## Cultivation

ZONES: Can be grown as an annual in all zones; short-lived perennial in zones 8 and higher. Full sun to light shade

SOIL: pH 4.5–8; fertile, well-drained garden soil

SIZE: 1½ to 2 feet tall; 1 foot wide

LIFESTYLE: Short-lived herbaceous perennial or annual

PROPAGATION: Sow the magical-looking seeds directly in the ground in mid-spring; germination takes 5 to 14 days. If your slug pressure is high or your springs are on the colder side, consider growing trays of calendula and transplanting starts. Space the plants 9 to 12 inches apart.

SITING AND GARDEN CARE: Calendula is an easygoing garden herb and plays well with others. It's a great companion plant, as it attracts beneficial insects such as hoverflies, predatory wasps, and robber flies. I plant calendula in between rows of tulsi, hibiscus, spilanthes, or salad greens because it attracts pollinators and protects the neighborhood from insect pests. True to its common name, pot marigold thrives in containers and is quite companionable with ornamental vegetables and herbs. It flowers more profusely in full sun but will tolerate a smidgen of shade throughout the day. Under too much shade, the herb will grow leggy and produce fewer blooms. In most gardens, the plants will self-sow if you don't mulch.

There are plenty of calendula varieties to choose from in hues of sunrise to sunset and all shades in between: orange, yellow, burgundy, and russet. Multi-petaled varieties offer garden bling (and extra edible petals), and those with increased resin are medicinally potent. One of my favorites is 'Alpha', a variety with plenty of resin and mixed double yellow and orange petals. You can use any of the calendula cultivars for food and medicine, but the yellow and orange types are standard for medicinal preparations.

PROBLEM INSECTS AND DISEASES: Slugs relish calendula seedlings. Aphids, whiteflies, mealybugs, leafminers, and leafhoppers can be a problem as well. Calendula is affected by aster yellows—a devastating viral-like disease that also affects echinacea. See page 73.

HARVESTING: Pick the flowers every two to three days to prolong the plant's flowering season. When you're harvesting the blooms, deadhead any that are past their prime and have started to develop seeds. If you let the plants go to seed, they'll stop making new flowers. Harvest the flowers in the heat of the morning after the dew has evaporated, and dry in a dehydrator or on screens or airy baskets. Tousle them about daily as they dry. Be sure the entire flower head is dry; the petals should be crunchy and the green base should be pliable but not moist in the center. Err on the side of over-drying. Depending on your climate and drying setup, it may take five to seven days to dry calendula.

## Medicinal Properties

PART USED: Whole flowers

MEDICINAL PREPARATIONS: Tea, tincture, infused oil, salve, lotion, body butter, broth, compress, poultice, vaginal douches and suppositories, and sitz baths

TINCTURE RATIOS AND DOSAGE: Fresh flowers (1:2 95%) or dried flowers (1:6 70%); both preparations 2–3 ml up to three times a day

TEA RATIOS AND DOSAGE: Infusion of 1 tablespoon dried flowers per 1 cup water up to three times a day

ACTIONS: Lymphagogue, antifungal, antibacterial, antiviral, antioxidant, anti-inflammatory, emmenagogue, cholagogue, and vulnerary

ENERGETICS: Warming and drying

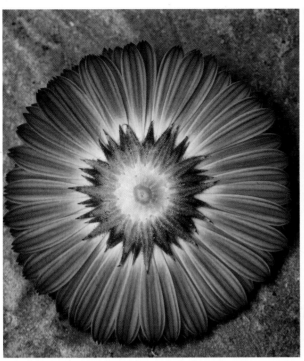 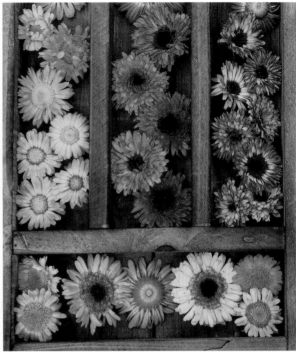

The underside of a calendula flower head—the green sticky structure (involucre) is highly potent, medicinally; calendula varieties **top left to right:** 'Alpha', 'Orange button', and 'Flashback'; **on bottom:** 'Princess'.

## Medicinal Uses

Calendula's notoriety has much to do with bottoms. The herb is *the* premier botanical in herbal diaper ointments, soothing baby bums with its anti-inflammatory, antimicrobial, and vulnerary (skin-healing) qualities. Calendula's wound-healing and tissue-repair actions are helpful internally in the digestive system. The flowers also support immunity through stimulating the lymphatic system. Calendula imparts joyfulness to the garden, and this hopeful buoyancy is infused into every cup of tea and pot of soup.

### REPRODUCTIVE SYSTEM

Calendula is helpful for a number of uterine and vaginal issues. The flowers can be prepared into a douche for bacterial vaginosis, yeast infections, or cervical dysplasia. Prepare the flowers as a sitz bath (a soaking tub filled with strong tea for immersing the pelvic and bottom regions) to heal perineal tears and abrasions after childbirth. Make a concentrated tea from the flowers along with garden sage and yarrow. Calendula salve and oil are common household remedies for healing sore, cracked nipples from nursing; it is safe for babies to ingest in small amounts (i.e., residual amounts on the nipples during breastfeeding).

### DIGESTIVE SYSTEM

The tea is a popular remedy for easing peptic ulcers, gastroesophageal reflux disease (GERD), and inflammatory bowel disease. Calendula helps reduce gastric and intestinal inflammation (from infection or irritation) through its vulnerary, anti-inflammatory, and antimicrobial actions. Combine the flowers with licorice, marshmallow, and meadowsweet in the treatment of GERD; see my recipe on page 326. In the case of peptic ulcers, the flowers can be taken concurrently with antibiotic therapy and continued for 2 weeks after finishing treatment.

### IMMUNE SYSTEM

Calendula is an outstanding tonic herb for stimulating and relieving stagnation of the lymphatic system, which can manifest as edema, or water retention, and weak immunity. Additionally, it's a traditional remedy for soothing acute or chronically swollen lymph nodes resulting from respiratory infections, localized infections, or tonsillitis. Calendula can be prepared into a tea or broth to build immunity. Astragalus is calendula's sidekick in these endeavors—you'll find the two teaming up in my Calendula Tulsi Chai Concentrate recipe on page 244 and the Herbal Immunity Broth Concentrate on page 174.

### TOPICAL USES

I keep calendula oil stocked in my refrigerator, as it's a handy topical remedy for a multitude of skin ailments and a useful binding agent for herbal poultices. The herb is an external remedy for practically every manner of skin complaint: rashes, stings, wounds, burns, sunburns, abrasions, swellings, eczema, acne, scars, scrapes, chicken pox, cold sores, and genital herpes sores. Match the appropriate topical preparation—oil, salve, compress, or poultice—with the skin condition according to the information on pages 155 and 160. I combine the blooms with chickweed, comfrey, and violet in salve form; see my recipe on page 158. When my daughter had chicken pox, I made a fresh poultice from calendula mixed with violet, plantain, and yarrow leaves and applied it daily. She had quite the outbreak and doesn't even have a single scar, thanks to this herbal poultice. Calendula is also a lovely herb for supporting the skin's luminance—see my recipes for Whipped Calendula Body Butter on page 242 and Floral Serum on page 364.

### NERVOUS SYSTEM

Calendula is one of my favorite wintertime teas. I find it uplifting when I'm feeling the long-dark-night-blahs and gray-day-blues. Most modern herbalists don't use calendula as one of their primary antidepressant herbs, but it was traditionally used by early European herbalists in this capacity, and I've seen it help many folks with their mood over the years. Combine calendula with other cheering flowers such as rose, mimosa, or lavender for grief and sadness, or consider adding one of its brightening allies, lemon balm or lemon verbena.

## Culinary Uses

Pluck the edible ray florets from the tough green base and sprinkle them into salads, salsas, scrambled eggs, quiche, and frittatas. Enliven compound butters and homemade spreads with a smattering of the summery florets. Freeze the entire flowers into decorative ice cubes for herbal libations. Harvest the flowers—with their longer stems intact—for garnishing iced herbal teas. Not merely a fetching adornment, the petals are loaded with antioxidant compounds.

Simmer the dried flowers in soups and stews throughout the winter months as a tonic for the immune system. This traditional folk use hails from medieval Europe. Street peddlers sold the flowers from barrels and home cooks added the blooms to bread, syrups, broths, soups, and conserves. See my recipe for Thai Calendula Chicken Soup on page 239 and the Herbal Immunity Broth Concentrate on page 174.

> **PRECAUTIONS:** Do not use internally during pregnancy. As calendula is in the aster family, it may cause a reaction in people who are highly sensitive to plants like ragweed and chamomile; this possibility is rare, but sensitive individuals should proceed with caution when taking the herb for the first time. Rare incidences of allergic contact dermatitis have occurred with the topical use of calendula.

# Thai Calendula Chicken Soup

YIELD: 3 quarts

### SPICED SOUP BROTH

2 cups Herbal Immunity Broth Concentrate (page 174)

1½ quarts water

2 tablespoons grated fresh ginger

3 stalks lemongrass, sliced in rounds (fresh or frozen)

9 makrut lime leaves (fresh or frozen)

### SOUP

¼ cup red curry paste (or to taste, depending on the brand)

¼ cup warm water

2 tablespoons extra-virgin olive oil

5 carrots, sliced on the diagonal

½ yellow onion, diced

1 small leek, washed well and sliced into tender rounds

20 (280 grams) shiitake mushrooms, sliced thinly

4 cups coarsely chopped cooking greens, such as spinach or chard (from 1 large bunch)

7 garlic cloves, minced

*(ingredients continue)*

Whenever I feel a tickle in my throat and sense an impending cold, I stare down the virus with a spicy bowl of this piping hot Thai-inspired soup. In addition to traditional ingredients, my version also contains immune-boosting calendula flowers and astragalus root. Vegetarians can prepare this soup using vegetable broth and substitute a block (about 12 ounces) of baked marinated tofu for the chicken. You may need to make a special trip to the Asian grocers to find the lemongrass stalks and makrut lime leaves, which are often sold frozen—in which case, you can stock up on the leaves for future soups. The soup's heat depends on the type and quantity of red curry paste you use. If you don't have the Herbal Immunity Broth Concentrate (although it's worth making and yields the chicken you need for this recipe), you can substitute the Quick Herbal Broth variation I give on page 241.

1. Prepare the spiced soup broth: In a saucepan, bring the Herbal Immunity Broth Concentrate and the water to a boil. Turn the heat to low and add the ginger, lemongrass, and makrut lime leaves. Simmer, covered, on low heat for 10 minutes, strain, and set aside.

2. While the soup stock is simmering, in a small cup, dissolve the curry paste in the water, stirring vigorously.

3. In a 4-quart soup pot, heat the olive oil on medium-high. After a few minutes, add the carrots, onion, and leek and sauté for 5 minutes or until the onion turns translucent. Add the mushrooms and cook for another 3 minutes. Add the greens, garlic, and chicken and cook for about 2 minutes. Finally, add the coconut milk, curry paste mixture, sea salt, and reserved spiced soup broth and stir. Continue to heat until hot and thoroughly cooked, about 4 minutes.

4. Garnish each bowl of soup with the cilantro, scallions, and calendula flowers. Serve with a lime wedge and hot chili sauce, if desired.

*(recipe continues)*

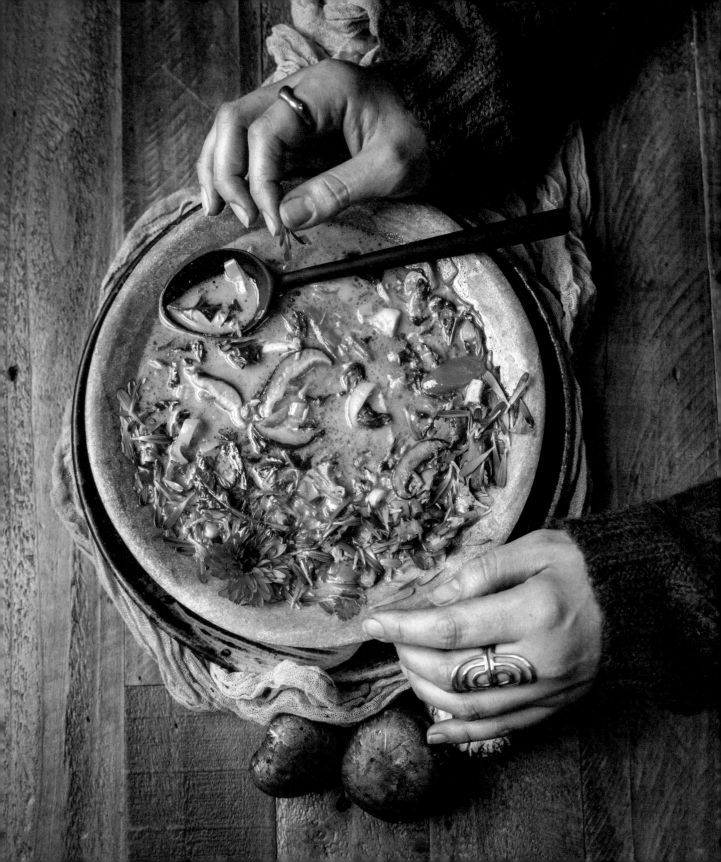

1 pound shredded cooked chicken (about 3½ cups, or use the chicken from the Herbal Immunity Broth Concentrate, page 174)

1 teaspoon sea salt, or more to taste

2 (13.5-ounce) cans full-fat coconut milk

GARNISH

1 cup coarsely chopped fresh cilantro leaves

4 scallions, sliced into thin rounds

5 fresh calendula flowers, florets separated from the flower head (*Calendula officinalis*)

Lime wedges

Hot chili sauce, to taste

**Tip:** 1½ pounds boneless chicken breasts will yield 1 pound of cooked meat.

## Quick Herbal Broth

1½ cups water

2 cups bone broth or vegetable broth

½ cup (10 grams) dried calendula flower (*Calendula officinalis*)

10 slices (12 grams) dried astragalus root (*Astragalus propinquus*)

---

Combine all the ingredients in a saucepan. Simmer, covered, on low heat for 10 minutes. Proceed with the rest of Step 1 on page 239, adding the ginger, lemongrass, and makrut lime leaves, and continuing to simmer for an additional 10 minutes; strain and set aside.

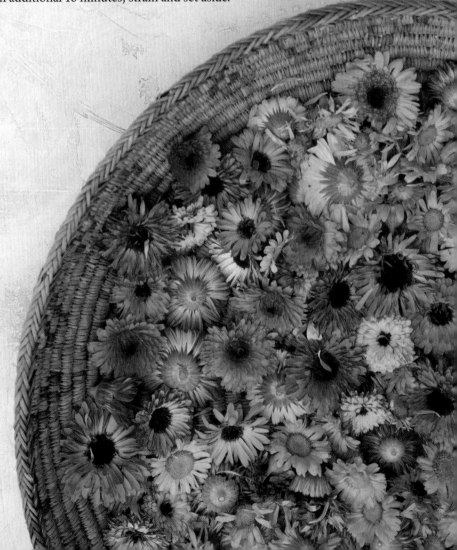

# Whipped Calendula Body Butter

YIELD: 9 to 12 ounces

½ cup (13 grams) very tightly packed whole dried calendula flower (*Calendula officinalis*)

3 fluid ounces cold-pressed and unrefined extra-virgin coconut oil, plus a tad more if needed

2 fluid ounces cold-pressed and unrefined jojoba oil

100 grams raw cold-pressed cacao butter (4 ounces by volume, melted)

If you're a newbie to homemade body care, body butters are an easy win. You're combining oils and plant butters and then whipping in air, which lightens the mixture. Compared to lotions, which readily soak into the skin, body butter is thicker and more moisturizing on dry skin—think elbows, feet, hands, stretch marks, and scars. Apply body butter after showering, when your warm skin is more receptive. It can be too rich to apply to the face, especially if you have oily skin or you're prone to acne and blackheads. If you have mature or dry skin that isn't particularly sensitive, then feel free to lavish the butter on your face.

1. Infuse the calendula into the coconut oil: Chop the calendula flowers finely, or grind in a spice grinder or clean coffee grinder. Put the calendula, coconut oil, and jojoba oil in a half-pint jar, stir, and seal loosely with a lid (**do not screw the lid tight, so air can escape**). Fill a small pot with water and put canning jar rings on the bottom of the pot. Place the jar on the rings and heat on the lowest stovetop setting for 3 hours. Do not allow the oil to go above 120°F (test periodically with a kitchen thermometer). You may need to turn off the heat from time to time and allow the oil to cool. After 3 hours remove the jar from the pot, take off the lid, and allow the oil to cool.

2. When the oil is still warm yet comfortable to touch, press and wring it thoroughly, squeezing out every last drop (see instructions for pressing oils on page 137). Compost the calendula flowers. Measure out 4 ounces of the strained oil. If you don't have quite enough, add a bit more coconut oil. If you have extra, reserve it for massage oil or an after-bath rubdown.

3. Place a large glass measuring cup in a small pot filled with water; use canning jar rings to elevate the jar from the bottom of the pot. Melt the cacao butter in the measuring cup over low heat. Add the 4 ounces strained calendula oil and stir until fully combined.

4. Remove from the heat, let cool for a few minutes, and then place the melted mixture, still in the measuring cup, in the freezer. Set a timer for 30 minutes. When the timer goes off, check to see if the butter has

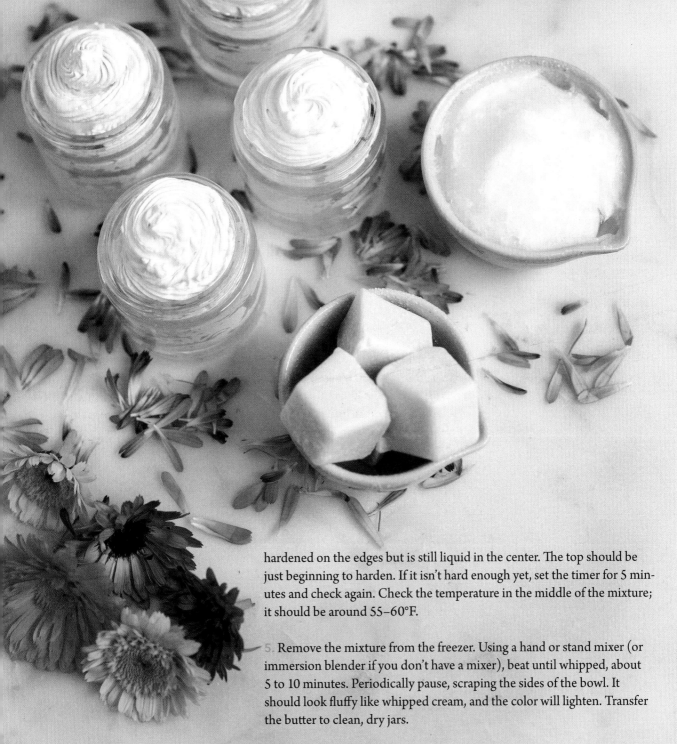

hardened on the edges but is still liquid in the center. The top should be just beginning to harden. If it isn't hard enough yet, set the timer for 5 minutes and check again. Check the temperature in the middle of the mixture; it should be around 55–60°F.

5. Remove the mixture from the freezer. Using a hand or stand mixer (or immersion blender if you don't have a mixer), beat until whipped, about 5 to 10 minutes. Periodically pause, scraping the sides of the bowl. It should look fluffy like whipped cream, and the color will lighten. Transfer the butter to clean, dry jars.

6. Keeps for 3 to 6 months unrefrigerated; check for signs of mold and rancidity. Store the back stock in the refrigerator for longer shelf life.

# Calendula Tulsi Chai Concentrate

YIELD: 4 cups (32 ounces) of concentrate, which makes 4 to 6 drinks

CHAI

5 cups water

4 medium cinnamon sticks (*Cinnamomum verum*), or substitute 20 grams cinnamon bark chips

12 dried astragalus root slices (*Astragalus propinquus*), or substitute 10 grams cut and sifted astragalus root

1½ tablespoons cut and sifted dried ginger root (*Zingiber officinale*)

2 teaspoons cardamom seeds (*Elettaria cardamomum*), hulled

1 teaspoon black peppercorns (*Piper nigrum*)

2 small star anise pods (*Illicium verum*)

2 whole cloves (*Syzygium aromaticum*)

⅓ cup whole dried calendula flower (*Calendula officinalis*)

1 tablespoon packed dried tulsi leaf (*Ocimum tenuiflorum*)

¼ cup organic cane sugar, honey, or stevia, to taste (optional)

TO SERVE

Crushed ice, for an iced chai

Choice of milk or cream (dairy or nondairy)

This herbal version of classic chai is loaded with immune support. Astragalus, calendula, and tulsi are herbal tonics for the lymphatic, nervous, and immune systems. Sip on this beverage during the winter months to help ward off colds and the flu. The aromatic botanicals in this chai blend—cinnamon, peppercorns, ginger, and cloves—keep the blood and lymph moving and are especially helpful for those who feel cold or sluggish. These pungent spices can be too heating and drying for hotheads and have the potential to aggravate heartburn, peptic ulcers, and gastrointestinal heat. During warmer weather, dilute the concentrate with ice and your choice of milk for a refreshing summertime beverage.

In a medium pot, combine the water with the cinnamon, astragalus, ginger, cardamom, peppercorns, star anise, and cloves. Bring to a boil, covered, and turn the heat down to simmer for 20 minutes. Turn off the heat and add the dried calendula flowers and tulsi leaf; stir. Infuse, covered, for 20 minutes and then strain. If you prefer sweet chai, add the sugar after straining; stir well. Let cool, and store the chai concentrate in the refrigerator. Use within 4 days.

FOR AN ICED CHAI: Pour the concentrate over a large cup of crushed ice with your choice of milk or cream.

FOR A HOT CHAI: Dilute the concentrate with an equal part water and heat. Serve with your choice of milk or cream.

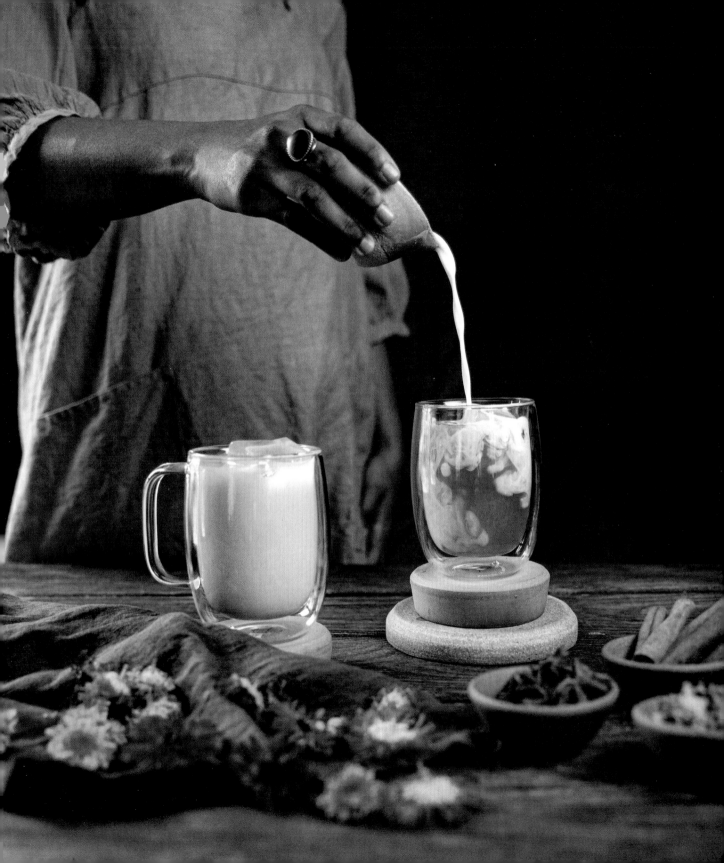

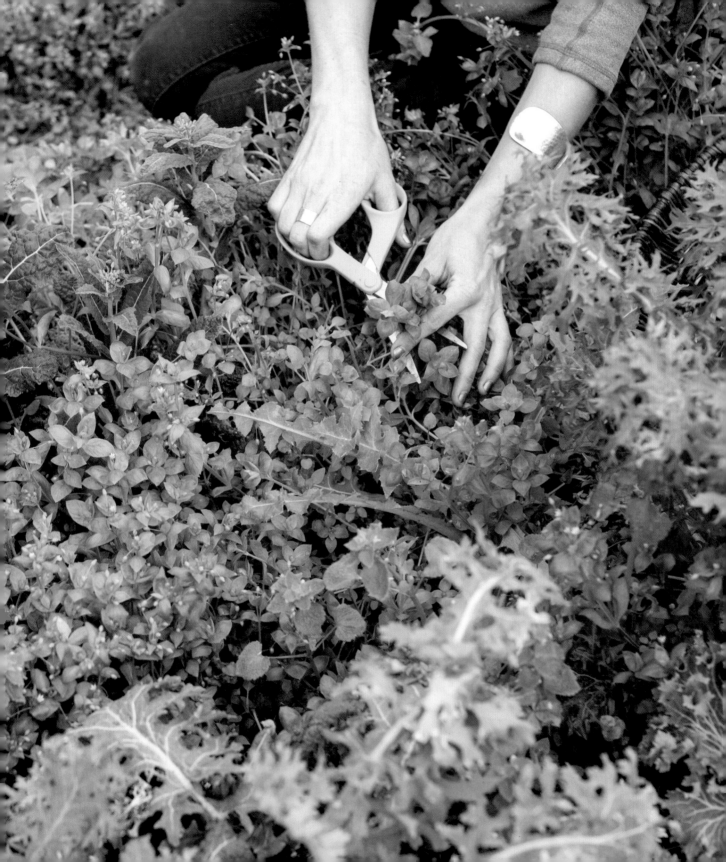

# CHICKWEED

SCIENTIFIC NAME: *Stellaria media*
CARYOPHYLLACEAE, pink or carnation family
AKA: starweed

Chickweed is one of my oldest green friends—we became acquainted when I was first learning about plants over three decades ago, and I'm as smitten as ever. This rambling weed is beloved by herbalists and chickens for its mild, succulent flavor. The herb's tiny white stellate flowers are the inspiration for its alternate moniker, *starweed*. Chickweed is a gentle medicinal belonging to the class of plants I call *food herbs*. These are plants that are both therapeutic and edible in larger quantities. Internally, it's a traditional blood cleanser and a nutritive tonic, and externally, the herb is a soothing and cooling remedy for hot and inflamed skin conditions.

Chickweed grows wild in gardens and near sidewalks, trailsides, and old manure and compost piles. Native to Europe, the plant has spread throughout the world and now grows in the Americas, Australia, Africa, and Asia.

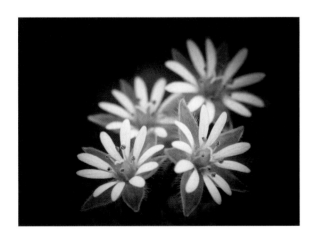

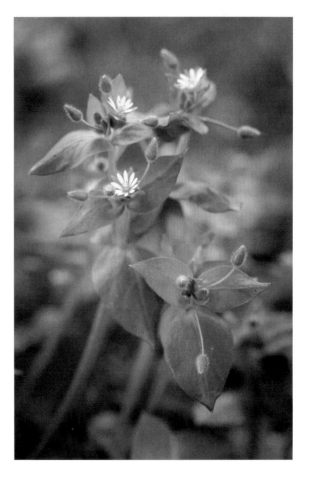

Chickweed growing as a groundcover under bolted cooking greens; this bed has been covered in spun polyester throughout the winter so the greens are further along in the season; chickweed has five petals that are cleft, so it appears to have ten tiny white petals; chickweed in flower

## Cultivation

ZONES: 2–13; full sun to partial shade

SOIL: pH 5.5–8; prefers rich, loamy soil with high moisture but is tolerant of a wide variety of soils

SIZE: 6 to 12 inches tall; 10 to 15 inches wide

LIFESTYLE: Annual, short-lived perennial

PROPAGATION: Sow the seeds on the surface of the soil in the early spring or fall, 1 inch apart. Seedlings emerge in 3 to 12 days at 53–65°F. Thin to 4 inches apart. The plant easily transplants.

SITING AND GARDEN CARE: You may, perhaps, scoff at the idea of planting chickweed, especially if it's a rampant weed in your garden, but I find the plant to be one of the most useful and productive herbs in my surroundings. And it's easy enough to manage and weed out of areas where it's misbehaving. For those of you with chickweed-less gardens, first, you must know that the herb will most certainly spread throughout your entire garden. However, chickweed can be strategically allowed to grow in a weed-and-crop polyculture: let it sprawl between planted crops as an edible groundcover where it can help reduce water loss, cool the soil, and suppress taller weeds. In the springtime, I encourage it to grow between rows of lettuce and cooking greens and harvest the quick-growing chickweed first until it dies back and enriches the soil, at which time the vegetables are ready to pick.

Chickweed grows in full sun to partial shade, depending on the season and climate. In warmer weather, it relishes a bit of shade, and in cooler weather, the plant prefers to sunbathe all day long. Chickweed is accustomed to cool, moist weather and shies away from the full summer sun. In four-season climates, the plant debuts in early spring and fall. In milder regions, chickweed grows throughout the winter.

Chickweed tends to hop into gardens via manure or compost, but to speed up the process, the plant easily transplants, and you'll have no problems finding willing neighbors to let you dig up some plants. I've done this

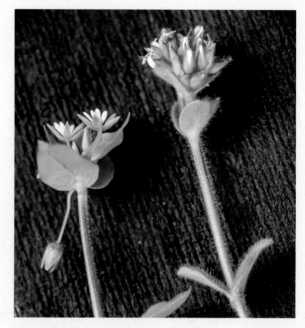

Chickweed (*Stellaria media*) on the left, with its single line of hairs, and mouse-eared chickweed (*Cerastium* sp.) on the right, with its uniformly hairy stem

with every garden I've created, impatient for the delectable greens. If you want a dense crop or you don't yet know how to identify it, grow the plant from seed. Sow the seeds directly on the surface of the soil in the early fall for a fall harvest and in the very early spring for a spring crop. The sprouts are cold-hardy, but young plants will grow more quickly under a cloche or spun polyester row cover. Amend the soil with extra compost or composted manure and you'll be rewarded with bigger leaves, as chickweed buffs up with a little nitrogen.

PROBLEM INSECTS AND DISEASES: None known

IDENTIFICATION AND HARVESTING: Chickweed has a handful of look-alikes, some of which are toxic or inedible, so it's crucial you are 100 percent sure of your identification before you harvest (this goes for all plants!). Use all of the traits here, combined, along with a local field guide, which will also show regional look-alikes, to aid in identification.

> ### Chickweed's Identifying Features:
>
> - Low-growing, sprawling annual with multiple stems. The stem is green or reddish and never woody.
>
> - Leaves do not have teeth, are smooth (without hairs), and grow opposite (directly opposite from each other on the stem). The leaves are generally as big as a pinky nail but can grow larger.
>
> - Tiny, star-shaped white flowers, growing in small clusters. Flowers appear to have 10 petals but are actually 5 deeply cleft petals.
>
> - A single line of white hairs growing on the stem (you may need to twirl the stem a bit in the light to see it), which switches positions on the stem at the leaf juncture, giving the line of hairs a spiraling or candy cane–like appearance.
>
> - Similar-looking plants include scarlet pimpernel (*Anagallis arvensis*), which has peach-colored (or sometimes blue) flowers and lacks the single telltale line of hairs, and the speedwells (*Veronica* spp.), which have blue flowers with four petals.
>
> - Chickweed's edible brethren, the mouse-ear chickweeds (*Cerastium* spp.), are similar in appearance but can readily be distinguished from chickweed by their uniformly hairy stems.
>
> - This is not an exhaustive list of look-alikes—use a local field guide to learn your regional look-alikes.

Garden or kitchen scissors are the best tools for harvesting chickweed. If you're harvesting the herb for food, cut back the top few tender inches, which will generally include leaves, stems, and flowers—all of which are edible and tasty. After receiving a "haircut," the plant will grow tender new shoots, making it possible to repeatedly harvest until the stems get too leggy and chewy. Below the tender tops, the plant can be quite fibrous. Look for densely growing patches of chickweed; the neighboring stems hold each other up, making harvesting much easier and quicker. When harvesting chickweed for medicine, it doesn't matter if it is fibrous. Cut the plant at its base to quickly harvest a sizable quantity. Triple wash the greens, as they can be sandy.

Dry on screens or open-weaved baskets. Dry chickweed quickly so it doesn't lose its color. It has a shorter shelf life than other herbs, lasting only six months to a year.

## Medicinal Properties

PART USED: Aboveground parts in flower (leaves, stem, reproductive parts)

MEDICINAL PREPARATIONS: Infusion, vinegar, pesto, salad, smoothie, juice, poultice, compress, salve, and infused oil

TINCTURE: Not recommended

TEA RATIOS AND DOSAGE: Infusion of 1 tablespoon dried herb per 1 cup water up to three times a day

ACTIONS: Diuretic, demulcent, anti-inflammatory, expectorant, galactagogue, alterative, nutritive tonic, gentle laxative, and vulnerary

ENERGETICS: Cooling and moistening

Chickweed's qualities are wasted in tincture form; the alcohol doesn't effectively extract the minerals or mucilage. Instead, consume it as food or prepare it as a tea or vinegar. Like other food herbs, the upper dosage isn't overly limited (if you can eat a whole plate of the herb, you certainly don't need to be dainty with the tea).

## Medicinal Uses

Chickweed is cooling, soothing, and anti-inflammatory both topically and internally. This sprightly herb is a traditional blood cleanser and a tonic, strengthening herb. Chickweed is a slow and steady companion. It's not going to move any mountains; instead, it will take the whole day to amble to the peak, stopping for snacks and panoramas. And it will have plenty of energy left over for the downhill trek. In other words, chickweed is one of those medicinals with mild actions, best taken daily for its slow but steady healing properties.

## NUTRITIVE TONIC

Chickweed's high iron levels make it a powerful ally in iron-deficiency anemia. To access the iron, ingest it liberally as a food and in tea or vinegar. To help build iron levels further, add stinging nettles to the tea or vinegar along with the tincture or syrup of yellow dock. Chickweed is safe to ingest while breastfeeding and is a traditional remedy for postpartum anemia and fatigue. It also increases breast milk production; however, it's not the most potent herb in this regard. Combine it with fenugreek, which helps increase breast milk through normalizing hormone function, and European vervain, if there's an emotional component involved.

## DIGESTIVE SYSTEM

With its soothing, cooling nature, chickweed is a common ingredient in herbal heartburn remedies and is equally beneficial for sore throats. Prepare a tea made from chickweed, meadowsweet, and marshmallow to soothe sore throats, peptic ulcers, and heartburn. The herb is a gentle bulking laxative, helping to move things along with its moisture and fiber.

## RESPIRATORY SYSTEM

Chickweed is a gentle moistening expectorant, useful as a tea for dry, hacking coughs and dry throat. Bronchitis, asthma, laryngitis, and sore throats from respiratory viruses benefit from chickweed's demulcent and anti-inflammatory effects. Chickweed isn't the most potent cough remedy and is best paired with other respiratory herbs, like mullein, licorice, and marshmallow.

## LIVER AND BLOOD TONIC

Herbalists use chickweed, along with red clover flowers and burdock root, as a daily tea for acne, psoriasis, and eczema. These herbs help to optimize the elimination of metabolic by-products via the bile and, in turn, the intestines through aiding and stimulating hepatic and digestive functions. Both burdock and chickweed are diuretics, aiding the kidneys in their work of detoxification and elimination.

## TOPICAL USES

Topically, chickweed is applied as a poultice, infused oil, salve, or compress. Its cooling, soothing, anti-inflammatory, and anti-itching qualities are helpful for rashes, chicken pox, poison ivy, contact dermatitis, insect bites, minor burns, eczema, and dry skin and lips. It's the main herb I use as a compress for conjunctivitis, along with chamomile flowers.

## Culinary Uses

I can honestly say that chickweed is my favorite wild edible. The greens are tasty enough to stand alone in a salad, or they can accompany lettuce and other wild greens, such as dandelion and violet. I use the chopped greens wherever lettuce would do: in tacos, burritos, sandwiches, and wraps. Come springtime, chickweed is on my daily breakfast menu, cozied up to scrambled eggs, nestled in omelets, or perched atop a bagel with an over-easy egg. One of my favorite ways to enjoy chickweed is in pesto; see my recipe on page 254. Substitute chickweed for the violet in my Violet Hummus recipe on page 410. Add chickweed to smoothies, or juice the greens. When my daughter was little, I would blend the greens with a bit of salad dressing, and she eagerly slurped it up by the baby spoonful.

Chickweed is easy to digest and nutrient-rich and is thus traditionally prepared as a first food after a long illness, stomach flu, or food poisoning. It's also a traditional weight-loss remedy, perhaps due to its beneficial qualities on digestion and cellular metabolism and high levels of fiber. Chickweed is chock-full of vitamins and minerals. According to studies by John Kallas of the Institute for the Study of Wild Plants, chickweed is higher in iron and zinc than any of the commonly cultivated greens such as spinach, collards, and kale. It has a fair amount of vitamin C and almost as much calcium as spinach.

> PRECAUTIONS: Avoid if you are prone to calcium oxalate kidney stones, due to the presence of oxalates in the leaves.

# Chickweed Crepes with Chickweed Pesto & Chickweed Garnish

YIELD: 7 (10-inch) crepes

1 cup unsweetened almond milk or grass-fed whole cow's milk

Heaping ½ cup (70 grams) arrowroot starch/flour

½ cup (64 grams) almond flour

½ cup (28 grams) lightly packed tender chickweed tops, plus more for serving

½ cup (28 grams) lightly packed baby spinach

3 large eggs

2 tablespoons coconut oil, plus more for the pan

¼ teaspoon salt

Chickweed Pesto (page 254), for serving

Sweet Potato Shiitake Filling (recipe follows), for serving

½ cup finely chopped chickweed tops, for garnish

With a dazzling emerald hue, these crepes rival the summer fields of the Scottish highlands. I'd like to tell you the rapture of chlorophyll is all chickweed, but in all honesty, it's the spinach that colors the crepe green. Amber Brown, my kitchen accomplice and paleo cook extraordinaire, came up with this recipe after I showed her a photo of spinach crepes and challenged her to dream up a chickweed version. When chickweed isn't in season, you can double the spinach in the recipe. Remember to only harvest the top few inches of chickweed and avoid the older, stemmy portions that are especially fibrous.

These crepes are grain-free and can be prepared with almond milk for a dairy-free version. They are sweet enough to play with breakfast fillings such as whipped cream and fresh berries or a bit of dark chocolate and almond butter. But you can also go the savory route, as I do here. Beyond the sweet potato filling on page 253, you could opt for curried potatoes with garbanzo beans and a splash of mint chutney or black beans and cauliflower rice with Mexican spices. If you have leftover sweet potato filling, enjoy it as a stand-alone meal the following day.

1. Combine the milk, arrowroot, almond flour, chickweed, spinach, eggs, coconut oil, and salt in a blender and blend until uniformly green and frothy, about 2 to 3 minutes. (Don't skimp on the blending time or the coconut oil might not fully incorporate into the batter.) Pause and scrape the sides of the blender as you go, removing any lumps that form.

2. Refrigerate the batter—still in the blender—for 10 minutes. After its chill time, give it another whirl in the blender to aerate the batter.

3. Heat a dollop of coconut oil in a 10-inch crepe pan or shallow skillet over medium heat. When the coconut oil is shimmery, ladle ⅓ cup of batter onto the skillet, tilting the pan quickly to swirl the batter so it evenly fills the pan.

*(recipe continues)*

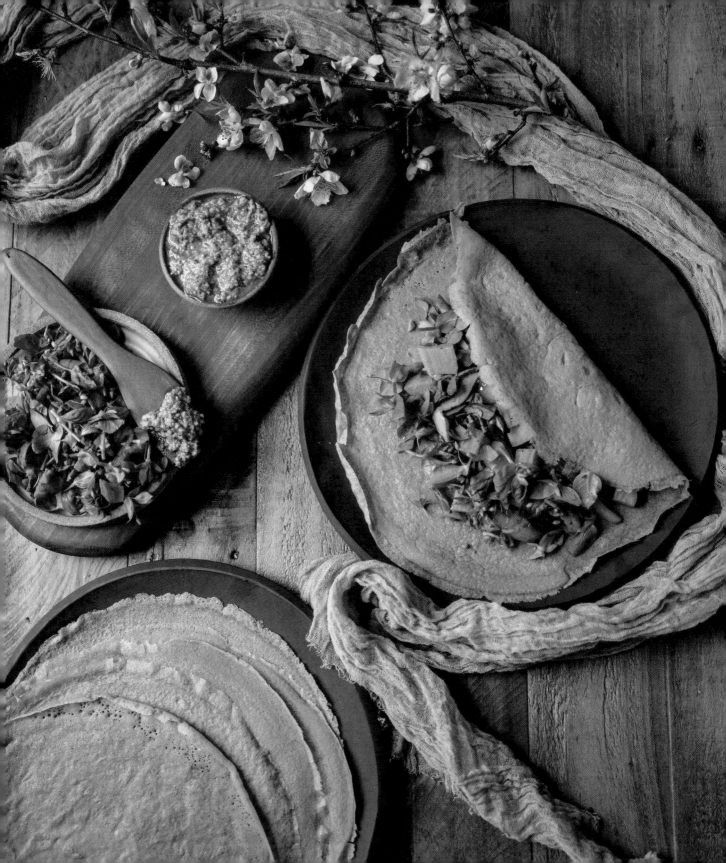

4. Cook until little bubbles appear on the surface and the edges of the crepe pull back and lift up slightly from the pan. (If you're using almond milk batter, this will take about 1½ to 2 minutes. Cow milk batter will cook a little quicker, about 1 to 1½ minutes.) Loosen the edge of the crepe with a spatula and carefully flip. Cook on the other side (about 1½ minutes if using almond milk and 1 to 1½ minutes if using cow milk). Place the crepe on a plate and set aside. Repeat until you've used all the batter, adding more coconut oil to the pan as needed.

5. To serve, spoon a dollop of chickweed pesto on the center of each crepe and then add the sweet potato shiitake mixture. Garnish with fresh chickweed tops.

## Sweet Potato Shiitake Filling

YIELD: Filling for 7 crepes

1 pound sweet potatoes (about 2 small or 1 large sweet potato), peeled and cut into 1-inch cubes

2 tablespoons extra-virgin olive oil

1 medium onion, cut lengthwise into long, thin slices

15 (142 grams) shiitake mushroom caps, cut into long slices

1 teaspoon sea salt

1. In a medium pot, steam the sweet potato cubes for about 15 minutes, or until tender.

2. Meanwhile, add 1 tablespoon of the olive oil to a large skillet and heat on medium. When the olive oil shimmers, add the onion and sauté for about 10 minutes, or until it is browning and becoming translucent. Add the shiitake mushrooms, the remaining tablespoon olive oil, and the salt; reduce the heat to medium-low and cook for another 8 minutes, or until the onion and mushrooms are cooked through. Turn off the heat, add the sweet potato cubes, and gently stir to combine, taking care to not break up the sweet potatoes (unless, of course, you like that kind of thing).

# Chickweed Pesto

YIELD: 2 cups

1½ cups (145 grams) whole walnuts

3 cups (105 grams) loosely packed fresh chickweed tops (*Stellaria media*) (tender stems and leaves from the upper few inches of the plant)

1 cup extra-virgin olive oil

½ cup (48 grams) grated Parmesan cheese

3 or 4 medium garlic cloves, peeled

2½ teaspoons lemon juice

½ teaspoon sea salt

Coarse black pepper, to taste

If you're new to eating garden weeds, this is your gateway dish! Chickweed's easygoing flavor is enhanced by the pungency of garlic and aged cheese. Dress up pasta, pizza, or grilled veggies with this nutrient-dense pesto. Our family loves it on zucchini noodles, topped with spring-fresh chickweed tips and steamed stinging nettles. Chickweed pesto is milder than basil pesto, which means you can do it up. For instance, go ahead and serve the pesto as a delicious dip for crackers or crudités. Now, if you're all in and want to take chickweed to the prom (try to beat me to it), this pesto is your ticket to the Chickweed Crepes dish on page 251.

1. Toast the walnuts in a preheated dry (non-oiled) skillet over medium heat, stirring frequently, for 1 to 2 minutes, until they are brown and aromatic. Do not leave unattended as the walnuts can burn quickly. Place the toasted walnuts immediately on a cutting board or plate to cool.

2. Thoroughly wash and drain the chickweed tops.

3. Combine all the ingredients in a food processor and blend until smooth. Taste, and adjust the garlic, sea salt, and black pepper as desired. Refrigerate in an airtight container for up to a week or freeze in ice cube trays for up to 6 months.

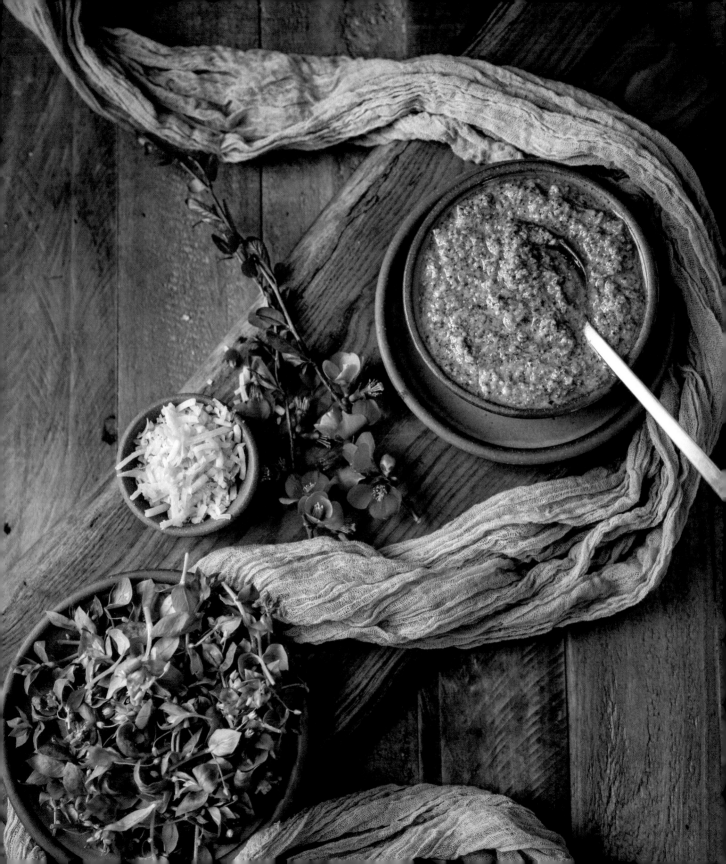

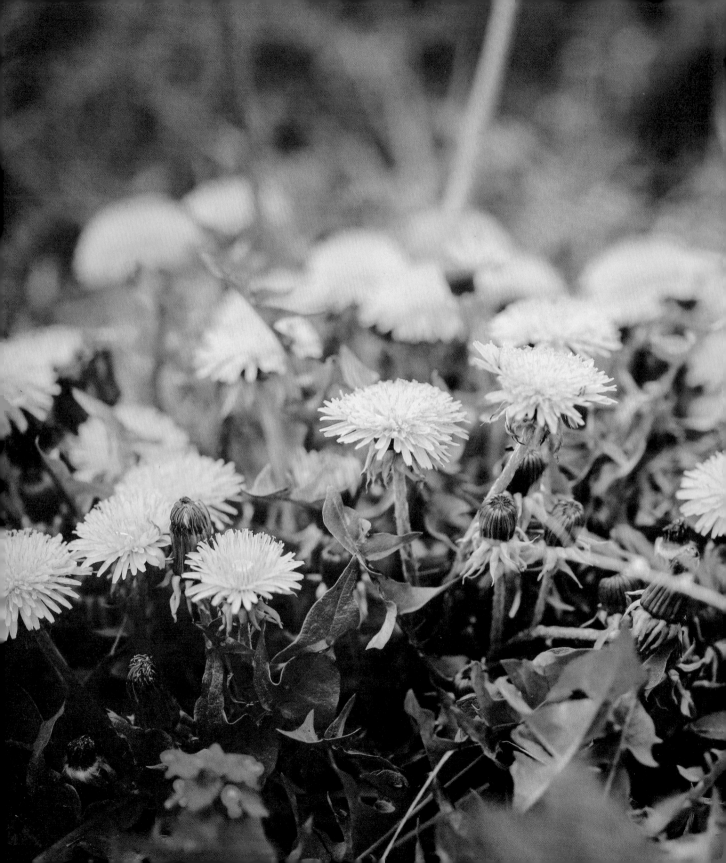

# DANDELION

SCIENTIFIC NAME: *Taraxacum officinale*
ASTERACEAE, sunflower or aster family
AKA: bitterwort, lion's tooth, blow-ball, *dent-de-lion*, *piss-en-lit*

In the early spring, dandelion's sunshiny blooms show up in our yards and bus stops with unrivaled moxie. By attempting to eradicate this starburst of a "weed" (good luck with that one, folks!), people are essentially killing off the most useful plant in their midst. Instead, lawn-lovers might learn to appreciate dandy's edible and medicinal uses. All parts of the plant are edible; the leaves are exceptionally high in vitamins and minerals, rivaling the likes of kale and collard greens. The leaves' toothy appearance inspired the French name for the plant, *dent-de-lion*, or "tooth of the lion," which transmogrified to *dandelion*. Dandelion root is a classic liver and blood tonic—used internally to soothe acne, eczema, and hives—and the leaves are also used medicinally as a bitter and diuretic. The French nickname for the plant, *piss-en-lit*—meaning "pee-in-bed"—is a testimony to its diuretic qualities. Dandelion is native to Eurasia and northern Africa but now grows all around the globe, thanks to human cultivation and botanical pluck.

What we commonly envision as a dandelion "flower" is actually a flower *head,* a composite of hundreds of minute individual flowers, or florets. Each golden strap-like "petal" is, in reality, a flower in its own right. Interestingly, many strains of dandelions produce seeds through asexual reproduction, which is to say that the seeds are clones of their parents. Each flower head opens and closes with the sun for three to four days, and then develops into dandy's signature seed heads—those familiar poufs of our childhoods.

Why grow dandelion? For starters, it ensures you'll have a steady supply of succulent roots and tender—and less bitter—greens for eating. And you'll have ready access to a crop of dandelion that you know hasn't been sprayed. Dandelion may be one of the most familiar plants on the planet, but it does have some look-alikes. So much so, that there are a bunch of plants called *false dandelion*. Growing your own crop is a way to confirm you have the right plant!

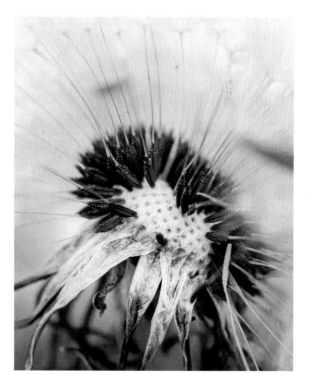

## Cultivation

ZONES: 3–9; sun to partial shade

SOIL: pH 5–8; moist, fertile, well-drained soil

SIZE: 10–18 inches tall; 6–9 inches wide

LIFESTYLE: Herbaceous perennial

PROPAGATION: Surface-sow (do not cover the seed) directly in the garden, one seed per inch. Germination takes place in 10 to 21 days at 50–75°F. Stratifying the seeds for one week prior to planting raises the germination rate to 90 percent. Thin to 8 to 10 inches apart.

SITING AND GARDEN CARE: Dandelion will grow best in fertile, moist soil but obviously tolerates a range of soil types, considering it will grow in sidewalk cracks! In hotter climates, the plant appreciates a bit of shade and will, as a bonus, reward you with milder-tasting greens. Cutting back the flowers will keep the plants from going to seed and spreading throughout your garden and will also encourage leaf production. The Italian varieties of "dandelion greens" are, in fact, the chicory (*Cichorium intybus*) plant.

PROBLEM INSECTS AND DISEASES: The leaves can develop powdery mildew.

IDENTIFICATION AND HARVESTING: Dandelion grows in open, disturbed ground, such as fields, gardens, lawns, farms, fencerows, and city lots. It is frequently sprayed with herbicide, so make sure you're picking from a clean location that isn't sprayed. Despite its familiarity, dandelion is a plant I see misidentified frequently. As with any plant, do not harvest if you're unsure of its identity.

### Dandelion's Identifying Characteristics:

- The scapes (flowering stalks) are hollow and leafless and exude a white "milk" (technically called *latex*) when cut.
- The scapes do not branch and are often tinged reddish.
- The scapes are topped by a single yellow flower head, which bears yellow ray florets—long strap-like structures that overlap.
- As the flower head opens, the lower row of phyllaries (green strap-like structures under the yellow florets) bends back toward the ground.
- The leaves are found only in the plant's basal rosette (clustering of leaves that emerge from a central point on the ground) and exude "milk" when cut; no leaves grow from the flower stem.
- The leaves are variably jagged-edged, bearing large pointed lobes and smaller teeth. Some leaves have large lobes, and some have teeth and shallow lobes.
- The leaf's central vein, or midrib, is pronounced, whitish to reddish, and protrudes from the underside of the leaf in a rounded hump. The midrib is *not* keeled or triangular in cross-section.
- The undersides of the leaves are hairless or bear wooly hairs that lie flat—these hairs, if present, are more commonly seen on the midrib.

Before dandelion (C) flowers, the herb closely resembles other aster family members, including cat's ear (*Hypochaeris radicata* [A]), chicory (*Cichorium intybus* [B]), wild lettuce (*Lactuca* spp.), and sow thistle (*Sonchus* spp.). All of these plants are also in the aster family and exude milky latex when disturbed. Thankfully, they are all edible, so if you confuse them, there aren't dire consequences. However, these dandy look-alikes aren't used medicinally like dandelion. (Note that other plant families exude white latex, including the spurge [Euphorbiaceae] and poppy [Papaveraceae] families.

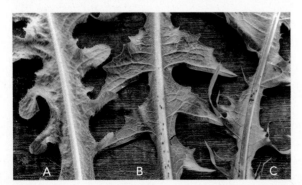

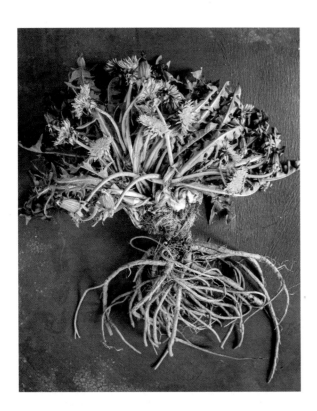

Both families contain some poisonous members, and their latex can be caustic. Moral of the story: when you see white latex in a plant, don't assume it's an edible aster family member.) You may have other dandelion lookalikes in your area, so do your homework with a field guide or knowledgeable local forager or herbalist. Or simply grow your own!

Dandelion leaves can be harvested for medicine whenever they're green and vital. Dry them on screens or in open baskets. If you're collecting the leaves for food, the early spring greens are less bitter. Larger, erect leaves growing in partial shade or rich, moist environments are the most tender and the least bitter. Garden beds often yield the best-tasting dandelion greens to be found. Harvest the flower heads for medicine in the morning after the dew has evaporated. For culinary use, pick them near the time when you'll be preparing them but before they close shop for the evening. Leave the flowers outside in the shade for a few minutes to let any hitchhiking insects depart. If you're collecting a boatload of blooms for dandelion wine or the like, you can freeze each day's harvest until you have enough stockpiled.

The roots can be harvested in the fall and spring. If the ground isn't frozen, you can collect them throughout the winter as long as you can still identify the plant. Sometimes plants will have a lone spindly taproot, and other times the roots will be gnarled, tough, and somewhat jaded (rotted). You're looking for the buff roots—filled out and turgid and not yet woody—but it can be hard to know about a plant's roots just by looking at the leaves. I recommend harvesting a mess of roots and then grading them: the woody ones can be dried for tea or made into a tincture and the tender roots can be prepared for food. As long as the root isn't discolored or rotten, it's still serviceable for medicine. The fall roots are much higher in inulin (about 40 percent), compared to the spring roots (2 percent). For more about inulin, see page 260.

## Medicinal Properties

PART USED: **All parts of the plant**

MEDICINAL PREPARATIONS: *Root:* Decoction, tincture, vinegar, bitters, and roasted herbal "coffee." *Leaf:* Infusion, vinegar, bitters, salad, nibble, and cooking greens. *Flower:* Infusion, garnish, and vinegar.

TINCTURE RATIOS AND DOSAGE: *Root and leaf:* Fresh (1:2 95%) or dry (1:4 60%); either preparation 2–4 ml up to three times a day

TEA RATIOS AND DOSAGE: *Leaf or flower:* Infusion of 2 to 3 teaspoons dried herb per 1 cup water up to three times a day. *Root:* Decoction of 2 to 3 teaspoons dried root per 1 cup water up to three times a day

ACTIONS: *Root:* Diuretic, bitter, hepatic, alterative, cholagogue, prebiotic, antirheumatic, and gentle laxative. *Leaf:* Diuretic, bitter, cholagogue, hepatic, and alterative.

ENERGETICS: **Cooling and drying**

## Medicinal Uses

Dandelion is a classic medicinal in our beloved food-herb tribe and can be used as a tonic remedy over a long period. Like other herbs in this class, the highest safe dosage is considerably higher than we find in nonfood medicinals. That said, dandelion is cooling and drying if taken daily. This is fine if you have plenty of moisture to go around, but if you run dry (have dry hair, skin, and sinuses), notice if the herb is drying your skin and sinuses. Add mucilaginous herbs, such as marshmallow and violet, into dandelion tea to help offset the herb's drying qualities. The root and leaves have some overlapping medicinal applications, but they are distinct medicines.

### LIVER AND BLOOD TONIC

Dandelion root is a traditional tonic for the liver and the blood and has long been used as an internal remedy for acne, psoriasis, and eczema. In a multitude of traditional healing systems, the health of the liver, the digestive tract, and the skin are intertwined and need to be addressed together. Dandelion can be combined with blood cleansers and liver and kidney tonics such as red clover blooms, cleavers, stinging nettles, burdock root, violet, chickweed, and yellow dock root for skin support.

### REPRODUCTIVE SYSTEM

The root is a frequent companion in formulas with reproductive herbal hormone tonics, such as black cohosh and vitex (see the Hormone Balancing Formula on page 232). Dandelion aids the liver in metabolizing and excreting excess reproductive hormones, like estrogen and progesterone. Accordingly, the root is used in tonic formulas to address menstrual cramps, endometriosis, infertility, cyclic breast tenderness, premenstrual moodiness, and ovarian cysts.

### DIGESTIVE SYSTEM

The fall-dug root is high in inulin, a type of indigestible, water-soluble fiber. Our digestive enzymes can't break it

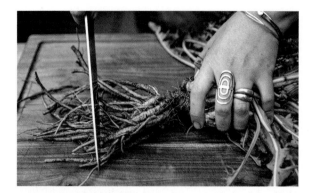

Chopping fresh dandelion root

down, but inulin feeds our intestinal flora (bacteria). It has been shown to decrease cholesterol, reduce hunger, and lessen constipation. The optimal way to ingest inulin is in food, but infusions and decoctions also extract the compound. Alcohol extraction and roasting destroy inulin. (Note that some people react to inulin with bloating and gastric upset. If you suffer from gassiness or IBS, proceed cautiously.) Dandelion root is a gentle laxative that works to stimulate digestive activity and can be used tonically to address chronic constipation, as it is non-habit-forming. Both the root and leaf stimulate bile production. It's best to take this bitter remedy 20 minutes before eating to effectively "prime" the digestive system and work in conjunction with your hormones and enzymes. Nibble on a leaf or take a few drops of tincture or vinegar for the bitter effect. A little goes a long way—you don't need high doses to reap the digestive benefits of the bitter flavor. See my recipe for Dandy-Orange Bitters on page 264.

### NUTRITIVE TONIC

Dandelion leaf is highly nutritious and is best ingested as a food, vinegar, or infusion to take full advantage of the array of vitamins and minerals.

### URINARY SYSTEM

The diuretic leaf can help reduce edema (water retention), alleviate premenstrual bloating, and lower blood pressure. (With high blood pressure, it's imperative to monitor blood pressure and seek the care of a physician before trying any herbal remedy.) Because it contains high levels of potassium, dandelion doesn't cause excessive potassium loss through the urine, as some pharmaceutical diuretics do. The root is also diuretic but to a lesser extent.

## Nourishing Skin Tea

With herbs that support the kidneys, liver, and cellular metabolism, dandelion tea can be sipped every day as a remedy for acne, psoriasis, and eczema. This formula is cooling and drying if taken daily. You can add 1 tablespoon each of marshmallow root and cinnamon bark chips to warm and moisten the formula. Other warming additions include cardamom and black pepper (add both sparingly, to taste), which will also improve the flavor of the tea, as it's a tad bitter on its own. It's crucial that you're consistent with the formula; it may take two months before you'll see the full benefits! It's also essential to address any underlying issues, like gut inflammation and intestinal flora imbalance, by following an anti-inflammatory diet (there are many to choose from) and eating fermented foods.

4 cups water

1½ tablespoons dried burdock root (*Arctium minus* or *A. lappa*)

1 tablespoon dried dandelion root (*Taraxacum officinale*)

2 tablespoons dried chickweed leaf (*Stellaria media*)

1 tablespoon dried nettles leaf (*Urtica dioica*)

1 tablespoon dried violet leaf and flower (*Viola sororia* or *V. odorata*)

In a small pot, combine the water, burdock, and dandelion roots. Bring to a boil, covered, then turn the heat down to simmer for 20 minutes. Turn off the heat and add the dried chickweed, nettles, and violet; stir. Infuse, covered, for 20 minutes and then strain. Adults, drink up to three cups a day. Sweeten with honey or maple syrup if desired.

## Culinary Uses

You can eat both the flower buds and the opened flower heads of dandelion; the buds are best when they are just beginning to emerge and are still close to the ground. Flower buds are typically cooked, as they're a bit chewy and bitter raw. The yellow florets can be pulled from the green base of the flower head and sprinkled onto salads and confections. The splashes of gold brighten quiches, omelets, herbed goat cheese, compound butters, and scrambled eggs. Dip the flower heads and floral buds in batter and fry as fritters or tempura—this isn't the healthiest dish, but it's a swoon-worthy treat for festive occasions. Chop and roast the sprightly young roots with other root vegetables.

The succulent spring greens are edible, both raw and cooked, but I'll let you know here and now: they are decidedly bitter. Sour and sweet flavors distract from the bitterness. Add a little vinegar or lemon to the greens, or top them off with a honey-sweetened salad dressing or sauce. As a bonus, the acids in the lemon or vinegar will help you assimilate the minerals in the greens.

Dandelion greens can be mixed with milder greens in salads or steamed with other vegetables, or they can be sautéed and added to a pizza or galette crust. See the recipe for Dandelion Galette on page 263. Wilted dandy greens are a popular Southern dish, prepared by pouring bacon grease over the greens, which softens them and removes some of the bitterness. The leaves are exceptionally nutritious, with higher levels of iron, riboflavin, and vitamin E than any of our commonly cultivated greens like spinach, collards, and kale. They are also high in fiber, beta-carotene, calcium, copper, and manganese.

> PRECAUTIONS: Because dandelion leaf is a powerful diuretic, it will compound the effects of pharmaceutical diuretics. Although rare, people have experienced contact dermatitis from the topical use of dandelion. People who are allergic to bee pollen or honey have a high likelihood of reacting to dandelion pollen and therefore should avoid ingesting the flower or any preparation from the flower that would contain pollen (i.e., the infusion).

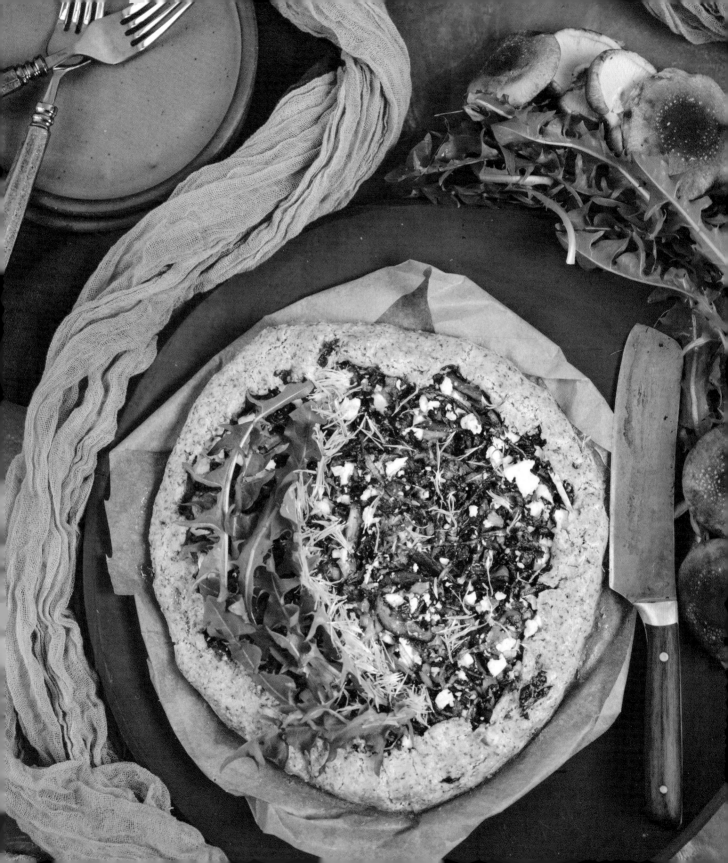

# Dandelion Galette

YIELD: 1 (8-inch) galette

### CRUST

5 tablespoons (71 grams) cold cultured unsalted butter

½ cup (64 grams) almond flour, plus a tad more if needed

½ cup (70 grams) arrowroot starch/flour

¼ cup (28 grams) grated Parmesan cheese

3 tablespoons (28 grams) ground flaxseed

¼ teaspoon sea salt

2 eggs

### TOPPING

2 tablespoons extra-virgin olive oil

1 leek, trimmed, washed well, and sliced into thin rounds

8 medium (80 grams) shiitake mushroom caps, sliced into long strips

2 garlic cloves, minced

¼ teaspoon sea salt

2 cups (85 grams) tightly packed, roughly chopped dandelion leaves

1 tablespoon balsamic vinegar

Freshly ground pepper, to taste

½ cup (85 grams) crumbled feta cheese

Handful of dandelion leaves and flower heads, for garnish

My kitchen collaborator, Amber Brown, first dreamt up the recipe for this rustic, grain-free crust for lamb's quarters, and we have since adapted it for dandelion. Substitute other cultivated or wild greens when dandelion is out of season.

**1. PREPARE THE CRUST.** Slice the butter into tablespoon-sized pieces and place them in the freezer for 5 minutes. Put the almond flour, arrowroot starch, Parmesan, flaxseed, and salt in a food processor. Pull the butter from the freezer and gradually add it to the food processor, pulsing until small pea-sized beads form. Add 1 of the eggs and pulse until a dough ball forms. Add more almond flour if needed if the dough is too wet.

**2.** Flatten the dough into a disc and refrigerate in an airtight container for about 30 minutes. Meanwhile, preheat the oven to 375°F.

**3. PREPARE THE TOPPING.** Heat a large skillet over medium heat. Add the olive oil. When the oil is shimmery, add the leek and cook for about 3 minutes. Add the mushrooms, garlic, and salt and cook for another 5 minutes. Add the dandelion leaves and cook until they are wilted, about 2 minutes. Stir in the balsamic vinegar and pepper. Turn off the heat.

**4.** Pull the chilled dough from the fridge and place it between 2 pieces of parchment paper. Roll it out until it's close to 12 inches wide and ¼ inch thick. Transfer the flattened dough, still on the parchment paper, onto a baking sheet. Remove the top piece of parchment.

**5.** Spread the dandelion mixture over the dough, leaving a couple inches at the edge. Sprinkle with the feta. Use the parchment paper to gently fold the edge of the pastry up and over the topping, creating a 1-inch border. Whisk the remaining egg in a small bowl and brush it over the border.

**6.** Bake for 25 to 30 minutes, or until the edges of the crust turn golden-brown. Gently lift with a spatula to check that the bottom is browned. Remove from the oven and cool for 5 minutes. Garnish with fresh dandelion leaves and flower heads.

# Dandy-Orange Bitters

YIELD: 1½ cups (12 ounces)

About ½ cup (56 grams) cut and sifted dried dandelion root, or 225 grams fresh dandelion root

Whole peel, including pith, from 1 organic orange, chopped

1¾ cups plus 2 tablespoons (15 fluid ounces) vodka or organic grain alcohol

This is a *dandy* all-purpose bitter for stimulating digestion. Take ½ dropper before meals, preferably 15 minutes prior to eating. Try a couple squirts as a bitter in mixed nonalcoholic drinks and cocktails. See these bitters in action in the Raspberry-Rose-Lime Bubbly recipe on page 365, the Orange Viola Mocktail on page 408, and the Pompeii, below.

1. Follow the general instructions for preparing tinctures on page 140. If you're using fresh roots, scrub the roots, rinse clean, and finely chop.

2. In a quart jar, combine the dandelion root, orange peel, and vodka. Cap and label. Infuse for 2 weeks, shaking periodically. Strain, bottle, and label as described on page 137.

# The Pompeii

SERVES 2

1⅓ cups fresh-squeezed orange juice (from 2 to 4 oranges, depending on variety and juiciness)

2 ounces vodka

1 tablespoon Raspberry-Rose-Lime Simple Syrup (page 189)

2½ teaspoons Dandy-Orange Bitters (recipe above)

2 cups ice, for serving

Here, we have a fruity libation with bright, citrusy tones. Leave out the vodka for an extraordinary mocktail.

Combine the orange juice, vodka, raspberry-rose syrup, and bitters in a jar, stir, and pour over 2 tall glasses of ice. Or, for an ombré effect, add one ingredient at a time and do not mix. Serve with an iced tea spoon.

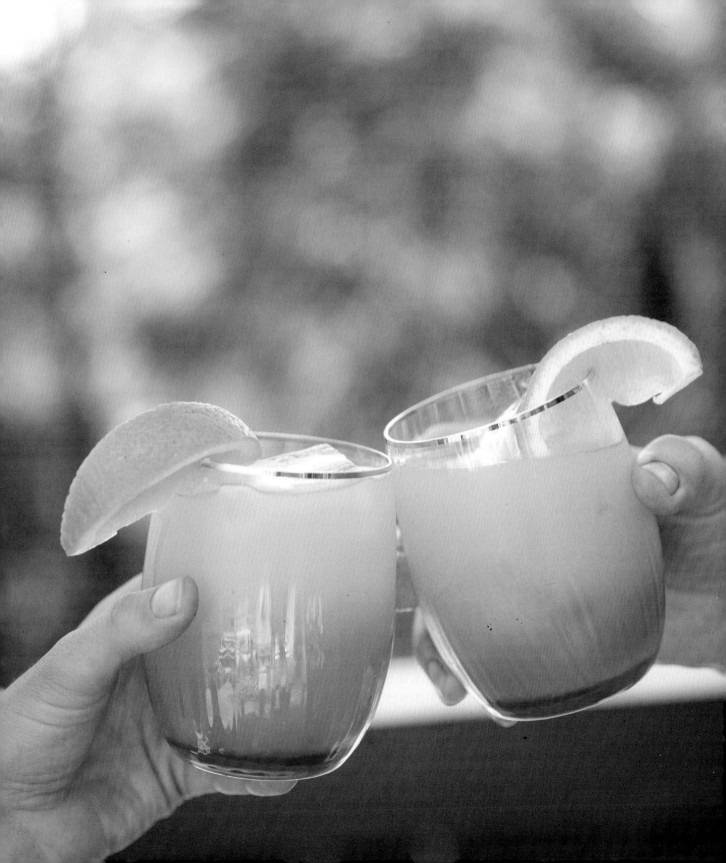

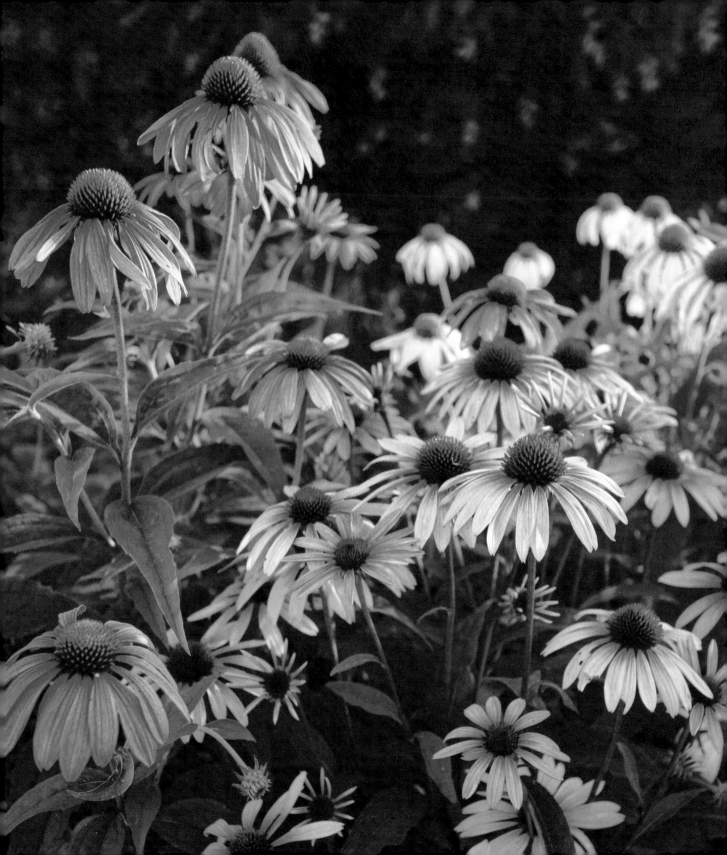

# ECHINACEA
## PURPLE CONEFLOWER

SCIENTIFIC NAME: *Echinacea purpurea*
ASTERACEAE, aster family
AKA: hedgehog coneflower, coneflower, *Echinacea angustifolia*: Kansas snakeroot and black-Sampson

Purple coneflower is a beloved perennial in flowerbeds, appreciated for its long-lasting blooms, drought tolerance, and ability to attract droves of pollinators for months on end. The roots, seeds, and fresh flowers and leaves are all medicinal and make a tingly-tasting, immune-stimulating tea or tincture. There are 10 species in the *Echinacea* genus, all native to central and eastern North America. The tribe has pinkish to purple blooms except for the paradoxical yellow coneflower (*Echinacea paradoxa*). The prickly, dome-shaped flower head inspired the plant's scientific name, which comes from the ancient Greek word *echinos,* meaning spiny, and relating to hedgehogs or sea urchins.

Many of these species are threatened or endangered due to habitat loss or overharvesting. Do not purchase wild-harvested coneflower. All contemporary knowledge of the herb has its roots in North American Indigenous traditions, where it is a key medicine. At least three species of coneflower are used, including *Echinacea angustifolia, E. pallida,* and *E. purpurea.* The Lakota, Cheyenne, Dakota, Omaha, and other Native peoples have long used the herb topically for many conditions, including burns, swellings, snakebites, infections, wounds, toothaches, and sores. Native peoples traditionally use the herb internally as a remedy for sore throats, bowel pain, and tonsillitis.

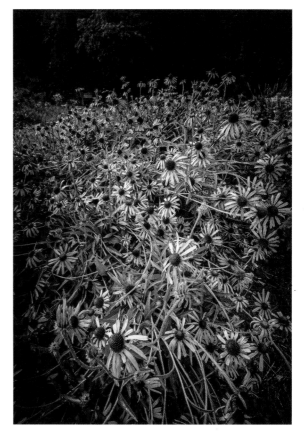

*Echinacea purpurea* and *Echinacea* cultivars growing at Robison Herb Gardens at Cornell Botanic Gardens; *Echinacea tennesseensis* growing at Herb Mountain Farm in Weaverville, North Carolina

## Cultivation

**ZONES:** 3–9; full sun to partial shade

**SOIL:** pH 6–8 (6–7 is ideal); fertile, well-drained soil

**SIZE:** 3–4 feet tall; 2–4 feet wide

**LIFESTYLE:** Herbaceous perennial

**PROPAGATION:** *Echinacea purpurea* roots can be divided in the spring or fall. The seeds will sprout without cold conditioning, but germination rates will increase with two weeks' stratification. Sow in flats or directly in the garden in early spring. Seeds germinate in 10 to 21 days at 70°F. Stratify other species of *Echinacea* for two to three months using the plastic bag method or sow outdoors in the fall. Space the plants 1 to 2 feet apart, depending on the species and cultivar. If you want to save seed and grow multiple species, know that they easily hybridize—you'll need to prevent cross-pollination if you'd like to save pure seed.

**SITING AND GARDEN CARE:** Echinacea is a laissez-faire garden companion, requiring little work to cultivate, yet yielding plentiful medicine after a few years. In the meantime, the herb will reward you with its long-lasting blooms and attract monarchs, fritillaries, skippers, and swallowtails into the garden. The nectar and the pollen feed honeybees and native bees, including bumblebees, leafcutter bees, and mining bees.

Plant echinacea where you can savor its glamor and entourage of pollinators. But remember its towering stature and plant it in the back of the border or against the fence. I find echinacea and wild bergamot to be a charming garden duo.

Coneflower is known to be a drought-tolerant native, but it will grow faster and bloom longer if you water it during dry weather. It will also flourish with spring side-dressing—fertilizing the plants will help them reach a harvestable size more quickly.

In the past decade, gardens have exploded with a swarm of new echinacea cultivars. You can now find blooms that are swan-white, cheddar-orange, and girly-pink. These delightful ornamentals should be left for the enjoyment of passersby and pollinators but shouldn't be used for their medicine—instead, plant the straight species for this purpose. Also, native pollinator experts caution gardeners that these novel varieties don't attract or feed native insects as well as the straight species.

*Echinacea purpurea* is the easiest of its brethren to grow for medicine. Other species are rare or endangered, and cultivating them can help broaden their population. Source your plants or seeds from native nurseries that take care to prevent crossing. Yellow coneflower (*E. paradoxa*) grows in limestone prairies in Missouri and Arkansas and is rare or endangered throughout its native habitat. *Echinacea angustifolia* is the second-most-cultivated coneflower for medicinal use and is the preferred species for some herbal manufacturers. I find *Echinacea purpurea* to be just as potent but much easier to grow in most gardens. *Echinacea angustifolia* is a native wildflower to the prairie states that feeds many native insects; I highly recommend planting it if you live in its indigenous range.

**PROBLEM INSECTS AND DISEASES:** Echinacea can become infected with aster yellows, a bacteria-like protozoan disease (see page 73). Because the disease is contagious and there is no known remedy, it's best to pull up any affected plants and remove them from the garden so the disease doesn't spread.

**HARVESTING:** Collect the flowers in full bloom, leaving plenty for the pollinators, and tincture while fresh. Harvest the seeds soon after the plants have bloomed and the seeds have formed. Using gloves, work the seeds free from the seed heads. Tincture fresh or dry in baskets. Wait to harvest the roots until the plants are at least three years old. Dig the roots in the late fall or early spring and scrub well. Tincture fresh, or chop and dry on screens or in loose-weave baskets.

## Medicinal Properties

**PART USED:** The whole plant. Root, seeds, and flowers are considered the most medicinal

MEDICINAL PREPARATIONS: Tincture, decoction, honey, syrup, oxymel, vinegar, compress, poultice, soak, and liniment

TINCTURE RATIOS AND DOSAGE: Fresh (1:2 95%) or dry (1:4 60%); either preparation 2–4 ml up to three times a day (6 doses a day is appropriate adult dosage in the first two to three days of an infection)

TEA RATIOS AND DOSAGE: Decoct 1 to 2 teaspoons dried root per 1 cup water up to three times a day

ACTIONS: Alterative, lymphagogue, anti-inflammatory, vulnerary, immunostimulant, antimicrobial, and sialagogue (stimulates salivation)

ENERGETICS: Cooling

## Medicinal Uses

I prefer the fresh tincture of echinacea to the dried, as I find it to be more potent. Each herbalist has their preference when it comes to the part of purple coneflower they use medicinally—I combine the root and seed tinctures in equal parts. Alkamides, also called alkylamines, are the constituents in purple coneflower that stimulate saliva and set your mouth to sparkle, and then settle into a numbing, tingly sensation. Spilanthes and prickly ash also contain alkamides. These compounds also play a part in these herbs' immune-stimulating qualities. If you don't experience the tingle, then the medicine isn't going to be strong!

### IMMUNE SYSTEM

I use echinacea as a short-term remedy for warding off colds and flu, particularly when a person has been exposed to an infection or feels the initial stages of sickness. Echinacea can also shorten the duration of an infectious illness. Many people stop taking it once they are sick, thinking it can't help anymore, but the herb stimulates many aspects of our immune system to help fight infection and thus can be taken throughout an infectious illness to heal more quickly. Echinacea helps relieve swollen lymph nodes and sore throats. Topically, it can be applied as a poultice, wash, or compress to wounds, sores, burns, infections, and boils. The root has similar oral uses to spilanthes (see page 374). In a meta-analysis (overview of multiple studies) of purple coneflower's efficacy in preventing colds, the placebo group was 55 percent more likely to contract a cold than those taking a standardized extract of purple coneflower.

Echinacea can also be helpful after injury or surgery to stimulate the cleanup crew—macrophages, which are specialized white blood cells that phagocytize (eat up) not only pathogens but also dead or damaged tissue. Echinacea, and herbal immune stimulants in general, can help clear the way for the regrowth of healthy tissue.

## Immune-Stimulating Formula

This blend is helpful as an internal remedy for fighting off imminent infections or bolstering immunity after exposure to pathogens. If there is a fever present, taking the tincture in a cup of hot water or tea will augment its diaphoretic (sweat-inducing) effect.

MAKES 4 OUNCES

2 ounces echinacea root and/or seed tincture (*Echinacea purpurea* or *E. angustifolia*)

1 ounce spilanthes leaf and flower tincture (*Acmella oleracea*)

1 ounce elderberry fruit or flower tincture or 1 ounce elderberry honey (*Sambucus canadensis*)

Note: Use fresh tinctures if possible (1:2 95%), but you can substitute dried tinctures or use different preparations for each tincture.

Combine all ingredients and store in a glass dispensing bottle. Dosage is 4 ml up to three times a day.

> PRECAUTIONS: Avoid squirting the fresh tincture directly in your mouth, as it can irritate the back of the throat. Use cautiously in autoimmune conditions; some individuals can experience a worsening of symptoms. Allergic reactions, especially with products containing the flowers and pollen, have occurred in a small subset of the population.

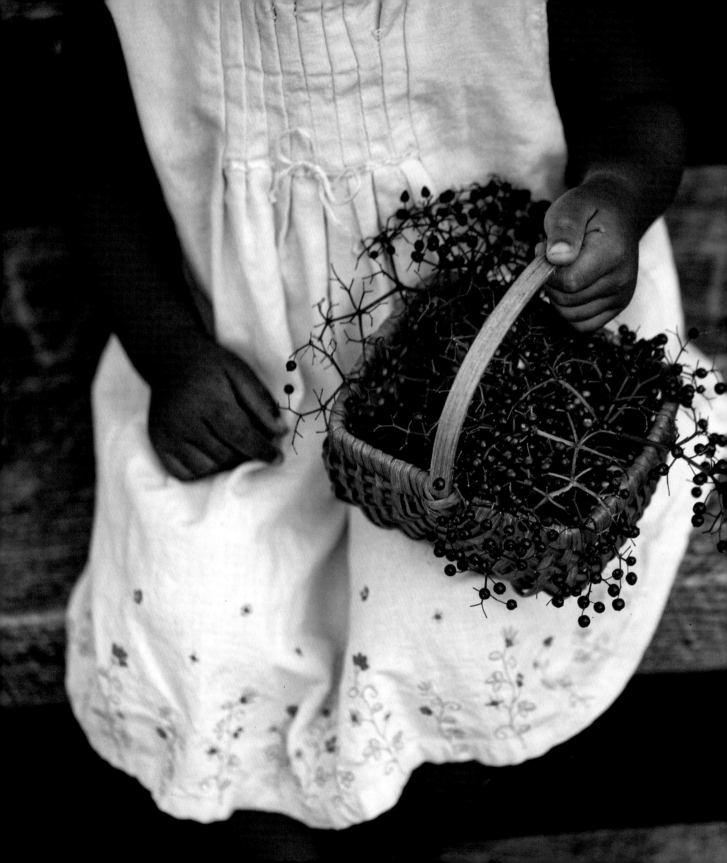

# ELDERBERRY

SCIENTIFIC NAME: *Sambucus canadensis*
ADOXACEAE, moschatel family (formerly in the Caprifoliaceae)
AKA: elder, pipe tree, bore tree, ellhorn, hylder

No herb is as steeped in folklore as elder. The Welsh kept a piece of its wood close to the body as a panacea against all sickness. In Scandinavia and England, elder is fabled to have housed Elda Mor (Hyldemoer), the Elder Mother, who was called upon to heal those suffering from sickness, especially children. In Scandinavia, legends held that if you slept under the tree on the summer solstice, you would be ferried to the Fey kingdom.

Elder is an edge plant, living at the intersection of land and water; forest and clearing; medicine and poison; winter and spring.

The antioxidant berries—rich in anthocyanins—are a familiar antiviral remedy but are also prepared into wine, jam, mead, shrubs, infused honeys and vinegars, and even pancakes. The flowers have similar medicinal use to the berries and are a common ingredient in cordials and cosmetics.

One of the easiest shrubs to propagate and grow, elder is fast growing and offers plentiful food and medicine. With its wandering roots, the shrub can quickly expand into a hedge or thick herbal fencerow. It provides nesting habitat for hummingbirds, warblers, and vireos and offers shelter for larger wildlife.

Elder's storied reputation is intertwined with a toxic constituent: sambunigrin, which is a type of cyanogenic glycoside. The concentration of sambunigrin varies by plant part and also by species. The roots and stems have the highest amounts, followed by the leaves and unripe berries. The flowers and ripe berries (technically, the seeds in the berries) have lower levels. Thankfully, cooking or drying elder destroys these compounds. These cyanogenic glycosides cause nausea and, in high enough doses, vomiting and diarrhea. This is why you'll want to pay attention to the part used and preparation when it comes to elder. Use only the flowers and berries internally unless you are an experienced herbalist. Don't consume fresh elderberry juice.

The botanical classification of the elderberry genus is in flux, which can be downright confusing. Contemporary herbalists primarily use the blue- and black-berried elders for food and medicine. I recommend planting a black or blue elderberry that's native to your bioregion, as it will likely thrive and optimally support biodiversity.

American elderberry (*S. nigra* ssp. *canadensis*; formerly *S. canadensis*) is native to central and eastern North America and Central America. It was once considered a distinct species from the black elderberry of Eurasia, but due to genetic studies, they are now thought to be the same species. Black elderberry (*S. nigra*) is native to Eurasia and northern Africa and now grows in gardens and the wild throughout much of the world. The blue elder (*Sambucus cerulea*, also classified as *S. nigra* ssp. *cerulea*) grows in western North America. Its fruit is deep blue, frosted with a white bloom, giving it a robin's-egg-blue hue. Blue elder is used for food and medicine like black elder. Red elder (*Sambucus racemosa*) varieties grow throughout North America and Eurasia and can be distinguished by their conical red berry clusters (some varieties are purple). They are considered more toxic than other elders and are traditionally eaten only after being cooked.

## Cultivation

ZONES: *Sambucus nigra* var. *canadensis*: 3–10; *Sambucus nigra*: 5–8; both grow in full sun to part shade

SOIL: pH 5.5–7.5; moist, rich soils with good drainage

SIZE: *Sambucus nigra* var. *canadensis*: 10–15 feet tall, 10–20 feet wide. *Sambucus nigra*: 18–25 feet tall, up to 15–20 feet wide. Both spread clonally and can form dense stands.

LIFESTYLE: Woody shrub

PROPAGATION: Elder is most easily propagated by stem cuttings. Take 10- to 15-inch hardwood cuttings in the fall after the trees have lost their leaves or in early spring before they leaf out. Stick the cuttings in potting soil and keep protected from the elements by placing the pots in a basement, garage, or indoors. Warmth will increase rooting. To plant seeds, sow the tiny seeds shallowly in the fall in outdoor trays or directly in the soil. Alternatively, stratify the seeds in damp sand for three months in the refrigerator using the plastic bag method. To plant seeds from your own bushes, collect the berries, separate the seeds from the pulp, and sow them straightaway in pots or trays that will be overwintered outdoors. When purchasing shrubs, look for varieties that are native to your region—they will be best suited to your climate.

SITING AND GARDEN CARE: Elder is a fast-growing shrub—flowering and fruiting at a young age—and will grow in most climates and soils. The plant prefers moist, fertile earth, so plant it in a wet meadow or near the edge of a stream, river, pond, or lake if you have such a spot. Elder is adaptable; it will also do just fine in regular garden soil, especially if you add generous amounts of organic matter and compost and mulch well. You'll need to keep its feet wet during dry weather.

Since I don't have any wet, semishaded areas in my landscape, I created a simulated wetland area in the lowest drainage point of my garden by adding copious amounts of compost, pine bark fines, and leaf mold. I planted elderberry bushes right away, which now tower over marshmallow, skullcap, blue vervain, boneset, and calamus, offering their herbal sidekicks dappled shade during the heat of the day. I prune the lower elderberry branches and pull out their suckers to give the herbs ample space in the understory. The whole area is mulched heavily and watered during dry spells.

Elder is a clonal plant—it sends forth new suckers from its roots at the base of the bush. If you plant it where space allows, you can let it expand into a hedge. Or dig the suckers up to transplant or share as gifts.

PROBLEM INSECTS AND DISEASES: Elder is relatively carefree in the garden. However, birds often beat humans to the berry harvest. It can sometimes be overrun by caterpillars or by the elder shoot borer (prune affected growth). The plant is susceptible to powdery mildew, leaf spot, canker, spider mites, and aphids.

HARVESTING: The lore of elder bushes reminds us to share gratitude with the plants, in thanks for their bountiful blessings, and ask permission before collecting.

Collect the flowering clusters when they're at their prime, and loosely place them in open-weave baskets. A stepladder is helpful for accessing the harder-to-reach blooms. Be careful bending the branches—they easily break. Don't crush or pile the flowers or they may oxidize. The flowers are often laden with a whole ecosystem of creepy crawlies; leave your harvest in the shade for an hour to let the insects depart. Visit the bushes repeatedly to keep up with the blooming season, and leave some flowers for the pollinators. The fertilized flowers will develop into berry clusters. The stems of the flowering and fruiting clusters are somewhat toxic—you'll need to remove them from your bounty. Pick out the larger stems and most of the tiny stalks; if a few "stemlets" find their way into your medicine, don't fret. It's a fiddly affair,

---

*Clockwise from top left:* Elder has opposite leaves that are pinnately compound; elderberry harvest in my simulated wetland herb garden; elderberries need to be removed from their fruiting stalks before consuming; elderflower harvest at Wild Abundance Permaculture and Homesteading School in North Carolina

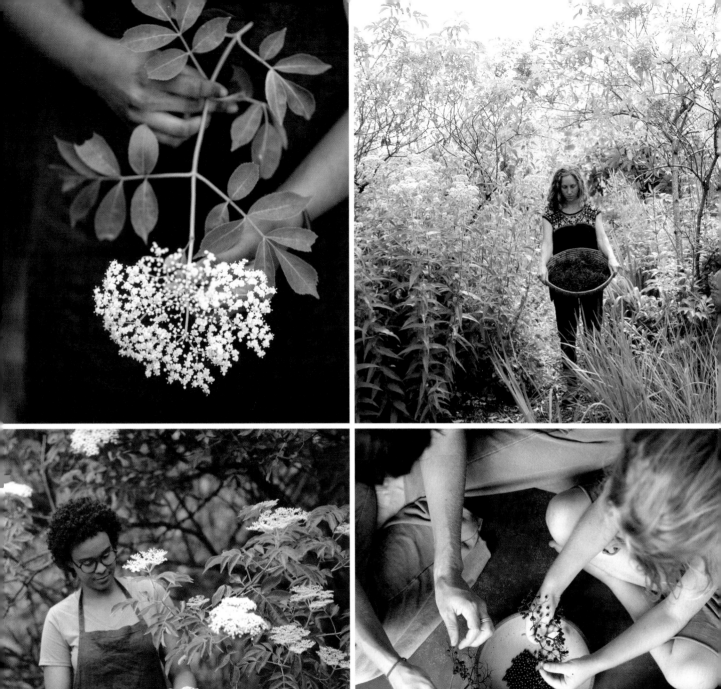

and a few stems won't be harmful. Store the dried flowers in glass jars to keep them fresh.

Harvest elderberries when most of the berries are ripe on a cluster—some will have fallen to the earth or found their way into a hungry beak, and there may be a few unripe berries. Err on the side of overripe. Place into wide bowls or baskets and take into the shade to process. Compost any unripe berries. The ripe fruit can be used for medicine making or cooking. They can also be frozen or dried.

If you're excellent at plant identification and you have a clean harvesting location, you may be interested in gathering wild elderflowers or berries. It's crucial to know that elder has several look-alikes. Consult a local field guide to learn which species of elder grow in your region and how to identify them and any similar-looking plants. **If you aren't paying close attention, you could mistake elder for the deadly poisonous water hemlock (*Cicuta* spp).** Water hemlock often grows in the same habitat as elder, but water hemlock is an herbaceous perennial with no woody parts, in contrast to elder's woody stems. The flower heads of water hemlock have a double umbel or inflorescence—small, secondary umbels growing from larger, primary umbels—whereas elder has a cyme (elder's flower stems don't all originate from the same place—they are more branched).

## Medicinal Properties

PART USED: Flowers and berries

MEDICINAL PREPARATIONS: Syrup, tincture, infusion, decoction, poultice, compress, mead, wine, honey, oxymel, shrub, and vinegar

TINCTURE RATIOS AND DOSAGE:

- Flowers: Fresh (1:2 95%) or dry (1:5 70%); either preparation 2–4 ml up to three times a day
- Berries: Fresh (1:2 95%) or dry (1:4 60%); either preparation 2–5 ml up to three times a day

TEA RATIOS AND DOSAGE:

- Flowers: Infusion of 2 teaspoons to 1 tablespoon dried flowers per 1 cup water up to three times a day.
- Berries: Decoction of 2 teaspoons dried berries per 1 cup water up to three times a day

ELDERBERRY SYRUP RATIOS AND DOSAGE:

- Immune tonic: 1 teaspoon (5 ml) three times a day
- Acute infections: 2 teaspoons (10 ml) every 2 hours at the first sign of a cold, flu, or other viral infection. If sickness takes hold, continue with 2 teaspoons (10 ml) five times a day during the acute stages of a viral illness

ACTIONS: Flowers: Diaphoretic, antiviral, anticatarrhal, astringent, anti-inflammatory, and diuretic. Berries: Diaphoretic, antiviral, antibacterial, antioxidant, diuretic, antirheumatic, anticatarrhal, anti-inflammatory, cardiovascular tonic, and immune stimulant.

## Medicinal Uses

The berries and flowers have overlapping uses. I find the flowers to be especially helpful for relieving sinus congestion stemming from allergies, sinus infections, the common cold, or the flu. They can also alleviate sinus headaches and earaches. The flowers have unique topical uses, described below. The berries are chock-full of antioxidant compounds and have more uses as a musculoskeletal anti-inflammatory and heart tonic than the blooms.

### IMMUNE SYSTEM

Elder is best known for its antiviral qualities, helpful for preventing infections as well as shortening their duration. In one random, double-blind, placebo-controlled study on the use of elderberry in influenza, participants took 1 tablespoon of elderberry syrup four times per day for five days. Symptoms were relieved, on average, four days earlier in those taking the syrup than in those taking the placebo. In vitro studies have shown elderberry to be active against several influenza strains.

Hot elderflower tea, along with yarrow and blue vervain, can help break a fever (see my recipe for "Influendsa" Tea on page 417). Elderberry syrup is a delicious way to bolster immunity throughout the winter. See the instructions for preparing herbal elderberry syrups on page 152.

## MUSCULOSKELETAL USES

Elderberry is a tonic anti-inflammatory for arthritic conditions and can be taken daily to relieve joint pain, tendinitis, and fibromyalgia.

## ANTIOXIDANT AND NUTRITIVE TONIC

The berries' high levels of anthocyanins protect blood vessel walls from oxidative stress, which helps prevent the development of atherosclerosis. Their antioxidant properties help protect cells against free radical stress and subsequent inflammation and mutation.

## TOPICAL USES

Elderflowers are a traditional ingredient in topical herbal remedies and natural body care products. A concentrated infusion can be used as an anti-inflammatory wash or compress to improve skin tone and soothe burns, eczema, psoriasis, insect bites, and hives. See my recipe for Floral Serum: Rose-Calendula-Elder Oil on page 364.

> PRECAUTIONS: The raw berries should not be consumed as they can cause nausea and vomiting. The leaves, root, and bark also have the potential to cause nausea and be purgative. The digestive upset varies by individual, part used, and dosage. See the precautions regarding a deadly look-alike in the Harvesting section.

# Antiviral & Immune-Stimulating Formula

This blend is helpful as an internal remedy for viral infections, as it contains immune-stimulating and antiviral herbs. Taking the tincture in a cup of hot water or tea will augment its diaphoretic (sweat-inducing) effect, which helps break fevers. If you can't find Japanese honeysuckle, substitute additional usnea tincture.

MAKES 5 OUNCES

1½ ounces echinacea root or seed tincture (*Echinacea purpurea* or *E. angustifolia*)

½ ounce usnea lichen tincture (*Usnea* spp.)

2 ounces elder fruit or flower tincture (*Sambucus nigra*)

1 ounce Japanese honeysuckle flower tincture (*Lonicera japonica*)

Combine all tinctures and store in a glass dispensing bottle. Dosage is 4 ml, three times a day. For persistent or virulent infections, the same dosage can be taken six times a day (keep this up for only two to three days).

# Culinary Uses

Elderberries can be prepared into jam, syrup, or wine. The berries are packed with nutrition and antioxidants—they contain iron, potassium, vitamins A and C, anthocyanins (which gives them the midnight purple hue), and quercetin (a bioflavonoid that helps with allergies and asthma). As noted on page 271, the seeds and unripe berries contain cyanogenic glycosides, which can cause nausea and vomiting. Do not eat them raw. Drying or cooking the berries renders them safe to consume.

Elderflowers can be safely eaten when cooked. Pull them from their stems and sprinkle them into crepes, pancakes, muffins, banana bread, and cupcakes. They can be used to season cordials, liqueurs, natural sodas, simple syrup, kombucha, water kefirs, and teas. Elderflower fritters are a spring delicacy—dip the flower clusters in batter and fry them until crisp and browned.

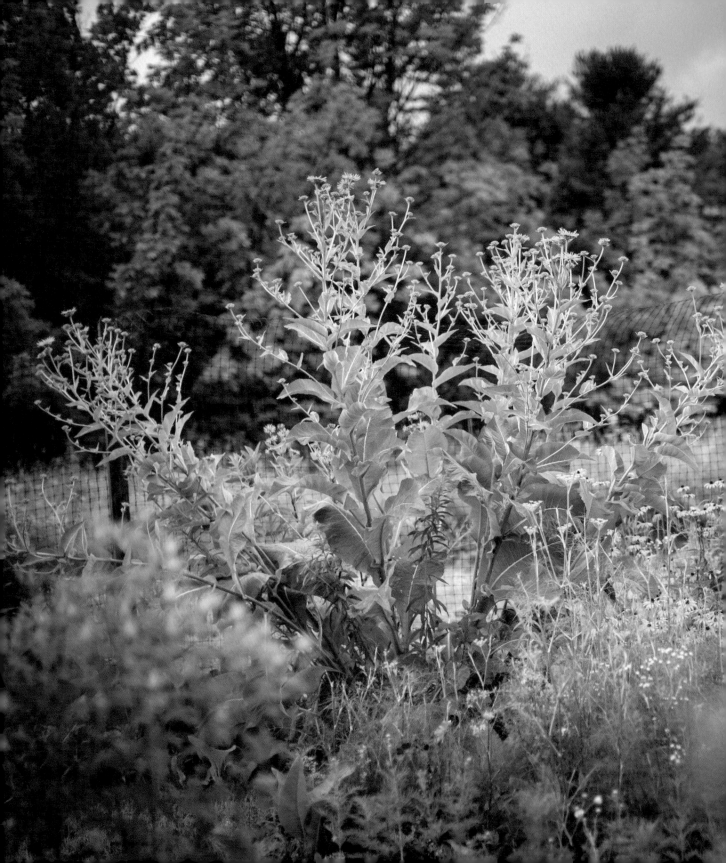

# ELECAMPANE

SCIENTIFIC NAME: *Inula helenium*
ASTERACEAE, aster or sunflower family
AKA: elecampagne, elfwort, horseheal, elf-dock, scabwort

A mainstay in the cottage herb garden, elecampane reliably charms passersby with its sprightly yellow flowers, resembling small unkempt sunflowers. The undersides of elecampane's gigantic leaves are textured with an intricate maze of veins, topped by a velvety dusting of woolen hairs. For centuries, the gnarled roots have been used as a digestive and respiratory folk medicine, with a compelling medley of sweet, bitter, and spicy flavors. The herb is native to Eurasia and has naturalized in the northern reaches of North America, where it's a feral denizen of fields and waysides.

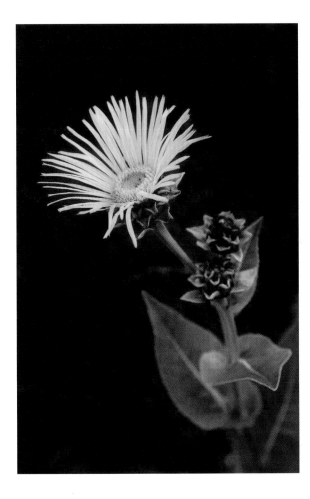

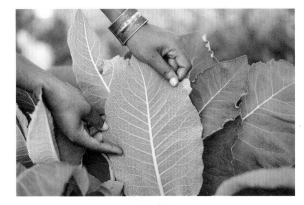

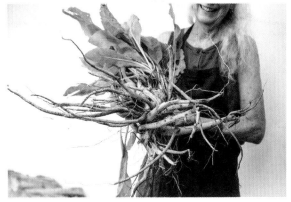

Elecampane growing in 7Song's herb garden in Ithaca, NY; the underside of an elecampane leaf—notice the pronounced veins and fuzzy texture; the roots are harvestable after two years

## Cultivation

ZONES: 3–8; full sun to partial shade

SOIL: pH 5–7.5 (optimal 6.2); rich, loamy soil

SIZE: 4 to 7 feet tall; 2 to 4 feet wide

LIFESTYLE: Long-lived herbaceous perennial

PROPAGATION: Sow the seeds on the surface of the soil; they need light to germinate. Seedlings emerge in 7 to 15 days at 65–70°F. Space 2 feet apart. Divide the roots after the fall of the second year. If you plant it from seed, elecampane will be vegetative (growing leaves only) the first year and will flower the second year and every year thereafter.

SITING AND GARDEN CARE: Elecampane is one of the most spectacular herbs for the garden, enchanting herbalists and pollinators alike. Plant this towering medicinal against a fence or wall or in the back of a border, where it can strike a statuesque pose without overshadowing its neighbors. Elecampane prefers full sun in colder climates but appreciates partial shade in hotter climates. Too much shade can cause the plant to grow leggy, and the plants will require staking. Elecampane is a fan of cooler weather and languishes when the summer temperatures are consistently high. If you live in a seriously hot and humid climate, the plant will look scrappy for most of the growing season. If you're growing elecampane for personal use, two to three plants will yield plenty of medicine, especially if you rotate your harvest and replant the root crown.

PROBLEM INSECTS AND DISEASES: Elecampane is generally free from disease and pests; however, slugs can take advantage of tender young leaves. I believe the plants can develop aster yellows disease (see page 73), but I haven't seen this confirmed in a lab.

HARVESTING: Harvest the roots in the fall or spring after two full growing seasons. After the third year of growth, the roots begin to get woody, often with decayed portions. Elecampane is a long-lived plant, and repeated harvesting and replanting of the root crown will result in a more youthful root system with less decay and woody portions. Older, knotted roots are still medicinal, but they require more care to cut out the unusable parts. Be sure of your identification in the garden, as elecampane can be confused with the deadly poisonous foxglove when the plants aren't in flower.

## Medicinal Properties

PART USED: Root

MEDICINAL PREPARATIONS: Tea, tincture, vinegar, infused honey, syrup, cordial, and candied roots

TINCTURE RATIOS AND DOSAGE: Fresh root (1:2 95%) or dry root (1:4 60%); either preparation 2–3 ml up to three times a day

TEA RATIOS AND DOSAGE: Decoction of ½ to 1 teaspoon dried root per 1 cup water up to three times a day

ACTIONS: Expectorant, circulatory stimulant, antibacterial, antifungal, diaphoretic, alterative, carminative, emmenagogue, diuretic, and aromatic bitter

ENERGETICS: Warming and drying

## Medicinal Uses

I became acquainted with elecampane when I was studying with 7Song, my first herbal teacher, in New York, where the plant grows wild, adorning windswept fields and overgrown stone walls on long-forgotten homesteads. Thoroughly smitten, I embarked on a lifelong affair with this scruffy herb, exploring every aspect of its medicinal uses.

I am not alone in this affinity for elecampane. It's one of those herbs with a profusion of therapeutic qualities, figuring prominently in the botanical folklore of Europe. Elecampane's name derives from that of the Greek goddess Helen and the Latin *campania*, meaning "field." Legend has it that when Helen of Troy was abducted, she shed copious tears upon the ravaged earth. Wherever a tear fell, an elecampane plant sprouted.

Elecampane was a culinary and medicinal pillar in European herb gardens and persists today around the ruins of old monasteries, where it once was grown as an ingredient for cordials. It was a treasured medicinal herb of the early Greeks, Welsh, and Celts.

## CIRCULATORY TONIC

Elecampane tea is an excellent warming daily tonic for folks who run cold, especially if they are prone to excess mucus in the respiratory tract, sluggish digestion, and frequent respiratory infections.

## DIGESTIVE SYSTEM

The roots are bitter with pinches of sweetness and spiciness, making elecampane a useful carminative and digestive bitter (of the warming kind) for indigestion, gassiness, and poor assimilation or absorption of nutrients. Many cultures have used the herb to ease nausea, belching, and indigestion. Chinese herbalists use the roots of elecampane and its cousin *Inula racemosa* as digestive tonics to allay queasiness, bloating, and diarrhea.

## RESPIRATORY SYSTEM

The roots are a stimulating expectorant, helpful for expelling thick, heavy mucus from the recesses of the lungs. Elecampane can be ingested as a decoction, infused honey, syrup, or tincture for that purpose. The herb is also antibacterial, helping to overcome and prevent bacterial respiratory infections. The roots are a traditional remedy for bronchitis, pneumonia, and asthma. Furthermore, its digestive qualities assist in the queasiness caused by nighttime postnasal drip.

## Warming Respiratory Tea

This stimulating and warming formula is helpful for respiratory conditions with thick mucus that's difficult to expectorate. The person may complain of a stuck feeling in the lungs. Omit the licorice while pregnant or nursing, and in cases of edema, high blood pressure, or heart or kidney disease.

4 cups water

1 tablespoon (5 grams) dried elecampane root (*Inula helenium*)

2 (10 grams) cinnamon sticks (*Cinnamomum verum*)

2 teaspoons (3 grams) dried licorice root (*Glycyrrhiza glabra* or *G. uralensis*)

2 teaspoons (3 grams) dried ginger root (*Zingiber officinale*)

¼ teaspoon (1 gram) hulled cardamom seeds (*Elettaria cardamomum*)

Combine the water and herbs in a small pot. Bring to a boil, simmer, covered, for 20 minutes, and then strain. Adults, drink one to three cups daily as needed.

## Culinary Uses

The Romans mixed elecampane's sweet and spicy roots with dates, raisins, and honey and enjoyed the blend as a digestive dessert. Lore tells us that elecampane candy was a favorite treat of Augustus Caesar's daughter, Julia. The root continues to be used in cordials and liqueurs, and it makes one of my all-time favorite herbal honeys. The honey deepens in flavor as it ages—I have a jar that is almost two decades old and still aromatic and medicinal.

> PRECAUTIONS: The external use of elecampane sometimes results in allergic contact dermatitis (due to the sesquiterpene lactones), although this is rare. Avoid the herb in pregnancy. Those with aster-family allergies should exercise caution when first trying elecampane. Elecampane is quite recognizable when in flower. However, when only the basal leaves are present, it can be confused with mullein, comfrey, or foxglove. **Because foxglove is deadly poisonous, you must correctly identify elecampane (true for all plants!).**

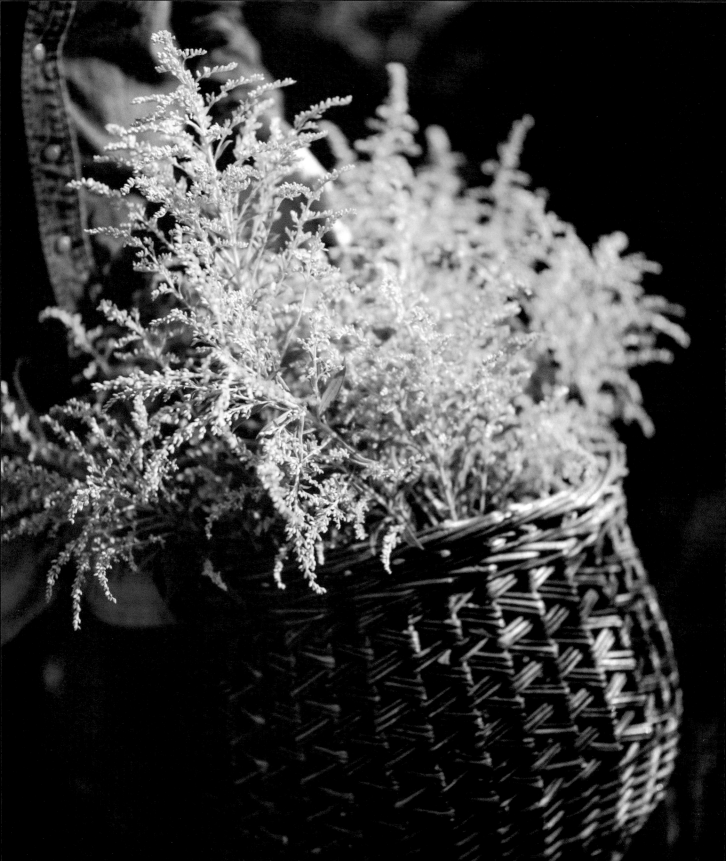

# GOLDENROD

SCIENTIFIC NAME: *Solidago* spp.
ASTERACEAE, aster family
AKA: goldrute, woundwort, Aaron's rod, and solidago

Each fall, goldenrod lights up meadows and fields with a refreshing blend of ruggedness and jubilation. Goldenrod's piney-tasting leaves and flowers are a reliable remedy for urinary, digestive, and respiratory complaints. The goldenrod tribe encompasses 100 species of late-blooming, knee- or hip-high herbaceous perennials. It's not just sunshine that goldenrod lends to the landscape—the plants increase biodiversity by attracting native pollinators and beneficial insects. Goldenrod has enriched our lives for centuries as a medicine, dye plant, and beverage tea. Although most species are native to North America, a few species are native to Eurasia and South America. European goldenrod (*Solidago virgaurea*) is a folk medicine for lessening bleeding and diarrhea and healing wounds, earning it the name *woundwort*. Goldenrod's resiny flavor nicely melds with both vinegar and honey. Meadowsweet and goldenrod make a lovely pair in mead or a naturally fermented homemade soda.

The plant grows wild in meadows, fields, open woods, trailsides, and waysides but can also play nice in the garden if you pay close attention to the species you plant and its location. Freshly picked goldenrod flowers lend a cheery splash of gold to bouquets, and the dried flowers are lovely in wreaths and everlasting bouquets. The blooms are used to dye silk and wool, lending a golden to olive-green color, depending on the type of mordant employed.

Goldenrod has been wrongly accused of causing hay fever simply because of its close association with the actual culprit: ragweed (*Ambrosia* spp.), which flowers at the same time. Goldenrod is insect-pollinated and doesn't release its pollen into the air; therefore, you'd need to stick your nose right in its face to induce any kind of histamine reaction.

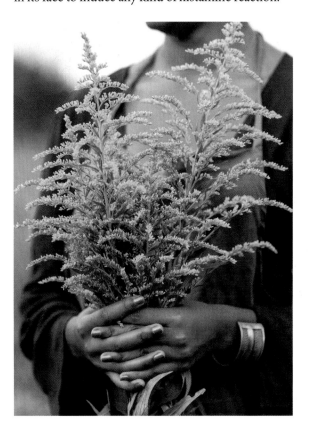

Harvest goldenrod when most of the flowers are still in bud and have not yet opened

## Cultivation

**ZONES:** Varies by species; look for natives to your bioregion (there are many to choose from in zones 3–9); full sun to partial shade

**SOIL:** Varies by species; soil requirements vary from dry to moist

**SIZE:** Varies by species, but generally 2 to 5 feet tall; some goldenrods spread aggressively by runners and some species modestly clump and expand in girth annually

**LIFESTYLE:** Herbaceous perennial

**PROPAGATION:** Stratify the seed for three months before planting and sow on the surface of the soil; do not bury the seed. Take softwood cuttings, consisting of four to six nodes, in the late spring. Divide the roots in spring.

**SITING AND GARDEN CARE:** Until recently, North American gardeners scoffed at inviting this "weed" into the tended landscape. Meanwhile, in Europe, goldenrod received a warm welcome in the garden and has been planted widely for upward of three centuries. After European plant breeders developed showy cultivars fit for the finest of cottage gardens, the opportunistic plant jumped the confines of cultivation and spread into European fields and meadows. Gardeners in North America are now recognizing goldenrod's desirability as an ornamental and medicinal. Gardening provides many nuggets of wisdom if we can simply manage to keep our garden gates unlatched.

The plant flowers in the late summer to early fall, at a time when most gardens could use some perkiness. Observe the pollinators flocking to the golden sprays and you will appreciate how important a role it plays in sustaining local insect populations. Goldenrod supports over 100 species of caterpillars. The nectar is popular with many butterflies, including monarchs. It also attracts garden beneficials such as praying mantises, ladybugs, assassin bugs, damsel bugs, syrphid flies, and parasitic wasps.

With a diversity of species to choose from and native habitats ranging from bog, to alpine meadow, to maritime dunes, you can be sure to find a goldenrod that will thrive in almost any niche. Goldenrod is a mainstay in meadow gardens and is especially delightful when growing next to its familiar, purple-blooming sidekick ironweed (*Vernonia* spp.). For massing, consider planting fast-spreading species, such as rough-stemmed goldenrod (*S. rugosa*), showy goldenrod (*S. speciosa*), tall goldenrod (*S. altissima*), and Canadian goldenrod (*S. canadensis*).

If your gardening space is limited, try one of the more demure clumping species, such as sweet goldenrod (*S. odora*) or any of the varieties described below. In a trial of goldenrod species conducted by the Chicago Botanic Gardens, *S. rugosa* 'Fireworks' was a choice cultivar, with its resistance to powdery mildew, slowly spreading habit, and explosive display of golden panicles. Other leaders include the hybrids 'Baby Sun' and 'Goldkind', both with tight clumping habits and generous floral displays. 'Golden Fleece' (*S. sphacelata*) is a late-flowering variety with heart-shaped leaves. For the partial shade garden, consider the variegated 'Variegata', which is a modestly spreading species rather than a clumping one.

**PROBLEM INSECTS AND DISEASES:** The plant is often affected by powdery mildew and rust. See the choice cultivars listed above, which have demonstrated resistance against both diseases.

**HARVESTING:** If you're new to plant identification, stick with garden-grown goldenrod and avoid harvesting wild goldenrod because there are toxic look-alikes that can be difficult to distinguish. There is a large group of plants variably called groundsel, life root, staggerweed, ragwort, and a slew of other regional names (*Senecio, Jacobea, Packera*, and other genera) that can be confused with wild goldenrod. Some members of this group have harmful pyrrolizidine alkaloids (PAs), which can cause irreparable damage to the livers of both humans and livestock. See page 200 for more on PAs.

Harvest flowering stalks with healthy-looking leaves that haven't been affected by powdery mildew or other diseases when they're just beginning to bloom. If powdery mildew is a big problem in your area, consider harvesting the leaves earlier in the season before the mildew takes hold. Just make sure of your identification, as you won't have the characteristic flowers present. Harvesting at the beginning of flowering ensures that your dried blooms retain their yellow hue. (If you harvest the plants in full bloom, the flowers will mature into their fluffy seed heads as they dry, resembling dull puffs instead of golden cheer!) I leave half the flowering stems intact for the pollinators and for the plant's regeneration. Hang the stalks to dry, and strip the leaves and flowers from the stem when they are crisp.

## Medicinal Properties

PART USED: Flowering herb (leaves and flowers)

MEDICINAL PREPARATIONS: Tea, tincture, vinegar, infused honey, oxymel, syrup, mead, and cordial

TINCTURE RATIOS AND DOSAGE: Fresh (1:2 95%) or dry (1:4 60%); either preparation, 2–4 ml up to three times a day

TEA RATIOS AND DOSAGE: Infusion of 1 to 2 teaspoons dried leaves and flowers per 1 cup water up to three times a day

ACTIONS: Diuretic, anticatarrhal, anti-inflammatory, antimicrobial, astringent, carminative, vulnerary, and diaphoretic

ENERGETICS: Slightly warming and very drying

## Medicinal Uses

Much of what we know about goldenrod's medicinal uses comes from Native American peoples who traditionally use various goldenrod species for a variety of ailments, both topically and internally. The herb is a

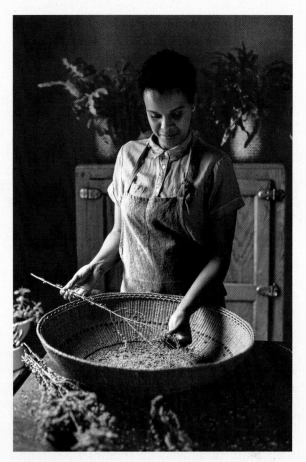

Stripping goldenrod leaves and flowers from the stem after drying

classical dermatological aid for sores, infections, burns, and wounds. Internally, the herb alleviates many urinary, respiratory, and digestive ailments. The book *Native American Ethnobotany* lists the medicinal uses of over 20 goldenrod species by over a dozen Native groups, with many overlapping uses between species. Although any species of goldenrod can be employed medicinally, aroma, taste, and medicinal qualities vary. The medicinal applications are similar between species; learn the individual nuances by tasting and smelling the leaves of any species you grow. Some species are more pleasant as a beverage tea, and some are more astringent. I detect hints of resin and seaside in the fragrance, a sublime blend of salt and balsam. The species that are more astringent (puckery and drying) are higher in tannins and will be more serviceable internally to slow diarrhea and topically to disinfect, soothe burns, and slow bleeding. Sweet goldenrod (*S. odora*) possesses honeyed hints of anise or licorice and is prized as a beverage tea.

### RESPIRATORY SYSTEM

Goldenrod is a premier decongestant, effectively alleviating upper respiratory congestion stemming from allergies, sinusitis, flu, or the common cold. In my experience, it's one of the most potent herbs for drying the sinuses. Combine it with sage to prepare a strong infusion that can be used as a gargle or mouthwash to ease sore throats, thrush, and laryngitis.

### URINARY SYSTEM

Goldenrod addresses urinary tract infections with its diuretic, antimicrobial, and anti-inflammatory properties and can be combined with marshmallow root, corn silk, uva-ursi, and goldenseal to prepare a tea for this purpose. (See the recipe on page 290.) The diuretic quality of the herb is also helpful in assuaging edema, gout, and kidney stones.

### TOPICAL USES

Goldenrod has long been used by Native American peoples and Europeans as a wash or poultice to help heal wounds, burns, open sores, and cuts. The vulnerary uses of the plant inspired the scientific name *Solidago,* which means "to make whole." The Kawaiisu use a decoction of the leaves of *S. californica* to treat boils and open sores and skin irritations. Various species of the herb have been used as a wash for thrush and as a toothache remedy.

## Free and Clear Sinuses Formula

This blend is helpful as an internal remedy for sinus congestion due to allergies, head colds, or sinus infections. It is very drying and decongesting and therefore isn't ideal for the beginning stages of a cold (when runny mucus helps expel pesky viruses) or for those who run dry.

**MAKES 4 OUNCES**

2 ounces goldenrod leaf and flower tincture (*Solidago* spp.)
1 ounce elder flower tincture (*Sambucus canadensis*)
½ ounce yarrow flower tincture (*Achillea millefolium*)
½ ounce nettles leaf tincture (*Urtica dioica*)

Use fresh tinctures if possible (1:2 95%), but you can substitute dried tinctures or use different preparations for each tincture. Combine all tinctures and store in a glass dispensing bottle. Dosage is 3–4 ml up to three times a day.

> **PRECAUTIONS:** Goldenrod can be overly drying as a beverage or tonic tea for people with a dry constitution, as it is diuretic, astringent, and decongestant. Short-term usage shouldn't be a problem. Do not use in pregnancy. Although rare, it has caused allergic contact dermatitis after both handling and oral administration. Those with Asteraceae allergies should exercise caution with goldenrod. Be sure you are harvesting the right species because there are deadly look-alikes (see Harvesting section on page 282).

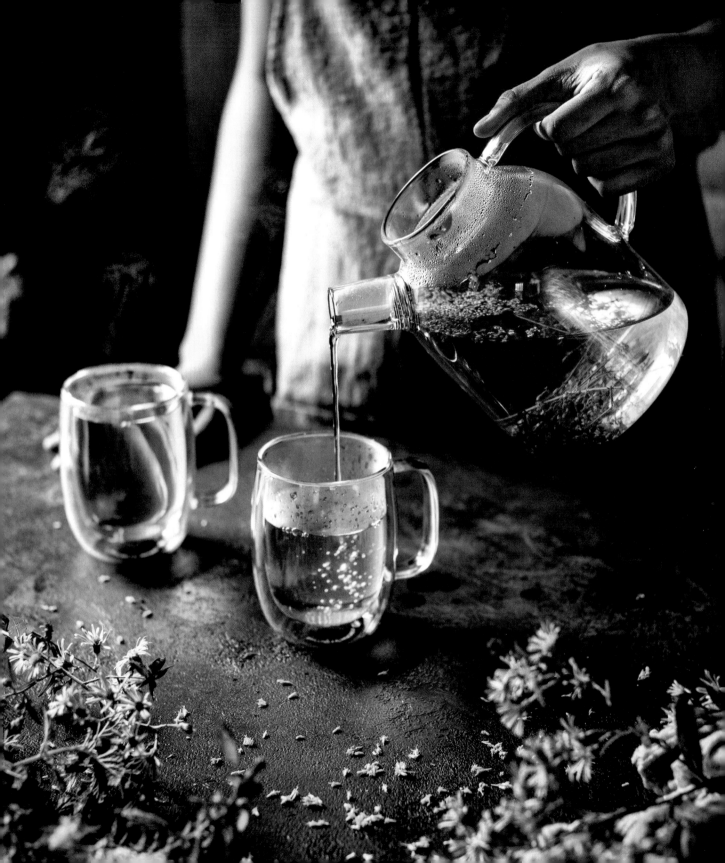

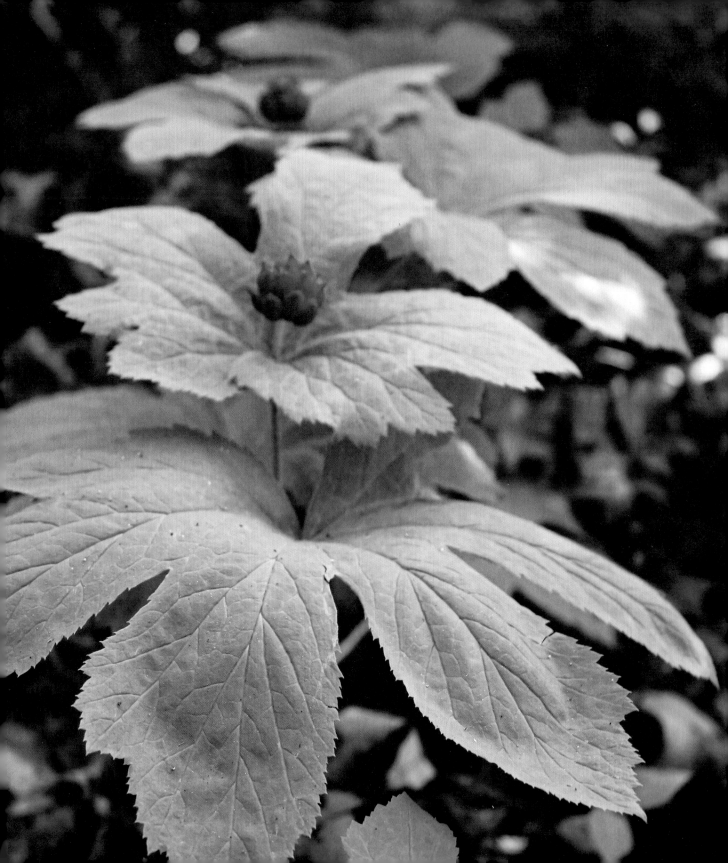

# GOLDENSEAL

SCIENTIFIC NAME: *Hydrastis canadensis*
RANUNCULACEAE, buttercup family
AKA: yellowroot and ground raspberry

Goldenseal is an iconic forest medicinal, renowned as a digestive and respiratory remedy for centuries. Contemporary use of the herb has its roots in Indigenous practices. The Cherokee use the rhizomes for increasing the appetite, alleviating indigestion, and topically as an anti-inflammatory. Iroquois healers have long used goldenseal to address digestive issues such as diarrhea and gassiness, along with liver and gallbladder complaints.

Goldenseal flowers lack petals but compensate with frilly white stamens; these hard-working male parts produce pollen *and* attract pollinators. The crimson fruit resembles a raspberry but, alas, is inedible. The plant is native to the deciduous forests of central and eastern North America but is now rare across all of its indigenous range due to centuries of overharvesting and habitat loss. Please do not gather goldenseal from the wild or purchase the wild-gathered herb; instead, grow your own or buy cultivated roots.

Naturalist and storyteller Doug Elliott describes the rhizomes as "a brilliant yellow that can hardly be surpassed by the blossoms of any wild flower." Botanically speaking, rhizomes are underground stems, but, in goldenseal's case, they're often called "roots." I'll use the terms interchangeably here. The golden rhizomes bear scars—left from the stems of bygone years—which resemble the wax seals on old-fashioned envelopes, inspiring the name gold-en*seal*. The root is a rousting bitter and is highly antimicrobial, both internally and topically. It clears the sinuses, soothes dental infections, and assuages inflammation. While goldenseal's roots are the most potent and widely used part of the plant, the leaves and stem are also medicinal, although slightly weaker than the roots. This is welcome news, as the plant is so precious—you can make use of the entire plant.

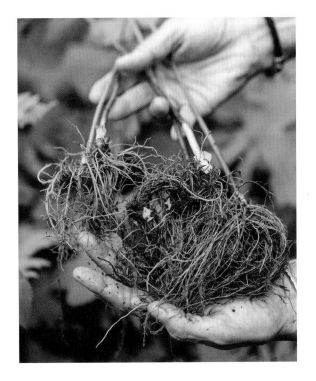

Goldenseal is a forgiving plant—this patch is growing in acidic soils amended with leaf mold in a young forest; goldenseal "roots" (rhizomes and rootlets)

## Cultivation

ZONES: 3–8; partial shade to full shade (70–75 percent)

SOIL: pH 4.5–7.5 (5.5–6 optimal); moist, fertile soil, rich in leaf mold, with ample drainage

SIZE: 10–12 inches tall; spreading plant forms colonies

LIFESTYLE: Creeping herbaceous perennial

PROPAGATION: Propagate the herb from seed or rhizome (spreading roots) divisions. Most people prefer to start with rhizome divisions because it takes many years for seed-grown plants to become a harvestable size, but seeds are a more economical option. Goldenseal seeds won't abide drying out and therefore should be planted soon after you receive them. The seeds require a period of warm, moist stratification (late summer and fall) followed by a period of cold, moist stratification (winter and early spring). Plant the fresh seeds in the late summer to early fall directly in prepared forest beds or in trays placed outdoors in the shade. In the first year, the plants will only produce cotyledons, or seed leaves; in the second year, they'll form true leaves. In the wild, goldenseal takes five to seven years before it flowers, but with a bit of coddling in the form of augmented soil fertility and bed preparation, plants can flower after only a few years.

When purchasing rhizomes, look for sellers who are using cultivated plants and not wild plants. Plant healthy ½- to 1-inch rhizome pieces (with intact rootlets) just below the surface of the soil, with any visible buds pointing upward. If your piece doesn't have a visible bud, don't fret—goldenseal also has hidden (adventitious) buds. To save your own seeds, harvest the fresh fruit, wash the pulp from the seed, and promptly plant as described above. Space plants 8 inches apart.

SITING AND GARDEN CARE: Goldenseal is one of the easiest woodland medicinals to cultivate. Even if you only have a small woodland to work with, you can likely grow a small colony of the herb. It will even grow in containers or clayey soil as long as you amend the soil with ample organic matter. If you're blessed with

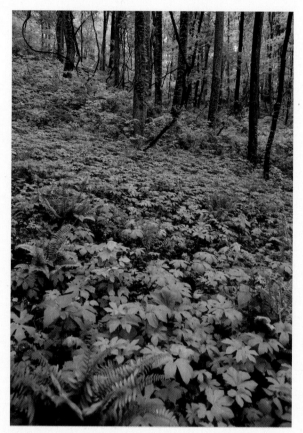

Forest-grown goldenseal growing in North Carolina

a hardwood forest to plant in, plant on north-facing or east-facing slopes, if possible. More importantly, look for indicator trees, which let you know you've got a suitable site. In central and eastern North America, look for black locust, tulip tree, beech, oak, maple, yellow buckeye, and basswood. Understory plants will also point to good goldenseal turf—look for ginseng, black cohosh, blue cohosh, trillium, Solomon's seal, bloodroot, and jack-in-the-pulpit. Outside the herb's native range, look for alder, oak, maple, beech, and linden as good indicator trees.

If the forest soils are poor, dig in amendments like pine bark fines, leaf mold, or aged compost. Make forest beds 3 feet wide, demarcated with fallen logs to protect from foot traffic, and loosen the soil before planting.

Be sure to cover the beds with a mulch of fallen leaves, and weed a few times throughout the growing season. Watering during dry spells will encourage quicker growth.

PROBLEM INSECTS AND DISEASES: Slugs can devour the plants and eat the fruit. Root-knot nematodes and spider mites are other possible pests. Cultivating the herb under shade cloth leaves goldenseal vulnerable to a slew of fungal diseases.

HARVESTING: As the plant has been overharvested, do not gather it from the wild or buy wild-gathered roots. Wait until the plants have begun flowering and fruiting—usually between three to five years—before digging the roots. Harvest the rhizomes in the late fall, after giving the plants a chance to set fruit and disperse their seed. If you have a lush colony, you can thin it by spot harvesting. Using a digging fork, gently pry the rhizomes from the soil, taking care to keep the rootlets intact. Spread the roots on a screen and spray them clean, picking out debris from the fine rootlets as you go. Chop the rhizomes into smaller pieces for medicine making or drying. Dry the roots on screens.

Gather the leaves and stems when they're looking vital and fresh but after the plants have set fruit. This way, earlier in the season, you can collect seed or the plants can self-sow, and the plants will have had ample time to photosynthesize. You'll want to collect the leaves as late in the season as possible but when the leaves are still perky. Spread the leaves on screens or in a dehydrator to dry.

## Medicinal Properties

PART USED: Rhizomes, roots, leaves, and stems (rhizomes and roots are the most potent medicinal parts)

MEDICINAL PREPARATIONS: Infusion (leaves), decoction (rhizome and roots), tincture, capsules, powder, poultice, wash, soak, douche, sitz bath, and gargle

TINCTURE RATIOS AND DOSAGE:

- Rhizomes and roots: Fresh (1:2 95%) or dry (1:4 60%); either preparation 2–3 ml up to three times a day
- Leaf: Fresh (1:2 95%) or dry (1:4 60%); either preparation 3–4 ml up to three times a day

TEA RATIOS AND DOSAGE:

- Rhizome: Decoction of 1 teaspoon dried rhizome and root per 1 cup water up to three times a day
- Leaf: Infusion of 2 teaspoons dried leaves per 1 cup water up to three times a day

ACTIONS: Bitter, antimicrobial, alterative, astringent, anticatarrhal, anti-inflammatory, and emmenagogue

ENERGETICS: Cooling and drying

## Medicinal Uses

Goldenseal possesses a few notable alkaloids (a class of bitter medicinal compounds), including *hydrastine* and *berberine*. In vitro studies conducted on berberine have demonstrated antimicrobial actions against a range of bacterial, fungal, and protozoan pathogens.

### DIGESTIVE SYSTEM

Goldenseal is a traditional remedy for peptic ulcers and diarrhea, especially when the cause is infectious in nature. In small doses, it's a bitter stimulant and digestive aid, but, in most cases, I prefer gentler and more common bitters, like dandelion leaf. The root can be prepared as an astringent and antimicrobial mouthwash for periodontal disease, loose gums, dental infections, and tooth decay. One of the easiest ways to use goldenseal in this capacity is first to brush the teeth with toothpaste and then apply goldenseal powder to a wetted toothbrush and brush once again. Rinse lightly so the powder can linger.

## RESPIRATORY SYSTEM

Goldenseal is a helpful remedy for sinus congestion characterized by thick yellow-green or yellowish discharge—usually this occurs toward the middle or end of a respiratory infection. In contrast, the root is not helpful at the beginning of respiratory infections when mucus is typically thin and runny and the sinuses are red with inflammatory heat. (Thin mucus escorts viruses out of the body with sneezing or blowing and may be annoying but is the body's way of taking care of invaders.) Warm goldenseal tea, along with mint and garden sage, and a pinch of salt, makes a useful gargle for sore throats.

## REPRODUCTIVE SYSTEM

The root is prepared as a douche and wash to remedy vaginal yeast infections and bacterial vaginosis (BV). Douching can irritate the vagina and disrupt healthy populations of vaginal flora, so it's only advised when there is a persistent infection present. At the first sign of BV or a yeast infection, insert a vaginal probiotic (beneficial bacteria) suppository (these are available online or in health food stores). Often, this will be enough to reset vaginal flora balance, and no further treatment will be necessary. If symptoms persist, antimicrobial medicinals can restore balance by reducing pesky populations of yeast or bacteria. To prepare an herbal douche, garden sage, calendula, marshmallow root, and lavender flowers can be combined with goldenseal and prepared as a concentrated tea. Follow up with a vaginal probiotic suppository.

## URINARY SYSTEM

The root is a classic urinary tract remedy due to its antibacterial, astringent, and anti-inflammatory qualities—see the recipe below.

## TOPICAL USES

Goldenseal—with its antimicrobial, astringent, and anti-inflammatory qualities—can be prepared as a wash or compress to alleviate skin conditions such as cuts, scrapes, insect bites, impetigo, ringworm, and athlete's foot.

# Urinary Tract "Back on Track" Tea

This tea blend addresses the symptoms and the root cause of urinary tract infections (UTIs). The herbs in this formula provide relief through their demulcent, astringent, and anti-inflammatory actions. They are also antimicrobial and diuretic, which helps flush out bacteria. Corn silk is one of the primary remedies I turn to for urinary tract inflammation and pain, as it is highly cooling and soothing, along with being demulcent and diuretic. You can dry your own by saving the silk when shucking organically grown sweet corn. Uva-ursi is, in my experience, the most useful antimicrobial and astringent herb for UTIs.

Drink the tea at room temperature to augment the diuretic effect of the botanicals. At the same time, it's wise to take an immune stimulant like echinacea or spilanthes to enhance the body's innate immune efforts. You can also drink unsweetened cranberry or blueberry juice. If the infection fails to clear up after a few days, consult your health care provider—antibiotics may be necessary. If you develop a fever or lower back pain, you may have a kidney infection; seek immediate medical attention, as this serious condition can damage the kidneys.

4 cups water

1½ tablespoons dried uva-ursi leaf (*Arctostaphylos uva-ursi*; see Note)

1 tablespoon dried marshmallow root (*Althaea officinalis*)

2 teaspoons dried goldenseal rhizome and root (*Hydrastis canadensis*)

3 tablespoons dried corn silk (*Zea mays*)

1 tablespoon dried goldenrod leaf and flower (*Solidago* spp.)

*Note:* If the uva-ursi leaf is whole, crush it with a mortar and pestle or grind in a coffee grinder.

In a small pot, combine the water, uva-ursi, and the marshmallow and goldenseal roots. Simmer, covered, for 20 minutes. Turn off the heat and add the corn silk and goldenrod. Infuse, covered, until the tea cools to room temperature, then strain. Adult dosage is three cups a day. Drink at room temperature. Do not use for more than four days because the astringency is too irritating to the digestive tract.

## Antibacterial & Immune-Stimulating Formula

This blend is helpful as an internal remedy for bacterial infections, as it offers both antibacterial and immunostimulating actions. If you can't find Japanese honeysuckle, substitute an additional ounce of usnea tincture.

MAKES 4 OUNCES

1 ounce goldenseal root and rhizome tincture (*Hydrastis canadensis*)

1 ounce spilanthes leaf and flower tincture (*Acmella oleracea*)

1 ounce Japanese honeysuckle flower tincture (*Lonicera japonica*)

½ ounce echinacea root or seed tincture (*Echinacea purpurea* or *E. angustifolia*)

½ ounce usnea lichen tincture (*Usnea* spp.)

Use fresh tinctures if possible (1:2 95%), but you can substitute dried tinctures or use different preparations for each tincture. Combine all the tinctures and store in a glass dispensing bottle. Dosage is 3–4 ml up to four times a day.

> PRECAUTIONS: High doses of goldenseal should only be taken for one to two weeks, as it can irritate the digestive tract. The herb can be overly cooling and drying to sensitive individuals. Other contraindications include kidney failure, acute stomach inflammation, pregnancy, and during lactation. If you have high blood pressure, use cautiously and consult your health care provider.

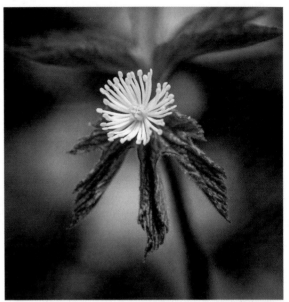

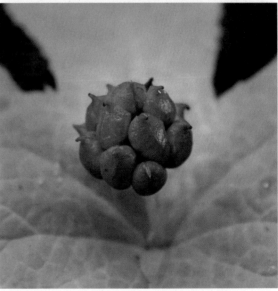

Goldenseal flowers lack petals—the frilly white structures are stamens, or the male floral part; goldenseal fruit

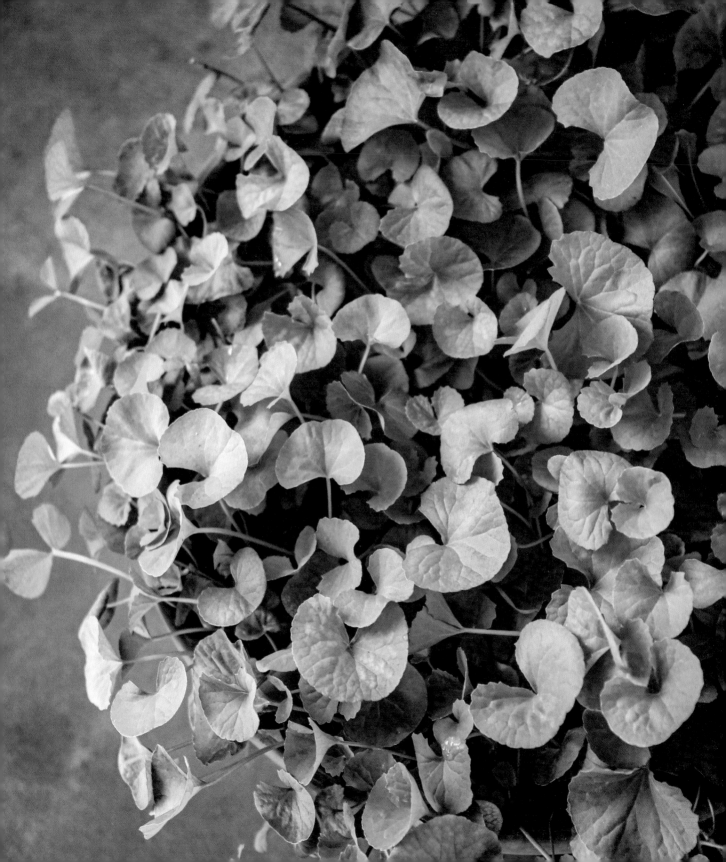

# GOTU KOLA

SCIENTIFIC NAME: *Centella asiatica*; formerly *Hydrocotyle asiatica*
APIACEAE, carrot family
AKA: brahmi, Indian pennywort, *Mandukaparni* (Sanskrit)

Gotu kola came onto my radar when I lived in Florida. Here was an herb that was both edible and medicinal, with a tally of medicinal uses bordering on legendary, that takes the sweltering heat and humidity in stride. Gotu kola is grown throughout southern Asia as a perennial medicinal potherb and salad green. Revered in India and China as a rejuvenating tonic for over 2,000 years, the herb is considered one of the best for promoting clarity, focus, and a peaceful, calm nature. Gotu kola, also called *brahmi,* is one of the easiest tonic herbs to grow both in the garden and in containers.

Native to wetlands of Asia and Africa, gotu kola has naturalized in the subtropics and tropics throughout the world, including Africa, the Middle East, and Hawai'i. With its cordate leaves and low-growing stature, the herb doesn't look like most familiar members of the carrot family such as parsley, dill, or fennel. Still, gotu kola shows its family resemblance when you crush a leaf and inhale its carroty aroma.

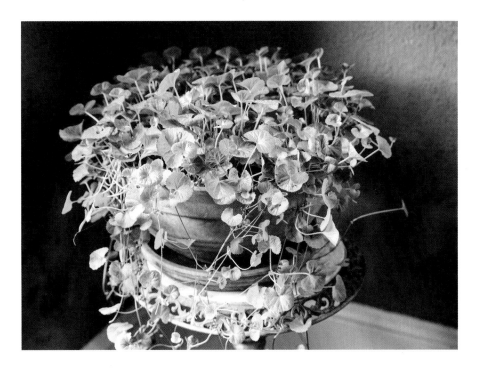

Gotu kola makes a lovely cascading houseplant

## Cultivation

**ZONES:** 3–7 as a frost-sensitive annual; perennial in zones 8–13; full sun to partial shade (especially in hot or dry climates)

**SOIL:** pH 6–7.5; moist but well-drained, rich soil

**SIZE:** 6 inches tall; indefinitely wide

**LIFESTYLE:** Herbaceous perennial

**PROPAGATION:** Gotu kola is most easily propagated from division (technically, dividing the stolons, or running stems). The runners root at the node, so it's easy to dig up a small portion of the rooted plant, separate it from the rest of the plant, and move the rooted portion to a new spot. Sow the seeds on the surface of the soil and lightly tamp into the soil, as they germinate better with light. The seed sprouts in three to four weeks at temperatures of 70°F or warmer. Sow heavily, as low germination rates are typical. Plant your starts in the garden, 9 to 12 inches apart, after the danger of frost has passed.

**SITING AND GARDEN CARE:** Gotu kola prefers moist soils with good drainage. That may sound like a contradiction, but picture a patch of moist sandy soil adjoining a small seasonal pond, under the dappled light of broad oaks, and you'll understand gotu kola's idea of good times. I've planted the herb under a tipi-type trellis of a passionflower vine, where the shade from the passionflower holds in the moisture and blocks the midday sun. Try growing gotu kola in a wooden whiskey barrel, retired bathtub, or a shallow, broad pot. To increase the drainage of your soil mix, add coarse sand or pine bark fines. Water the plants so the soil is continuously damp but not waterlogged.

In warmer climates, full morning sun and afternoon shade suit the plant just fine. In Southeast Asia, farmers plant gotu kola as a low-growing groundcover under shrubby crops. Where summer temperatures are mild, you can plant the herb in full sun if you keep it regularly irrigated.

In the colder reaches of its range as a perennial (areas with milder winter freezes), gotu kola benefits from some winter protection, such as heavy mulch, an unheated greenhouse, or placement in a protected location. In climates with hard freezes (zones 7 and lower), it is grown as an annual. Plant divisions in the garden after the last frost, letting the plants spread over the growing season. In the fall, before the first frost, dig up small clumps to overwinter indoors or in a heated greenhouse—these plants will serve as a reservoir for new divisions to plant outside come springtime.

I bring my potted gotu kola plants inside every winter to a window that receives bright, indirect light and then take them outside when the temperatures warm in the spring. When overwintering gotu kola indoors, you'll need to keep an eye on the plants, as they easily wilt and are bothered by spider mites and mealybugs—two common houseplant pests. Gotu kola makes one of the most luscious herbal houseplants, and I enjoy its presence in my office, where it keeps me company throughout the winter as I'm writing about medicinal herbs. When my inspiration sputters, I nibble on a few leaves to get my mojo back.

**PROBLEM INSECTS AND DISEASES:** Slugs are inordinately fond of gotu kola, and aphids can sometimes be a problem, too. Spider mites and mealybugs often bother container-grown plants.

**HARVESTING:** I harvest gotu kola with the haircut method, using scissors to cut off all, or most of, the leaves. It quickly grows a new batch of tender leaves, typically offering at least three cuttings per growing season. Stray reproductive bits are often included in the harvest and can be used medicinally with the leaves. Dry on screens or in loose baskets, or process immediately for tincturing. If you're harvesting the greens to eat, repeated harvesting encourages the production of tender new growth, which is less fibrous and more pleasant to eat.

## Medicinal Properties

**PART USED:** Primarily leaves but may also include small amounts of the stem, flowers, and fruit

**MEDICINAL PREPARATIONS:** Tea, tincture, infused oil, garnish, nibble, potherb, infused ghee, milk decoction, powder, broth, poultice, compress, green smoothie, and fresh juice. Gotu kola is a food herb, so the dosage can be quite high and still be considered safe. Traditional Ayurvedic dosages of the fresh juice are 2 to 3 teaspoons (10–15 ml) two times a day.

**TINCTURE RATIOS AND DOSAGE:** Fresh (1:2 95%) or dry (1:5 50%); either preparation 2–5 ml up to three times a day

**TEA RATIOS AND DOSAGE:** Infusion of 1 to 2 teaspoons dried leaves per 1 cup water up to three times a day

**ACTIONS:** Vulnerary, diuretic, anti-inflammatory, antioxidant, antianxiety, nervine, antibacterial, alterative, and secondary adaptogen

**ENERGETICS:** Slightly cooling but overall fairly neutral; it is considered tridoshic (balancing to all three doshas, or constitutions) in Ayurvedic medicine

## Medicinal Uses

Gotu kola has been used medicinally in Asia for over two millennia as a tonic in the treatment of memory loss, stress, worry, and foggy thinking. The Western understanding of the herb hails entirely from Ayurvedic medicine and folk uses in Southeast Asia.

### NERVOUS SYSTEM

Gotu kola is favored in India as an herbal ally to increase clarity and focus in meditation and to promote a tranquil nature. In Ayurvedic medicine, it is considered a rejuvenating tonic for overall vitality. It is often combined with ginkgo to improve memory and concentration and is especially favored by students for this purpose. Because gotu kola is an herb that aids concentration while simultaneously increasing a calm nature, it's one of the most common natural remedies for attention deficit hyperactivity disorder (ADHD). The herb is helpful, in general, for people who have trouble concentrating or who feel scattered or indecisive. For this purpose, I combine gotu kola with rosemary, tulsi, calamus, milky oats, and garden basil.

Gotu kola isn't considered a true adaptogen in the strictest sense, but its tonic tradition speaks to its use for increasing vitality, reducing stress, balancing the immune response, and supporting overall well-being. It's generally safe for a wide variety of constitutions.

### TISSUE REPAIR

Famous for its historical use in treating leprosy in India, gotu kola has a long tradition of use, both internally and topically, for healing burns and wounds and minimizing scarring. Gotu kola is the primary herb I use for promoting tissue repair after surgery or injury such as sprains, bone breaks, bruising, burns, and wounds. Gotu kola appears to promote wound healing through its anti-inflammatory, antioxidant, and antibacterial qualities, in addition to stimulating keratinization and epidermal repair.

For this purpose, it can be ingested as a tea, a tincture, or a food. Or you can sneak the herb into the diet in broths, vinegars, smoothies, and vegetable juices. An added benefit of its internal use is the ease it brings to the emotional and physiological stress of bodily trauma. Calendula is another herb that I frequently pair with gotu kola; the flowers also promote tissue repair.

### TOPICAL USES

Gotu kola is also used topically as an infused oil, compress, soak, or poultice to heal a variety of skin conditions, including insect bites, rashes, seborrheic dermatitis, herpes sores, eczema, psoriasis, and dry, irritated skin. The dried herb can be infused into sesame or coconut oil and rubbed into the scalp to calm the mind, promote sleep, and promote hair growth.

## Focus & Clarity Tea Blend

This tea is both calming and enlivening, promoting mental clarity and focus. It can be enjoyed by children and adults, but be sure to adjust the dosage for children (see page 133).

4 cups water

2 tablespoons dried gotu kola leaf (*Centella asiatica*)

1 tablespoon dried tulsi leaf and flower (*Ocimum tenuiflorum*)

1 tablespoon dried milky oats (*Avena sativa*)

2 teaspoons dried peppermint leaf (*Mentha x piperita*)

In a small saucepan, bring the water to boil. Turn off the heat, add all the herbs, and infuse, covered, for 30 minutes, then strain. Adults drink up to three cups a day.

## Recovery Tea Blend

This tingly tea helps promote tissue repair after surgery or injury. Drink it as is or transform it into a sipping broth by adding a touch of tamari and toasted sesame oil. To minimize inflammation and encourage healing, ingest ample protein and beneficial fats in the diet and also focus on antioxidant foods such as berries, dark leafy greens, winter squash, beets, black beans, and black rice.

4 cups water

3 tablespoons dried gotu kola leaf (*Centella asiatica*)

3 tablespoons dried calendula flower (*Calendula officinalis*)

1 tablespoon dried nettles leaf (*Urtica dioica*)

2 teaspoons dried spilanthes leaf and flower (*Acmella oleracea*)

In a small saucepan, bring the water to boil. Turn off the heat, add all the herbs, and infuse, covered, for 30 minutes, then strain. Adults drink up to three cups a day.

## Culinary Uses

Gotu kola greens are consumed, both raw and cooked, in many Asian countries, including Bangladesh, Thailand, Indonesia, and Sri Lanka. Many herbalists—widely known for their peculiar penchant for nibbling anything green, flavorful, and medicinal—munch on a leaf or two when passing by the plant. Folklore tells us that chewing on a few leaves daily keeps the mind fresh for a long and vital life. Add a few leaves as flavorful medicinal additions to salads, or throw a pinch of leaves into your soups and stews, imparting a mild parsnip-like flavor. Gotu kola can be added to herbal broths with seaweed, astragalus, and calendula, making a fine food for recuperating from injury or surgery. Add a smidge of leaves to green smoothies or juices. The flavor of the juiced greens companionably pairs with juices containing apples, ginger, lemon, and kale. Green drinks made from fresh gotu kola leaves are sold on the streets in many tropical Asian countries as a healthy energy tonic.

> PRECAUTIONS: Avoid in pregnancy or if attempting to conceive. Although rare, some people react with dermatitis to topical use. In Ayurveda, there are precautions that high doses may lead to headaches.

Harvest gotu kola with scissors and it will quickly send up a flush of new leaves

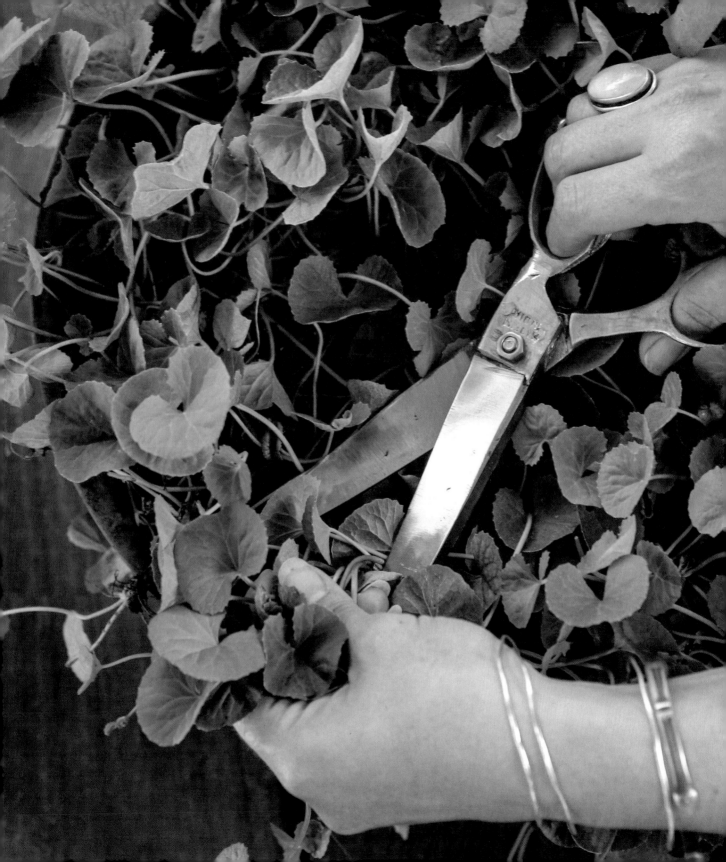

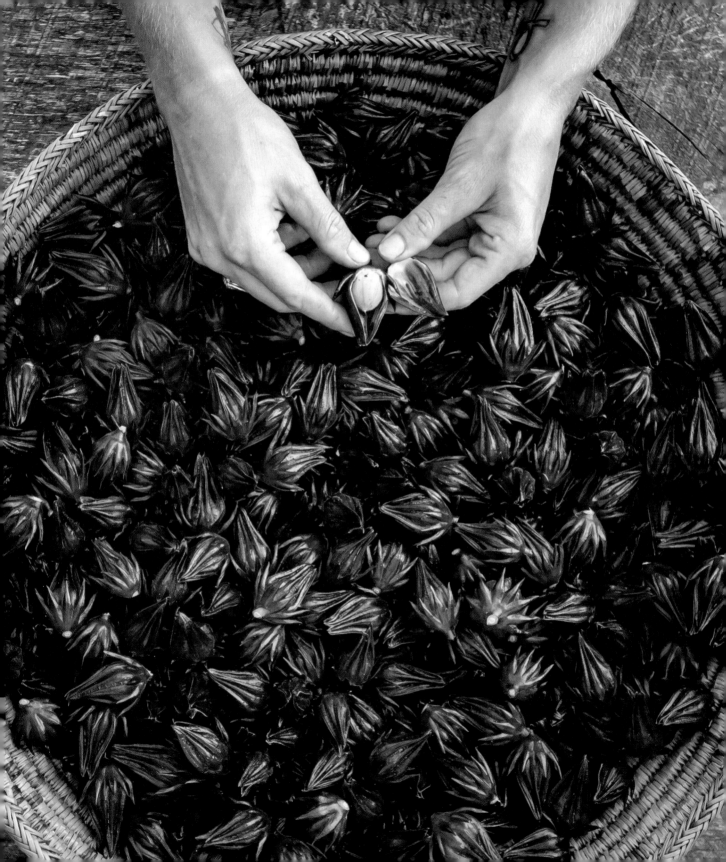

# HIBISCUS
## ROSELLE

SCIENTIFIC NAME: *Hibiscus sabdariffa*
MALVACEAE, mallow family
AKA: hibiscus, sorrel, rosella, roselle hibiscus, flor de Jamaica, rosa de Jamaica, Jamaican sorrel, Indian sorrel, Florida cranberry, and lemon bush

There are several hundred species in the *Hibiscus* genus, many of which are medicinal or edible, but only roselle (*Hibiscus sabdariffa*) produces a fleshy red edible crown, or "fruit." Botanically speaking, the crown is the plant's developing calyx (joined sepals) and receptacle (floral base), but they are commonly sold as "flowers." Hibiscus is enjoyed as a refreshing crimson beverage throughout the world and is especially prevalent in the tropics as a food crop and medicinal herb. Roselle's garnet-hued crowns are prepared into jams, chutneys, conserves, and alcoholic fermented beverages. Hibiscus can also be grown as an annual in colder climates by planting the right variety and getting a head start on the season.

Roselle has been cultivated for thousands of years as a food, medicine, and fiber crop in northern Africa. Enslaved Africans brought the plant to the Caribbean in the 1700s, and the crop radiated throughout the African diaspora. Most of what we know about the plant's medicinal uses originates with traditional African medicine. Hibiscus became briefly popular as an edible ornamental in Florida in the 1800s, giving rise to the name *Florida cranberry*. It's now cultivated worldwide throughout the tropics and has been adopted as a food and medicine by a number of cultures.

Certain species of hibiscus have edible flowers or leaves, but they aren't all considered edible or medicinal. Since *Hibiscus* is a large and varied genus, each species' traditional usage needs to be considered on an individual basis, and we can't generalize as a whole about the group's usefulness. Throughout this profile, I am only referring to *H. sabdariffa* unless otherwise specified.

Cranberry hibiscus, or false roselle (*Hibiscus acetosella*), looks like a red-headed roselle. It has edible burgundy, maple-like leaves that are sour, slightly mucilaginous, and boldly complementary to green lettuces in salads. The plant is a tantalizing ornamental, lending a tropical bling to the landscape.

Rose of Sharon (*Hibiscus syriacus*) is an ornamental shrub, native to eastern Asia, which is grown throughout warmer temperate regions of the world. It has edible flowers, which are slightly mucilaginous but pleasantly sweet in flavor. Gently pull the petals free from the reproductive parts and add them to salsas and fruit salads. Any of the varieties and colors of *H. syriacus* are edible—just be sure you have this species, as several other shrubs share the same common name.

Chinese hibiscus (*Hibiscus rosa-sinensis*) is a shrub native to southeastern Asia, grown throughout the tropics for its ornamental flowers, which vary in color from cream to peach to the classic crimson. Both the flowers and tender young leaves are edible. In Central America and the Caribbean, Chinese hibiscus flowers and leaves are used to stanch excessive menstrual flow.

Removing hibiscus crowns from the green ovary after harvest

## Cultivation

ZONES: 9–13 as a short-lived, frost-tender perennial; grown as a frost-tender annual in colder climates; full sun

SOIL: pH 5–8 (6.8 is optimal); fertile, moist, yet well-drained loam

SIZE: Annual plants: 3–4 feet tall, 3–4 feet wide; perennial shrubs in the tropics can reach 6–9 feet tall and 5 feet wide; size varies by cultivar

PROPAGATION: Scarify the seeds and then soak overnight before planting. Plant the seeds in 6-inch pots, as the seedlings do not like to be transplanted and consequently do not tolerate being "stepped up." The seeds can also be directly sown in the garden after scarification and soaking. Germinates in five days to two weeks at 75–85°F. Plant the seeds at the same time you plant tomato starts, and transplant the seedlings in the garden after the danger of frost has passed, taking care not to disturb the finicky roots. Take semi-hardwood cuttings in summer. Space 3 feet apart.

SITING AND GARDEN CARE: Despite roselle's tropical nature, it can be grown as an annual in temperate climates if you plant the right variety and get a head start on the season. Weed assertively when the plants are young, as they can become stunted with heavy competition. Once they reach a respectable stature, they can fend for themselves with less coddling. The hibiscus varieties available in nurseries and garden supply centers showcase glamorous blooms, but our dear roselle's flowers aren't as flashy, so the plant isn't commonly sold. You may be able to find roselle hibiscus plants at a local nursery specializing in herbs or useful plants, but you may simply need to grow it from seed.

Roselle's flowering rhythm is aligned with daylight cycles. Specifically, it is a "short-day" plant, which means it begins flowering in the early fall. This timing isn't optimal if you live in an area that regularly freezes. The narrow window between flowering and frost allows for slim pickings, if you're lucky enough to obtain any harvest at all. The good news is that certain varieties flower earlier, such as Thai red roselle, which typically begins flowering in July. Thai red roselle has a compact form compared to other members of its species and bright red, glossy stems. It is the variety featured in most of these photos. I recommend purchasing the seed from Southern Exposure Seed Exchange. In my experience, other seed sellers do not always have the right variety. For gardeners who live outside the tropics, having the right variety makes all the difference between an abundant and a nonexistent harvest. In the tropics, where roselle grows into a short-lived woody shrub, it isn't essential to grow specific varieties, as the plants can flower throughout the fall and winter months without fear of frost.

As hibiscus matures, it takes on a vase-shaped, erect habit, leaving the ground layer open for lower-growing plants. Prune the lower branches and plant petite herbs like gotu kola or spilanthes underneath. Calendula and hibiscus also make outstanding neighbors, with boldly complementary colors and companionable statures. Roselle is wind tolerant and can withstand temporary waterlogging. The plants produce fewer flowers and fruit with heavy applications of nitrogen, but they still appreciate fertilization via compost or aged manure. Mulch heavily to retain soil moisture and water in drier climates. Roselle is in full reproductive glory right up until the first icy fingers of frost settle upon the garden. You can extend the harvest by throwing a frost blanket or row cover over the plants during light freezes.

PROBLEM INSECTS AND DISEASES: Root-knot nematodes can be a problem in warmer climates; rotate plantings to avoid infestation. Scale insects and aphids can also affect the plants.

HARVESTING: When the yellow-pink petals fall off, the receptacle (flower base) and calyx (sepals) remain on the stem, appearing as fleshy scarlet crowns. This crown is the primary part of the plant used, both medicinally and as a food. Harvest the crown while it is still pliable and crimson, a few days to a few weeks after the petals have fallen off. I like to wait until the calyx is 2 inches long to maximize the yield when harvesting for tea. When the

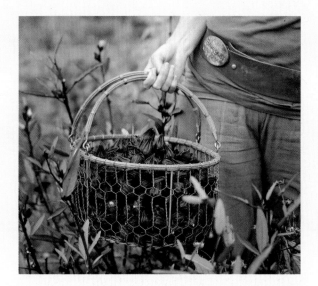

crowns reach this size, you'll need pruners or garden scissors to cut them from the stems. If you're preparing hibiscus as a food, pick the calyx when it's smaller, as it's less fibrous.

After you pick the calyx, separate it from the green ovary in the center. The ovary resembles a green ball nestled in the crown. When the ovary is young, it is mucilaginous and edible and can be included in foods made from the hibiscus calyces. As it matures, it becomes woody and must be removed. If you're drying hibiscus, always remove the ovary because it easily molds and can ruin the harvest.

Ovary removal can be tedious and is best achieved by corralling unsuspecting herbalist buddies. Ingenious herbalists in the Caribbean have devised makeshift hibiscus pokers to get the job done. Flower production is encouraged by regularly harvesting the crowns. The acidic juices can be irritating, and you may want to wear gloves when processing an abundant harvest. Small batches shouldn't cause a problem for most people. If you're drying hibiscus for tea, coarsely chop the calyces and spread them in a single layer on loose baskets or screens. Hibiscus has a propensity to mold in humid climates, so you may want to place the calyces in a dehydrator or dry them with extra heat and airflow.

## Medicinal Properties

PART USED: Calyx (red fleshy sepals); these are commonly described and sold as "flowers" or "petals."

MEDICINAL PREPARATIONS: Tea, honey, syrup, powder, chutney, vinegar, wine, popsicles, jam, fire cider, and margarita

TINCTURE RATIOS AND DOSAGE: Not recommended, as the minerals, vitamins, and mucilage aren't effectively extracted by alcohol

TEA RATIOS AND DOSAGE: Infusion of 2 teaspoons of the "flowers" per 1 cup boiling water; infuse for 1 hour or decoct for 10 minutes; up to three times a day. Higher doses are fine since hibiscus is a food herb.

ACTIONS: Diuretic, hypotensive, anti-inflammatory, cardiotonic, astringent, cholesterol lowering, antioxidant, antimicrobial, and demulcent

ENERGETICS: Cooling

## Medicinal Uses

Roselle has been used medicinally in many cultures for its diuretic, hypotensive, and antimicrobial properties. In Mexico, roselle is highly regarded as a natural liver and kidney tonic and traditional weight-loss herb. With its demulcent and soothing qualities, roselle preparations assuage colds, mouth sores, and sore throats. The herb has demonstrated antibacterial actions against a variety of bacteria in studies.

With its high levels of vitamin C, minerals, soluble fiber, and antioxidant flavonoids, hibiscus tea is one of the most healthful beverage teas on the planet. And considering its widespread popularity as a food around the globe, it has a high degree of safety and can be consumed daily to maintain health and lower the risk of developing cancer and cardiovascular disease—two of the biggest killers in industrialized nations. Plus, it's wildly delicious and can be woven into food and drinks with endless creative and colorful flair.

## CARDIOVASCULAR SYSTEM AND ANTIOXIDANT QUALITIES

Hibiscus has beneficial effects on the cardiovascular system through its ability to lower blood pressure and reduce excess cholesterol (although not all people respond to hibiscus's ability to lower cholesterol). High in antioxidant anthocyanins, hibiscus has been the focus of studies for its anti-inflammatory, cardioprotective, neuroprotective, and hepatoprotective (heart, nervous system, and liver, respectively) qualities. Anthocyanins are a type of flavonoid that lend blue, purple, and reddish tints to many vegetables, flowers, and fruits. These potent antioxidant compounds are helpful as a preventive against free-radical stress in the body, which in turn lessens the risk of cancer, heart disease, and inflammatory conditions in general.

In an overview of animal and human studies conducted with hibiscus tea, researchers determined that the herb was as effective in lowering blood pressure as the blood pressure medication captopril. These studies also demonstrated favorable effects on lipid profiles, including reduced total cholesterol, low-density lipoprotein cholesterol (LDL-C), triglycerides, and increased high-density lipoprotein cholesterol (HDL-C).

## Culinary Uses

Hibiscus has achieved high acclaim in tropical regions around the globe for its refreshing qualities. It's popular in the Caribbean and Central America as an iced herbal tea mixed with sugar; this drink is called *sorrel* in the islands and *agua de flor de Jamaica* in Mexico. Hibiscus is also widely favored in Africa and South America as a beverage tea, medicinal herb, and food. In many parts of the world, roselle "fruits" are sold fresh at markets.

Hibiscus stars in more of my recipes than any other herb. It's highly nutritive and easily prepared in hundreds of different ways. The tart young leaves can be eaten raw or cooked, and they are a favorite food in many tropical cuisines. The leaves are high in soluble fiber—like okra and oatmeal—and are thus helpful for supporting healthy intestinal flora and reducing excess cholesterol. The flavor of the calyx is often likened to rhubarb or cranberry. It can be eaten raw or cooked. Its sour taste, coupled with its natural pectin content, readily lends itself to jams, pies, sauces, and chutneys. Infused in honey, hibiscus makes a lovely garnet-colored treat with a delectably fruity flavor. During the summertime, hibiscus honey is a frequent muse for our garden cocktails. You can prepare a hibiscus honey lemonade or add the crimson honey to sparkling water for a rose-hued festive libation that's suitable for the whole family.

As an herbal iced tea ingredient, it's marvelous with mint, lemon balm, and meadowsweet. Hibiscus also makes delicious popsicles, especially when sweetened with fruit or fruit juice. (See my recipe for Hibiscus-Strawberry Ice Pops on page 309.) Another way to enjoy roselle in the summertime is to make crimson tart ice cubes out of the concentrated tea. With its bold color and tart flavor, hibiscus chutney is one of my favorite condiments. Hibiscus makes a lovely "cranberry" sauce for autumnal harvest feasts.

Nutritionally, hibiscus contains vitamin C, calcium, iron, magnesium, potassium, and heart-friendly compounds. Boiling the calyces for 10 minutes optimally extracts the minerals, flavonoids, and vitamin C.

> **PRECAUTIONS:** Roselle is generally considered safe, although its sour nature can aggravate heartburn. Hibiscus has been shown to increase the urinary excretion of acetaminophen (Tylenol), which lessens the drug's efficacy. As a precaution, wait three hours after taking acetaminophen before ingesting hibiscus. Hibiscus reduces the absorption of chloroquine (an antimalarial, amebicide, and immunosuppressive pharmaceutical). As a diuretic and hypotensive herb, hibiscus could potentially compound the effects of pharmaceuticals with similar actions; however, no studies have examined this compounding action.

*Clockwise from top left:* Hibicus bloom; 'Thai Red Roselle' growing in my North Carolina garden; roselle's developing calyx and receptacle, or "crown"; cranberry hibiscus, or false roselle (*Hibiscus acetosella*), has edible tart leaves

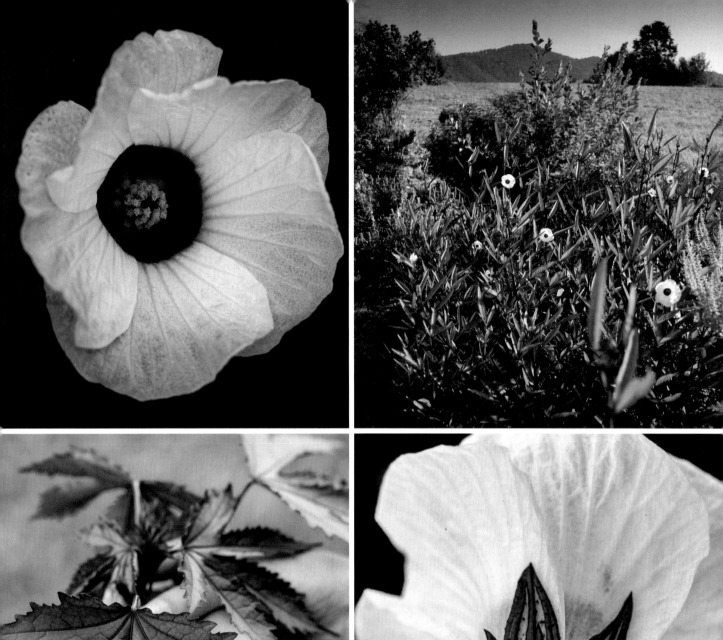

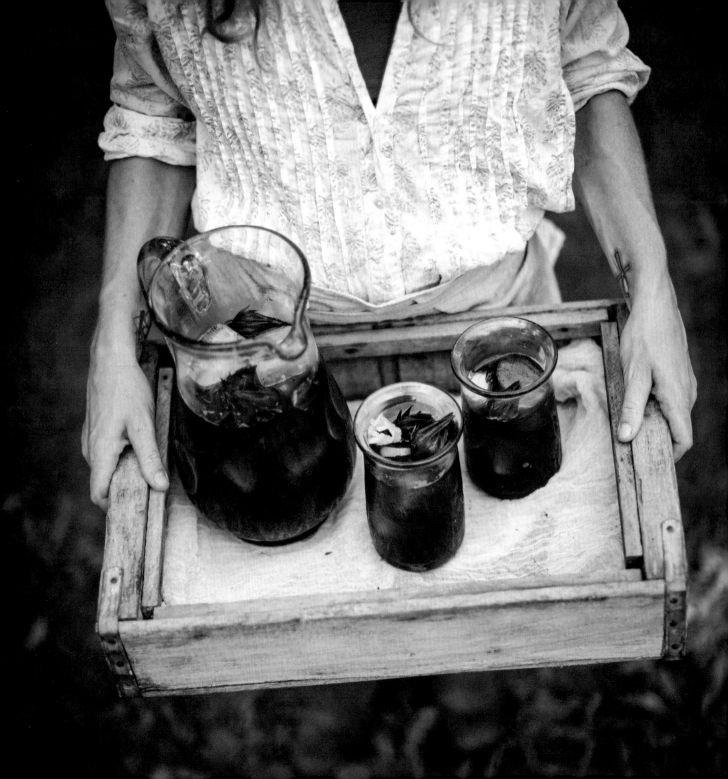

# Hibiscus Limeade

YIELD: ½ gallon

2 cups water, plus more as needed

1 cup (25 grams) packed dried hibiscus flower (*Hibiscus sabdariffa*)

¾ to 1 cup whole cane sugar or coconut sugar, to taste

½ cup fresh lime juice (from 5 to 6 limes)

4 cups ice, for serving

Lime wedges, for serving

This ruby limeade is refreshingly tart and sweet. Hibiscus and lime are companionable, sour in a complementary fashion. If you've ever had a hibiscus agua fresca in a traditional Mexican restaurant, served alongside spicy fare, you're already familiar with the thirst-quenching powers of this herb. Feel free to add a shot of vodka or tequila to your glass.

1. In a small saucepan, bring 2 cups of water and the dried hibiscus flowers to a boil. Turn down the heat to medium; simmer, covered, for 20 minutes. Strain into a large measuring cup, pressing the flowers with a spoon. You'll end up with less liquid than you started with, which is fine! Add the sugar to the hibiscus tea and stir until dissolved.

2. In a large pitcher or jar, combine the sweetened hibiscus tea and lime juice. Bring the final volume of limeade up to a half gallon by adding ice and cold water. Serve in ice-filled cups with lime wedges.

# Hibiscus-Raspberry-Rose Margarita

YIELD: 2 drinks

1 cup water

1½ tablespoons (3 grams) dried hibiscus flower (*Hibiscus sabdariffa*)

2 lime wedges

Crimson Cajun Salt, for the rim (page 171, or substitute a mix of coarse sea salt and chipotle powder)

2 ounces tequila

3 to 4 tablespoons Raspberry-Rose-Lime Simple Syrup (page 189), to taste

2 tablespoons fresh lime juice

2 cups ice, for serving

Some people have a sweet tooth. Others, like myself, are blessed with a tequila tooth. As a certified margarita fangirl, I can honestly say this is my favorite version ever. It's pretty hard to go wrong with hibiscus, raspberry, and rose, but once you add a spicy rim, the drink transforms into a libation that's truly blush-worthy.

1. Bring the water to a boil and add the dried hibiscus flowers. Simmer, covered, for 15 minutes. Strain the tea, pressing the flowers with a spoon.

2. Rub the rims of 2 margarita glasses with the lime wedges and dip into a shallow bowl of Crimson Cajun Salt.

3. In a pint jar, combine the strained hibiscus tea, tequila, Raspberry-Rose Syrup, and lime juice; shake until combined. Fill the glasses with ice and equally distribute the crimson liquid goodness from the pint jar.

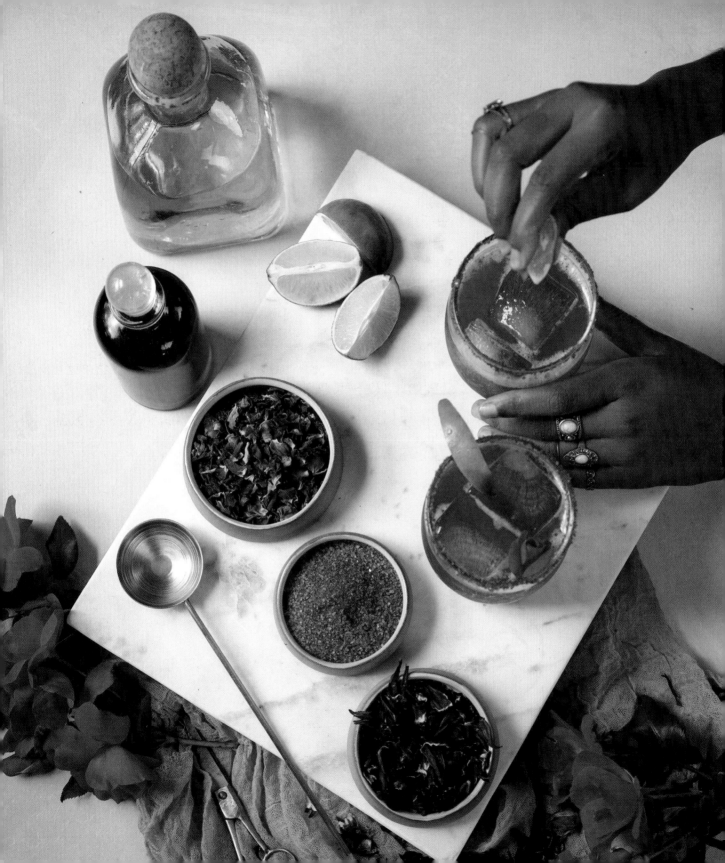

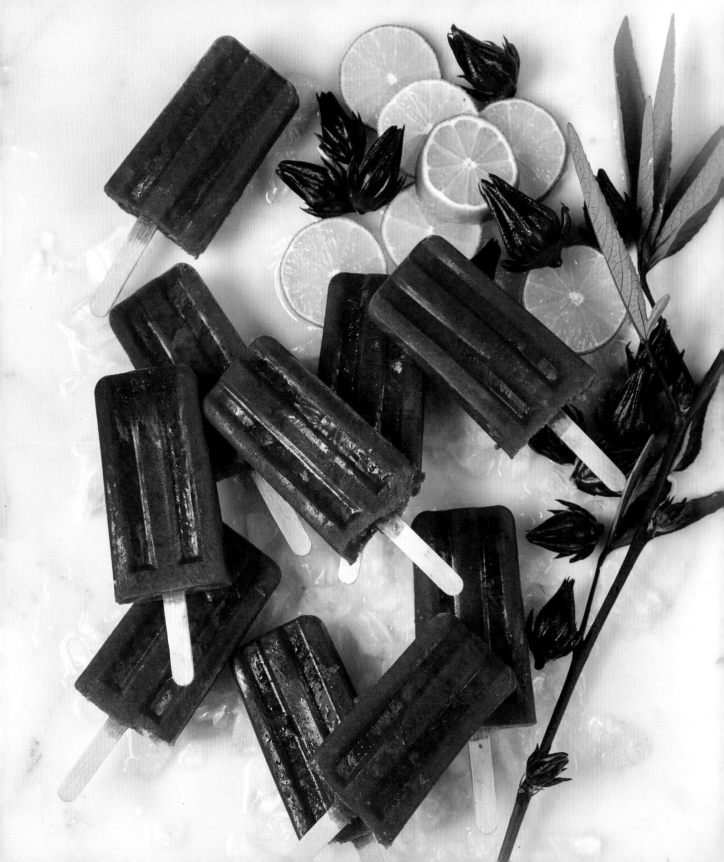

# Hibiscus-Strawberry Ice Pops

YIELD: 10 (3-ounce) ice pops

2 cups water

¾ cup (20 grams) packed dried hibiscus flower (*Hibiscus sabdariffa*)

⅓ cup pure cane sugar or coconut sugar

2½ cups frozen or fresh whole strawberries

2 teaspoons lime juice

Tart, fruity, and sweet, these pops are a crowd-pleaser. The hibiscus and strawberries are full of bioflavonoids and lend an antioxidant flair to a familiar frozen confection. Leave out the sugar if you're feeling tarty.

1. In a small saucepan, bring the water and dried hibiscus flowers to a boil. Turn down the heat to medium and simmer, covered, for 20 minutes. Strain into a large measuring cup, pressing the flowers with a spoon. You'll end up with less liquid than you started with, which is fine!

2. Add the sugar to the strained hibiscus tea and stir until dissolved. Transfer the tea to a blender and add the strawberries and lime juice. Blend until smooth and combined.

3. Pour the mixture into ice pop molds and freeze until firm, about 6 hours. If you're left with excess hibiscus mixture, you can enjoy it as a smoothie. Alternatively, adults might add some tequila and crushed ice to prepare a lushy-slushy.

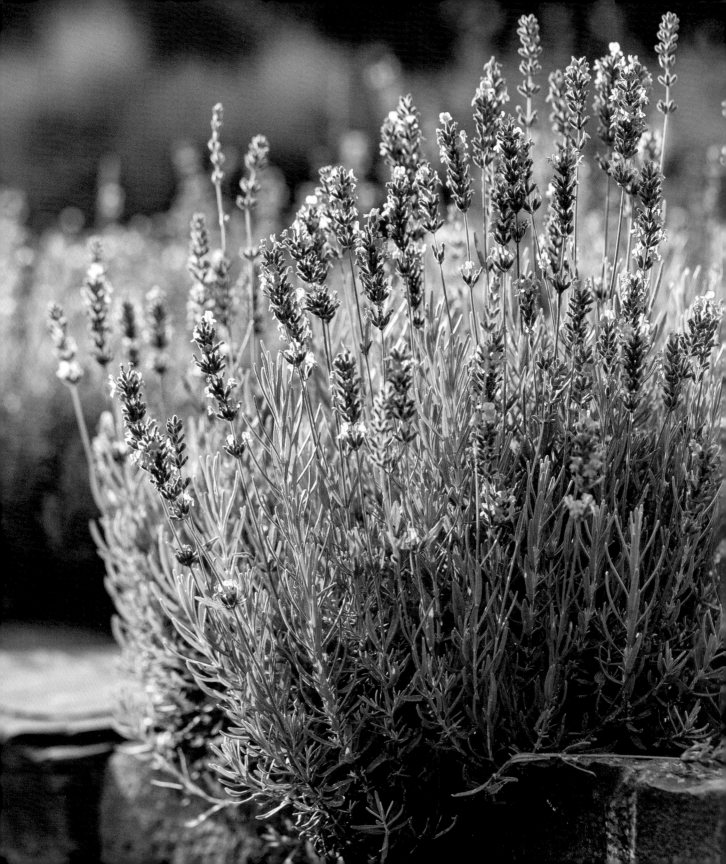

# LAVENDER

SCIENTIFIC NAME: *Lavandula angustifolia* (formerly *L. officinalis*)
LAMIACEAE, mint family
AKA: English lavender

If the garden herbs elected an ambassador to win over the hearts of vegetable gardeners, lavender would be the frontrunner, with its silvery foliage, purple floral wands, and clean and refreshing scent. The herb's common and scientific names originate from the Latin, *lavare,* for washing or bathing. In Europe, lavender has been infused into laundry water for centuries, and the Romans scented their baths with the herb. Anyone who has submerged in a lavender tub can attest to the olfactory allure, and the herb's antibacterial and antifungal qualities have obvious benefits when it comes to communal bathing. Lavender deters insects, including moths, flies, rodents, and mosquitos—fresh handfuls of the herb used to be strewn on the floor and hung in windows to keep the air smelling fresh and dissuade pests. (Imagine life when windows didn't have screens or glass and barnyard animals practically lived underfoot.) The herb is a beloved sachet botanical; I fill mesh bags with homegrown aromatics—lavender, white sage, and Arizona cypress needles—and place the sachets in my car, drawers, and closets.

There are close to 50 species of lavender—all in the *Lavandula* genus—and hundreds of named varieties. Native to northern Africa, the Mediterranean, India, and the Middle East, the lavender tribe is comprised of arid-loving small shrubs. English lavender (*Lavandula angustifolia*) is actually native to the Mediterranean and is the most common species used medicinally. The leaves and flowers have been used for centuries as a remedy for digestive issues, headaches, grief, and stress. In the following pages, when I refer to lavender's medicinal uses, I am only referring to this species. Some other species you are likely to see at your local nursery or may already have in your garden (but are not used medicinally). Spike lavender (*Lavandula latifolia*) hails from Spain and Portugal and is often used to scent soaps. Lavandin (*Lavandula* x *intermedia*) is a cross between English lavender and spike lavender. Lavandin essential oil is cheaper to produce than lavender and is thus widely used in cleaning products and cosmetics. Many of the ornamental lavenders are actually lavandin hybrids, prized for their numerous blooms, increased stature, and formidable vigor, including resistance to sudden wilts. Notable cultivars include 'Hidcote Giant', 'Grosso', 'Provence', and the newcomer 'Phenomenal', which overwinters in zone 4 or 5, keeping its foliage throughout the year.

Lavender (*Lavandula angustifolia*) growing at the Robison Herb Garden at Cornell Botanic Gardens

## Cultivation

ZONES: 5–10; full sun; cold-hardiness and heat tolerance varies by cultivar

SOIL: pH 6.5–8 (pH 7 is ideal); well-drained soil

SIZE: 2–3 feet tall; 2–3 feet wide; size depends on the cultivar

LIFESTYLE: Woody perennial

PROPAGATION: Named lavender varieties need to be propagated from layering or stem cuttings, as they will not come true from seed. Take semi-ripe cuttings of the plant in summer, following the directions on page 103. To plant from seed, lightly scarify the seeds, stratify them for 30 days in sand in the refrigerator, and then plant them on the surface of the soil; cover the seeds with a fine layer of sand. Germination occurs in two to three weeks at 70–85°F. Seeds will germinate without stratification or scarification but will take longer to emerge. Space plants 2 to 3 feet apart, depending on the strain. Proper spacing is essential, as airflow minimizes the risk of fungal diseases, which often affect lavender grown in humid climates. Plants grown from seed often wait to flower until their second year.

SITING AND GARDEN CARE: In New Mexico, you sometimes see hedges of lavender planted in wide swaths in the median. The herb is decidedly happier in Mediterranean climates—arid and bright are lavender's middle names—but it will tolerate humidity with a bit of pampering. First, you'll want to select a variety suited for your region; check with local nurseries and herb growers to see which ones they recommend. Plant lavender in full sun and give it a wide berth between other plants to dissuade diseases. If your soil is clayey, add coarse sand and pine bark fines to increase drainage. If you live in a coastal region, mulch with crushed oyster shells; inland, mulch plants with light-colored gravel. Mulching is crucial in humid climates because it keeps the soil from splashing onto the foliage along with soil-borne pathogens. Using lighter-colored materials helps maximize solar exposure.

Winter is often the death of lavender plants, so it's essential to choose a variety capable of surviving in your climate. Ample soil drainage will help avoid winterkill from sodden soils. Prune plants in the fall, which helps them to overwinter and encourages a profusion of fresh growth (and blooms) the following season. There are varieties of English lavender that can tolerate colder temperatures—'Hidcote,' 'Munstead,' and 'Royal Lavender' are a few of the lavenders that are hardy to zone 5.

PROBLEM INSECTS AND DISEASES: The potted herb can become infested by spider mites. Lavender is also affected by *Phytophthora* root rot, which starts with the foliage on a few stems wilting and then turning brown. Remove infected plants.

HARVESTING: Harvest the flowering stalks when the individual flowers begin to open, and bundle to dry. I prefer to harvest some leaves with the flowers and combine the two. If you'd like to go this route, cut the flowering stalks lower on the plant so there are leaves attached to the base of the stems. When dried, the leaves and flowers can be stripped from the stems and combined. The leaves can also be harvested earlier in the season and dried or prepared into medicine.

## Medicinal Properties

PART USED: Leaf and flower

MEDICINAL PREPARATIONS: Infusion, vinegar, tincture, poultice, compress, liniment, wash, infused oil, salve, condiment, and essential oil

TINCTURE RATIOS AND DOSAGE: Fresh (1:2 95%) or dry (1:5 70%); either preparation 2–3 ml three times a day

INFUSION RATIOS AND DOSAGE: Infusion of 1 to 2 teaspoons dried herb per 1 cup boiling water up to three times a day

ACTIONS: Nervine, hypnotic, analgesic, anti-inflammatory, antianxiety, antidepressant, antioxidant, antimicrobial, cholagogue, and carminative

ENERGETICS: Cooling and drying

## Medicinal Uses

The flavor of lavender tea is stronger than one might expect, being slightly bitter and astringent. A little goes a long way. Even though the herb helps promote relaxation, it has a stimulating quality, energetically, and can be helpful for releasing pent-up or "stuck" emotional states. If someone is brooding or just can't let something go, try a bit of lavender tea.

### NERVOUS SYSTEM

Lavender is a gentle sedative, alleviating anxiety, stress, depression, and insomnia. To help lift the spirits, try a tea of the herb combined with lemon balm, linden, and lemon verbena. Also see the Sunlight Breaking Through the Clouds tincture recipe on page 314. The herb is a friend to the grieving, along with the flowers of hawthorn, rose, and mimosa.

### DIGESTIVE SYSTEM

Lavender is slightly bitter and can help stoke the digestive fire and promote the release of bile and enzymes. Safe for children and elders, it eases intestinal gas and nausea, along with other gentle digestive herbs such as catnip, chamomile, and lemon balm.

### TOPICAL USE

A strong infusion of the flowers, combined with calendula, witch hazel, and chickweed, is made into a compress or bath to heal tears in the perineum from childbirth. Lavender-infused oil (the flowers and leaves steeped in an oil, such as jojoba or sesame oil) has a subtler aroma as compared to the essential oil but is a potent anti-inflammatory and soothing agent for bruises, sore joints, varicose veins, insect bites, and chafed skin.

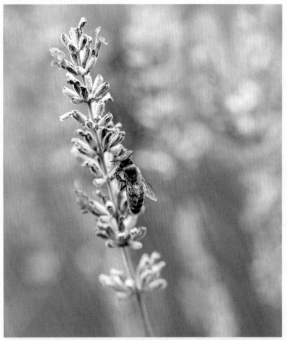

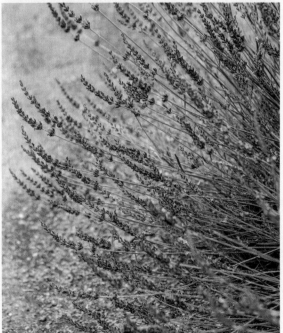

Lavender (*Lavandula angustifolia*) is popular with honeybees; lavender gracefully arches over garden pathways.

## Sunlight Breaking Through the Clouds Formula

This blend is helpful for depression, sadness, and grief. For optimal results, it should be taken daily. If you can't find mimosa tincture, substitute a tincture of rose petals or rosebuds.

MAKES 4 OUNCES

1 ounce lavender flower tincture (*Lavandula angustifolia*)

1 ounce St. John's wort flower tincture (*Hypericum perforatum* or *H. punctatum*)

1 ounce tulsi leaf and flower tincture (*Ocimum tenuiflorum*)

½ ounce lemon balm leaf and flower tincture (*Melissa officinalis*)

½ ounce mimosa flower or bark tincture (*Albizia julibrissin*)

Use fresh St. John's wort tincture. The other tinctures can be made from fresh or dried herbs. Combine all tinctures and store in a glass dispensing bottle. Dosage is 2 to 4 ml, three times a day. Note: St. John's wort shouldn't be combined with many pharmaceuticals because it increases the clearance of certain drugs through the liver. Do not take this formula if you're taking pharmaceutical medications for anxiety or depression. This blend is intended for mild to moderate depression and likely won't alleviate severe depression. Healing from mental illness requires a multifaceted and individualized approach, which may include talk therapy, nutritional strategies, pharmaceuticals, and exercise. (Herbs aren't always the answer.) Please seek a trusted mental health care provider, and seek immediate help if you are concerned that you might hurt yourself or others.

PRECAUTIONS: Rare incidences of contact dermatitis have occurred with the essential oil. Use cautiously with individuals with known mint-family sensitivities. Concerns about lavender essential oil having an estrogenic effect have been debunked. Use lavandin essential oil cautiously if taking pharmaceutical blood thinners.

LAVENDER ESSENTIAL OIL is used topically as an antimicrobial, anti-inflammatory, hypnotic, and anxiolytic. I keep a bottle of the essential oil on my nightstand and in my first aid kit, car, and travel bag. Lavender is one of the few essential oils that can be used topically without dilution (one to two drops only). Although extremely rare, some individuals react to the essential oil with allergic contact dermatitis. After cleaning and disinfecting scrapes and cuts, I use lavender as an all-purpose antimicrobial. It's also my go-to remedy for easing the itch and swelling of mosquito and chigger bites. Lavender can be applied topically on sunburn and on first-degree burns: add a couple of drops of the essential oil to a teaspoon of aloe vera gel (fresh, if possible) for a highly soothing home remedy. One to two drops each of lavender and peppermint essential oils can be diluted into a teaspoon of jojoba or coconut oil and rubbed into the temples for headaches. A couple drops on the pillow can help quiet a busy mind and promote deep sleep. Add a couple of drops of lavender essential oil, diluted in ½ cup of Epsom salts, into a bedtime bath for fussy children and adults.

## Culinary Uses

Lavender's bitter aromatics balance the sweetness of confections, which is why the herb is fancied in baked goods, like scones, cookies, and shortbread. A little goes a long way, so proceed tentatively, in small batches. Even then, the flavor isn't for everyone; some find the herb to be floral-cloying, soapy, or overly bitter. Lavender is an ingredient in the French herbal blend *herbes de Provence*, along with rosemary, thyme, basil, tarragon, marjoram, and other Mediterranean herbs.

# Lavender-Lemon Bundt Cake

YIELD: 1 (10-cup) Bundt cake or 2 (9-inch) loaves

### CAKE

10 ounces unsweetened coconut cream (see Note)

¼ cup (8 grams) dried lavender flower (*Lavandula angustifolia*)

4 teaspoons grated lemon zest (from 3 small lemons)

4 teaspoons lemon juice

5⅓ cups (620 grams) extra-fine almond flour

2 tablespoons plus 1 teaspoon (18 grams) coconut flour

2¼ teaspoons baking powder

1¼ teaspoons baking soda

¼ teaspoon salt

10 tablespoons (141 grams) unsalted butter, melted

1 cup (170 grams) lightly packed light brown sugar or coconut sugar

7 large eggs, at room temperature

Nonstick cooking spray

### RASPBERRY SUGAR DUSTING

2 tablespoons (10 grams) powdered freeze-dried raspberries (see Notes)

1 heaping tablespoon (10 grams) powdered sugar

*(ingredients continue)*

This cake is not only dense and moist but also ever so pretty. The flavor is elevated by the lavender and lemon, with the raspberry-sugar dusting and fresh berries lending a festive and light touch. Amber Brown, our resident recipe creator, and I modified her delectable grain-free cake recipe and dialed down the sweetness compared to most other cakes.

For the best results, weigh your ingredients. If you don't have a Bundt pan, you can bake this cake in two 9-inch loaf pans; the baking directions are the same.

1. In a small saucepan, heat the coconut cream until steaming but not yet bubbling. Turn off the heat, add the lavender flowers, and steep, covered, for 30 minutes.

2. Meanwhile, combine the lemon zest and juice in a small bowl; set aside.

3. In a medium bowl, whisk together the almond flour, coconut flour, baking powder, baking soda, and salt.

4. Preheat the oven to 350°F.

5. Strain the lavender cream through a fine mesh strainer or a straining cloth. Be sure to press out all the cream. Measure ¾ cup of the lavender-infused coconut cream and set aside. If you have extra cream, reserve it for tea.

6. In a large mixing bowl, use a whisk or mixer to beat the butter and brown sugar until creamy, fluffy, and well whipped, 4 to 5 minutes. Slowly add the eggs, lavender-infused coconut cream, and lemon juice and zest, beating until well incorporated, about 2 minutes. Working in batches and mixing by hand, fold the dry ingredients into the wet ingredients.

*(recipe continues)*

### TO SERVE

Fresh lavender flowering stalks

2 cups raspberries or seasonal berries

Whipped cream (optional)

**Notes:** For the powdered raspberries, start with ⅓ cup freeze-dried whole raspberries; grind to a powder in a food processor or spice grinder. Look for coconut cream in the baking or Asian food section of your grocery store. Alternatively, skim the thicker cream off a jar of full-fat coconut milk, reserving the coconut milk (thinner portion) for another use.

7. Spray a 10-cup Bundt pan with the cooking spray, taking care that the entire surface is coated (use a pastry brush, if necessary, to evenly coat the recesses of the pan). Spoon the batter into the pan, allowing it to fill the reliefs of the pan. Gently tap the pan on the counter a few times to remove air bubbles. Smooth the batter up the sides of the pan, so it's slightly higher on the sides than in the middle of the pan—this will help prevent doming as the cake rises.

8. Bake for 45 to 50 minutes, or until golden brown and a toothpick or knife inserted into the cake comes out clean and batter-free. Let the cake sit in the pan for 10 minutes to set. Shake the cake free from the edges of the Bundt pan before turning out onto a plate or cake stand. If the cake has domed during baking, you can trim it so it has a flat bottom. Allow to fully cool before serving.

9. Combine the raspberry powder and the powdered sugar in a small bowl.

10. To serve, surround the cake with berries and flowering lavender stalks. Using a sifter or tea strainer, sprinkle the raspberry sugar dusting over the berries and cake. Serve with whipped cream, if desired.

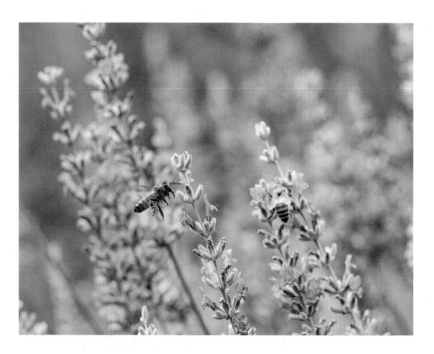

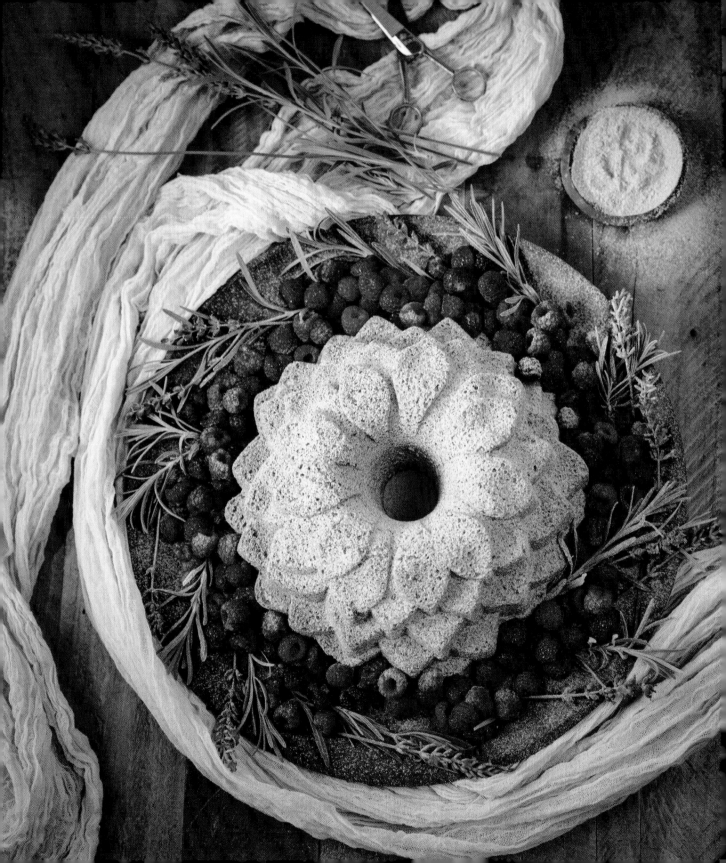

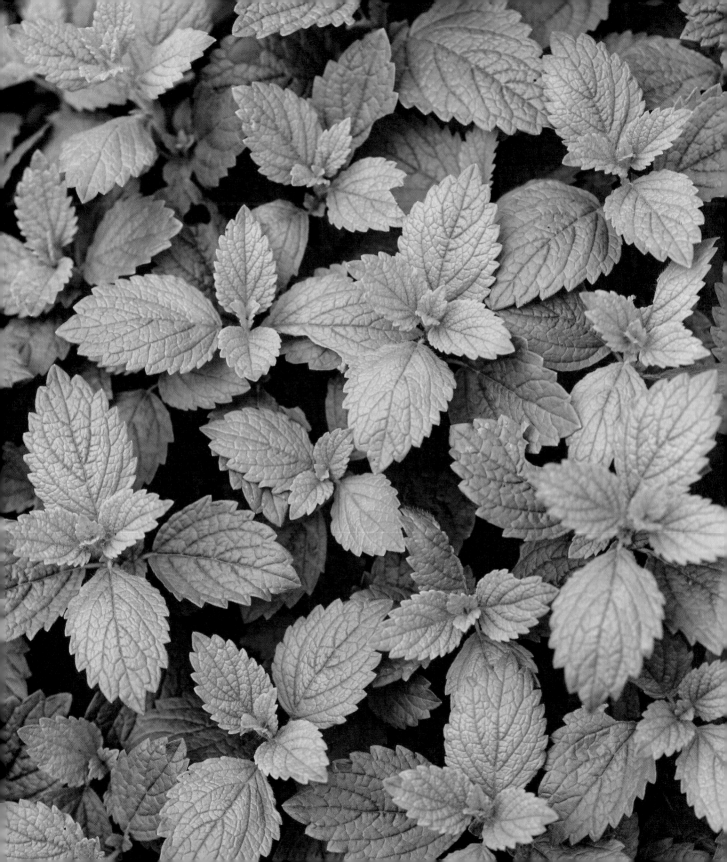

# LEMON BALM

SCIENTIFIC NAME: *Melissa officinalis*
LAMIACEAE, mint family
AKA: balm, melissa, sweet balm, common balm, balm mint

With its citrusy aroma and quilted lime-green leaves, lemon balm brightens our gardens and kitchens alike. This mint family medicinal is known as the "gladdening herb" for the uplifting qualities it brings to the spirit. Lemon balm is a pillar in the herb garden, amenable to human companionship and cultivation with its patient and easygoing nature. Children have a particular fondness for its sunny aroma and sour flavor. Bees are equally fond of the herb—so much so that the Greek word for bee, *melissa,* is another name for the plant. The origin of the word *balm* is similarly telling: it is derived from *balsam,* a plant or application with healing or restorative qualities. Lemon balm has long been thought to impart vitality and bestow longevity. Paracelsus, the Swiss alchemist, called the herb "the elixir of life."

Lemon balm is best known for its medicinal uses, namely as a digestive, nervine, and immune remedy, but it's equally at home as a culinary herb. The lemony-fresh leaves illuminate and elevate sorbets, ice cream, whipped cream, and compound butters. Come summertime, lemon balm is one of my favorites in herbal iced tea blends—it makes a splash in chilled pitchers with lemon verbena and mint. The plant is native to the Mediterranean and the Middle East but now grows throughout the globe.

Along with bees, lemon balm's blooms attract many small native pollinators, and it is considered a generalist nectary plant. The herb is also a classic companion—interspersed throughout the garden, it can help keep away problematic insects with its volatile compounds. Consider planting the clumping herb with low-growing medicinals and edibles, such as gotu kola, chickweed, and violet.

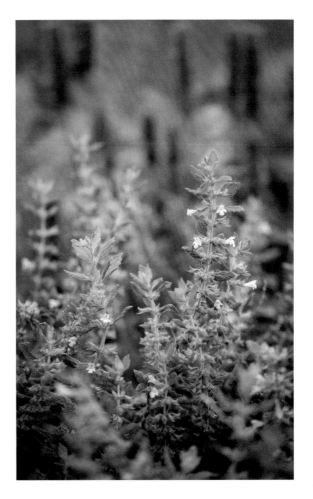

## Cultivation

ZONES: 4–10; full sun to partial shade

SOIL: pH 5–7.5; fertile soils with good drainage

SIZE: 1–2 feet tall; 1–2 feet wide

LIFESTYLE: Herbaceous perennial

PROPAGATION: Sow the seeds directly on the surface of the soil and lightly tamp in; seeds need light to germinate. A two-week stratification period will increase germination rates. Germination occurs in one to two weeks at 65–70°F. Roots can be divided into three or four divisions in the early spring or fall. Space plants 1½ feet apart.

SITING AND GARDEN CARE: It is scandalous to imagine an herb garden without lemon balm, considering its amicability and medicinal and culinary versatility. Cut back the flowering stems before they set seed or the plant will self-sow and become weedy. Mulch to keep dirt from splashing up on the leaves and spreading soil-borne diseases. If you live in a hot and humid climate, plant the herb in partial shade, and it will reward you with larger, more luscious leaves. If you live in a cooler region, lemon balm will grow buoyantly in full sun—its leaves may be smaller, but it will be highly aromatic. In the northern reaches of lemon balm's range, wet soils can kill the plants over the winter. Be sure to create ample drainage to prevent this.

PROBLEM INSECTS AND DISEASES: Lemon balm is generally carefree but can be affected by spider mites, powdery mildew, leaf spots, and rust.

HARVESTING: You can obtain several harvests by giving the plants a periodic haircut, leaving 6 inches of growth intact. Be careful not to pile up the harvest, as lemon balm is prone to oxidation and can turn an unsavory brown color. Hang in bundles or dry on screens. Lemon balm doesn't keep as long as other dried herbs. Let its aroma guide you in determining when your stored lemon balm is no longer potent. For culinary use, such as pesto, the tender new growth in the spring is ideal.

## Medicinal Properties

PART USED: Leaves and flowering tops

MEDICINAL PREPARATIONS: Infusion, tincture, vinegar, honey, oxymel, infused oil, salve, pesto, finishing salts, compound butter, and condiment

TINCTURE RATIOS AND DOSAGE: Fresh (1:2 95%) or dry (1:5 70%); either preparation 2–4 ml three times a day

INFUSION RATIOS AND DOSAGE: Infusion of 2 teaspoons to 1 tablespoon dried leaves per 1 cup boiling water three times a day

ACTIONS: Nervine, hypnotic, carminative, antiviral, antibacterial, antianxiety, antidepressant, antioxidant, and diaphoretic

ENERGETICS: Cooling and slightly drying

## Medicinal Uses

Lemon balm's gentle nature and pleasant taste and aroma make it a superb herb for adding to formulas to mask the flavor of bitter herbs and improve the overall flavor. It has long been used internally and topically to buoy the spirits and brighten the mind.

### NERVOUS SYSTEM

Lemon balm is both soothing and uplifting. Tea is the best form for its nervine qualities, as the herb's essential oils gently waft over the imbiber from the teacup. It is a gentle sedative, on par with mint, linden, and chamomile, and safe for children or those with chronic illness. Lemon balm assuages tension headaches, anxiety, insomnia, restlessness, and panic attacks. Combine it with milky oats, ashwagandha, and skullcap as a tonic herb for stress. Lemon balm, along with lavender and lemon verbena, is an ally for depression, especially seasonal affective disorder (SAD).

### DIGESTIVE SYSTEM

As a carminative, lemon balm soothes intestinal gas and bloating, especially when stress-related. Fennel, mint, and catnip are all fine companions for lemon balm in a digestive tea for all ages. When breastfeeding, you can sip on the tea to help calm restless babies and mollify colic: the herb's healing qualities pass into breast milk.

### ENDOCRINE SYSTEM

Lemon balm is used by herbalists to remedy mild hyperthyroidism, along with bugleweed and motherwort. It has demonstrated the ability to block thyroid-stimulating hormone (TSH) receptors and the binding of autoantibodies in Grave's disease using in vitro studies. (See the precautions below if you have hypothyroidism.)

### TOPICAL USES

The herb has long been used on wounds and insect bites to promote healing, most likely through its anti-inflammatory and antimicrobial qualities. Lemon balm and lavender play a starring role in the centuries-old herbal toner known as Queen of Hungary's Water. This garden cosmetic also features rose, calendula, rosemary, sage, elderflower, and comfrey infused in a base of vinegar or witch hazel extract. The fragrant elixir is an antioxidant and astringent toner—it is said to have kept the queen looking so sprightly that she attracted the attention of a suitor nearly 50 years her junior.

### ANTIMICROBIAL USES

Lemon balm essential oil has demonstrated antiviral, antifungal, and antibacterial properties. It can be used internally and topically for viral infections and appears to block viral replication in the body. The herb's topical antiviral activity against the herpes simplex virus (HSV) 1 and 2 has been demonstrated in a number of studies. One randomized, double-blind, placebo-controlled study demonstrated the efficacy of applying a concentrated lemon balm cream (70:1) on genital herpes (HSV-2) sores. Study participants applied the cream four times a day for five days and demonstrated a quicker recovery time, fewer symptoms, and less spreading of lesions.

## Lemony Tea Blend

This refreshing tea is uplifting and rejuvenating and can be enjoyed year-round as a pleasant beverage tea.

4 cups water

2 tablespoons dried lemon balm leaf and flower (*Melissa officinalis*)

2 tablespoons dried lemon verbena leaf (*Aloysia citrodora*)

1 tablespoon dried lemongrass leaf (*Cymbopogon citratus*)

In a small pot, bring the water to a boil. Turn off the heat, add the herbs, and infuse, covered, for 20 minutes. Strain, and enjoy warm or iced, garnished with lemon slices. Adults, drink up to three cups a day.

## Culinary Uses

Lemon balm leaves have a sour and aromatic minty flavor. Like citrus, lemon balm comfortably saddles up to sweet and savory dishes alike. Add the tender fresh leaves to finishing salts, herbal vinegars, compound butters, salsas, and pestos (see my recipe on page 173); or mince the leaves and add them to fruit salad, jam, cookies, scones, whipped cream, sorbet, or ice cream. In the summertime, add a few sprigs to a pitcher of water or a carafe of white wine and let infuse for one to two hours before enjoying. Not only is lemon balm a delightful culinary herb, it's also high in vitamins and minerals, such as calcium, magnesium, and potassium. Like other minty medicinals, its soothing qualities on the digestive tract carry over equally in food as well as in tea.

> **PRECAUTIONS:** The herb may lower thyroid levels; consult a medical practitioner and use cautiously in hypothyroidism and with thyroid hormone replacement.

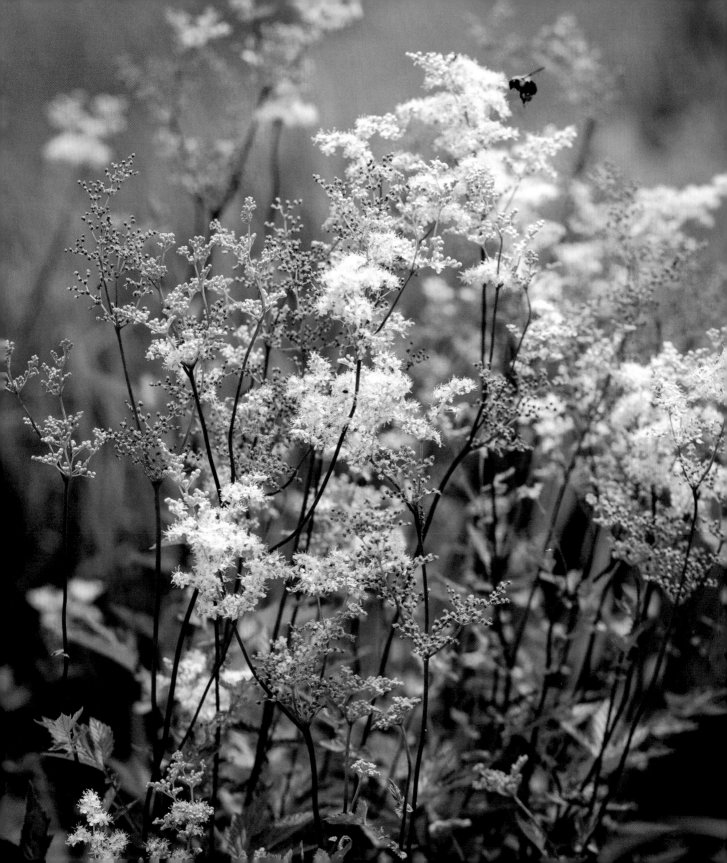

# MEADOWSWEET

SCIENTIFIC NAME: *Filipendula ulmaria*
ROSACEAE, rose family
AKA: queen of the meadow, dropwort, meadwort, meadsweet, lady of the meadow

With a creamy garland of billowy flowers reigning over ferny leaves, meadowsweet is rightly crowned "queen of the meadow." This herbaceous perennial favors moist soils and open ground yet is adaptable to a range of climates and garden sites. Native to wet meadows of Eurasia, the plant has naturalized in northeastern North America and is quite cold-hardy. The aromatic leaves and flowers taste of wintergreen tangled with black tea, with a bit of marshmallow thrown in. Meadowsweet is a traditional remedy for digestive and arthritic complaints and has long been used to flavor meads; hence its former name of "meadwort." Meadowsweet is a classical strewing herb. Back when most everyone had dirt floors and few windows, people strewed fragrant herbs about their domicile, releasing their pleasant aromas when they walked upon the fresh greenery. An added benefit was the deterrence of pests and pathogens.

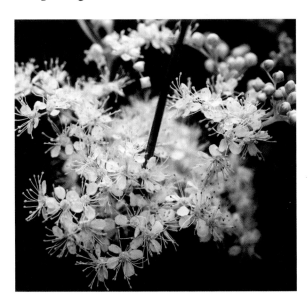

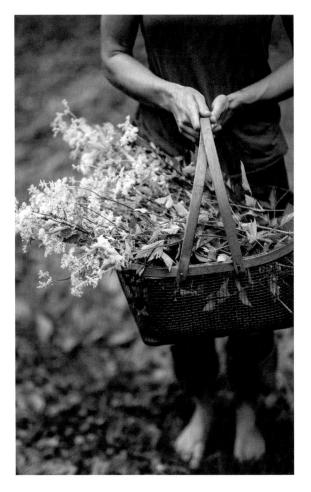

# Cultivation

ZONES: 3–8; full sun to partial shade

SOIL: pH 6–8 (7–7.5 optimal); moist, rich soil

SIZE: 3–4 feet tall; 2–3 feet wide

LIFESTYLE: Herbaceous perennial

PROPAGATION: Meadowsweet is much easier to grow from division than seed—any little piece of the root will take hold and grow a new plant. From one older plant, you can make at least 25 divisions. The seeds require a period of moist, warm stratification, followed by cold stratification, and finally a period of moderate temperatures to germinate. This can be accomplished by shallowly sowing the seeds in a flat or directly in the garden in the late summer and letting the elements work their magic. Alternatively, stratify the seeds in moist sand following the directions in the Herb Propagation Chart on page 108 and barely cover the seeds. Space plants 2 feet apart.

SITING AND GARDEN CARE: A wet meadow, streamside, or pond margin are perfect spots for meadowsweet. It will tolerate seasonal or intermittent flooding, but it won't tolerate constant standing water. If you haven't such a spot, try planting it in a low dip in the garden, mulch heavily, and irrigate during drought. If you live in a sultry climate, the herb will be happier with a little afternoon shade and a wet spot to dip its feet during the heat of the day. In cooler climates, meadowsweet will tolerate more sunshine and drier soils, and even regular garden soil will nurture the growth of beautiful, healthy plants. Alternatively, try growing it in a big container with a saucer underneath to keep in the moisture. Meadowsweet tolerates clayey soils, especially if amended with compost. If your soil is overly sandy, add clay and compost or aged manure to increase water retention. Several showy cultivars are sold: 'Flore Pleno', with lacey double flowers, and 'Aurea', with golden foliage. I would avoid using these for medicine. Other species of meadowsweet are similar looking, with closely

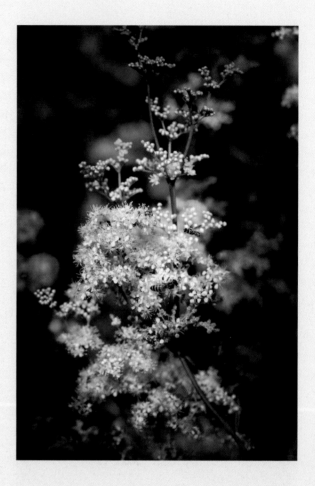

named cultivars, so make sure to check the scientific name when purchasing plants.

PROBLEM INSECTS AND DISEASES: Japanese beetles will leave their signature mark: lacy, skeletonized leaves. Powdery mildew and meadowsweet orange rust gall can also affect plants.

HARVESTING: Harvest meadowsweet when it's beginning to bloom by cutting the flowering stalks close to the base of the plant. Hang these longer stems in bundles, placing a cloth underneath to catch any blossoms that fall during the drying process. The plant will still have plenty of basal leaves left intact after harvesting the flowering stalk. Harvest a third to half of the basal leaves with garden scissors or pruning shears, and the plants will eventually send forth a flush of new leaves, which can be harvested a second time in the fall, before the first frost. After the flowering stems and basal leaves have dried, combine the two.

## Medicinal Properties

**PART USED:** Flowering herb (leaves and flowers)

**MEDICINAL PREPARATIONS:** Tea, tincture, vinegar, honey, oxymel, syrup, mead, elixir, cordial, and homemade soda

**TINCTURE RATIOS AND DOSAGE:** Fresh (1:2 95%) or dry (1:4 60%); either preparation 2–4 ml up to three times a day

**INFUSION RATIOS AND DOSAGE:** Infusion of 2 teaspoons to 1 tablespoon dried leaves per 1 cup boiling water up to three times a day

**ACTIONS:** Astringent, slightly demulcent, anti-inflammatory, antirheumatic, antiemetic, anodyne, antibacterial, diuretic, and diaphoretic

**ENERGETICS:** Slightly cooling and drying

## Medicinal Uses

The leaves and flowers have a pleasant wintergreen aroma and flavor and are used internally in tea or tincture form for inflammation, fevers, heartburn, and peptic ulcers. Most people, including finicky children, love the tasty tea. The wintergreen aroma and flavor are courtesy of the compound *methyl salicylate,* which is also found in a number of unrelated plants—wintergreen and certain birch trees, for example.

Meadowsweet contains a smorgasbord of salicylate compounds, including salicylic acid, methyl salicylate, salicin, and other related molecules. Most people associate the origins of aspirin with white willow, but the drug is actually named after meadowsweet, the first plant to yield isolated salicylates. In understanding how aspirin arrived at its name, it's helpful to remember that the older scientific name for meadowsweet was *Spirea.* (Add an *a* to *Spirea,* and voilà: *aspirin*!)

### DIGESTIVE SYSTEM

Owing to meadowsweet's anti-inflammatory, astringent, and demulcent qualities, it is used for inflammation in the gastrointestinal tract, including heartburn, peptic ulcers, inflammatory bowel disease (IBD), and nervous indigestion. It is one of my trusted remedies for heartburn, along with licorice, marshmallow, and calendula—see the recipe on page 326. It can be used concurrently with antibiotic therapy for peptic ulcers and offers its own antibacterial qualities against *Helicobacter pylori,* the bacteria associated with peptic ulcers. I have seen meadowsweet help nervous indigestion, especially in folks who react to stress with diarrhea and gastric pain. In this scenario, it can be combined with linden and chamomile, two gentle antianxiety herbs that also assuage nervous indigestion and gastrointestinal inflammation.

### MUSCULOSKELETAL SYSTEM

Meadowsweet is a classic remedy for arthritic conditions such as osteoarthritis, rheumatoid arthritis, and tendinitis. It can also be used for musculoskeletal injury and strain—combine it with skeletal muscle antispasmodics, such as black haw, skullcap, or valerian. The herb eases tension headaches stemming from musculoskeletal inflammation and tightness in the neck and shoulders.

### URINARY SYSTEM

British herbalists use meadowsweet as a mild urinary antimicrobial and diuretic for cystitis, edema (water retention), gout, and kidney problems.

## Gastrointestinal Inflammation Tea

This tasty tea blend is helpful for acid reflux and helps to reduce heartburn through the anti-inflammatory, astringent, and demulcent actions of the herbs. It's also soothing for sore throats and peptic ulcers. Please note that this blend is not appropriate for heartburn in pregnancy (instead, use slippery elm). Omit the licorice while nursing and in cases of edema, high blood pressure, or heart or kidney disease. If licorice is not advisable, use a DGL licorice (deglycyrrhizinated licorice) preparation (available at health food stores and many pharmacies) instead, and use the same proportions for the remaining herbs in the formula.

4 cups water

1½ tablespoons dried licorice root (*Glycyrrhiza glabra* or *G. uralensis*)

1 tablespoon dried marshmallow root (*Althaea officinalis*)

2 tablespoons dried meadowsweet leaf and flower (*Filipendula ulmaria*)

1 tablespoon dried calendula flower (*Calendula officinalis*)

In a small pot, combine the water, licorice root, and marshmallow root. Simmer for 20 minutes, turn off the heat, and add the meadowsweet and calendula. Infuse, covered, for 20 minutes, and strain. Adults, drink up to three cups a day.

## Minty Meadow Tea

This tea blend is a helpful digestion aid and reduces gassiness and bloating. It is kid-friendly—both tasty and gentle. The chamomile and mint are mild sedatives, appropriate for children. The tea blend can be prepared as a sleepy bedtime blend or enjoyed as an after-dinner-prebath ritual.

1¼ cups water

1 teaspoon dried peppermint or spearmint leaf (*Mentha* spp.)

½ teaspoon dried chamomile flower (*Matricaria recutita*)

½ teaspoon dried meadowsweet leaf and flower (*Filipendula ulmaria*)

Bring the water to a boil. Turn off the heat, add the herbs, and cover for 20 minutes. Strain and drink warm. Adults, drink up to three cups a day. See page 133 for calculating dosage for children.

## Culinary Uses

I like to combine meadowsweet with sassafras root, black birch bark, and a touch of cloves to make root beer–flavored mead and naturally fermented sodas. To make a homemade root beer soda, prepare an herbal simple syrup from those same herbs and add sparkling water. Goldenrod and meadowsweet also make a lovely pairing in mead or as a naturally fermented homemade soda.

> PRECAUTIONS: Use cautiously with people who have aspirin or salicylate sensitivity. The herb can be too drying for tonic use in individuals with a dry constitution. Take separately from iron supplements (meadowsweet will decrease the absorption of iron). Avoid with blood thinners or monitor coagulation values under the care of a cardiologist (the evidence for meadowsweet's effect on coagulation is inconclusive).

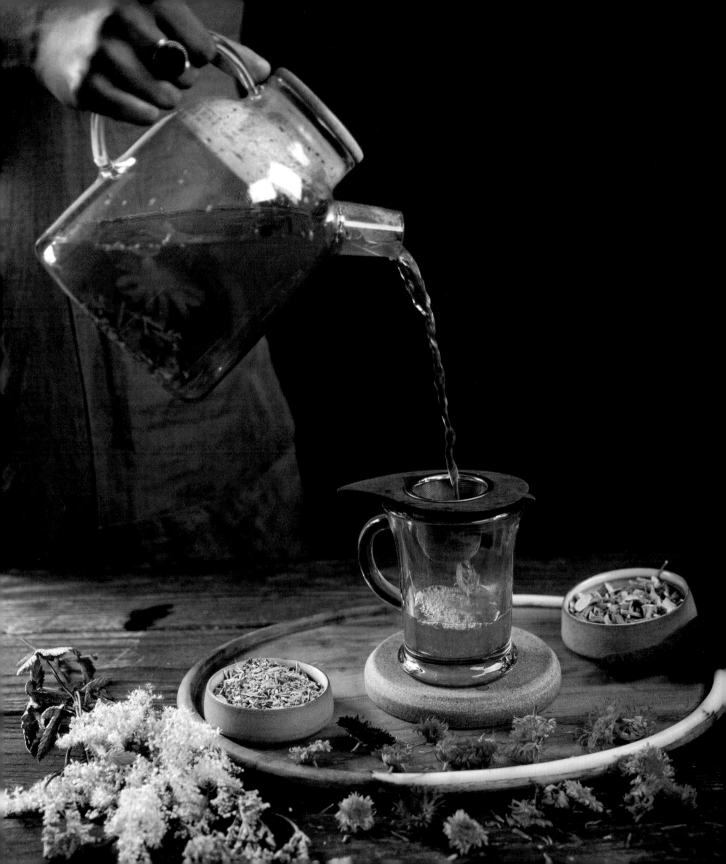

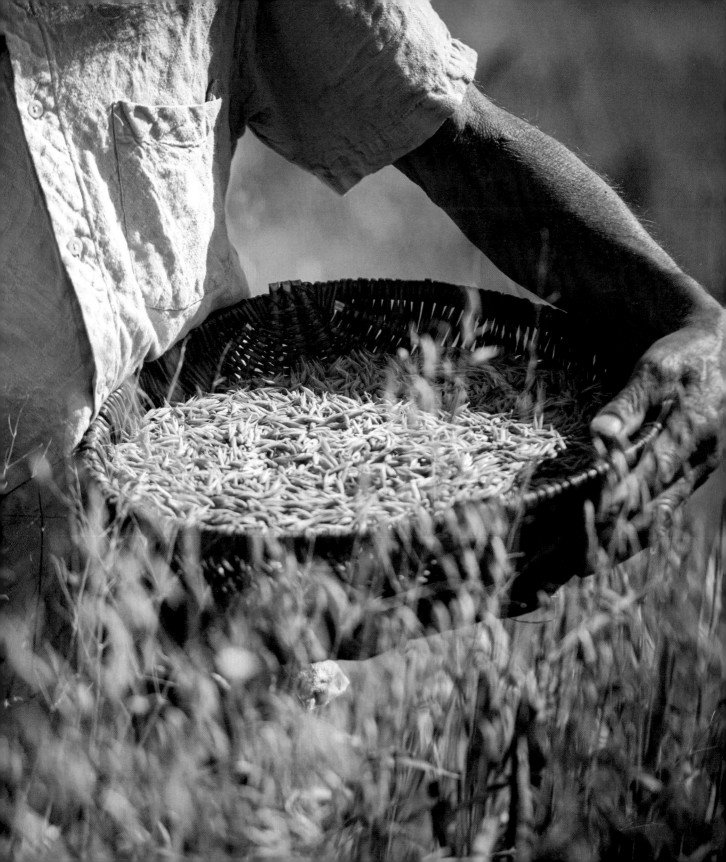

# MILKY OATS

SCIENTIFIC NAME: *Avena sativa*
POACEAE, grass family

Imagine you are in a small vessel held aloft by a billowing sea of grass, swishing peacefully with a gentle afternoon breeze, illuminated with the golden light of the setting sun. This is the calm and restorative energy that oats impart. Best known as a food crop, oats are commonly eaten as a grain, but they are also a medicinal herb and a cover crop, grown for their rapid growth and vigor. Native to Europe, oats have been in cultivation for over 2,000 years; today, they are grown around the globe. In fact, humans and oats have become so intertwined that the plant now solely exists by our side—it is only found in cultivation (or thereabouts) and no longer grows in the wild.

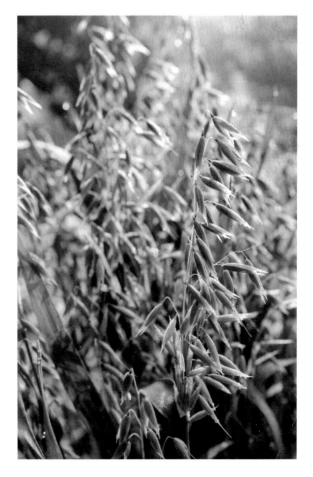

This grassy herbal companion provides three distinct remedies, each with its own medicinal use. Oatmeal (the pressed seeds of oats) is a highly medicinal food, rich in minerals and soothing soluble fiber. A familiar first aid remedy, oats are prepared in baths and poultices to soothe inflamed and irritated skin. Milky oats, the unripe "milky" seeds, are a nourishing tonic for the nervous system, assuaging anxiety and insomnia. Oatstraw, the plant's leaves and stem, is rich in minerals and provides gentle support to the nerves. We tend to think of oats as being relegated to the farm, but they're actually an easy and practical herb to grow in the home garden, especially if your primary goal is to harvest milky oats and oatstraw.

## Cultivation

ZONES: 3–10; full sun

SOIL: pH 5.5–7; well-drained fertile soil is preferable but will tolerate sandy and clayey soils

SIZE: 3 to 4 feet tall; 6 inches wide

LIFESTYLE: Annual

PROPAGATION: Sow oats directly in the field or garden in the spring or early fall (see the notes below). Purchase oat seed in bulk quantities from organic vegetable seed companies; regular oat seed is fine for milky oats harvest (no special medicinal variety exists). Plant oats two weeks before the *average* date of the last freeze in the spring (not the same as the absolute last possible date of freezing). When planting oats, I make long furrows with the edge of a hoe and sow the seed densely approximately 2 to 3 inches apart and ½ inch deep. You can alternate rows with a leguminous cover crop (see the notes below). Cover the seed with soil and keep moist until germination, which occurs in 7 to 10 days when the soil is warm. For larger-scale plantings, use a handheld or push broadcast spreader, and then cover the seed using a hard rake. Sow at the rate of 3 to 4 pounds per 1,000 square feet or 40 pounds per quarter acre.

SITING AND GARDEN CARE: Even if you have a modest-sized garden, you can still grow oats medicinally; a small patch is all that is needed to make a large quantity of medicine. Oats aren't especially finicky about where they grow; however, they don't appreciate waterlogged soils and instead prefer fertile soils with good tilth. The grass needs a fair amount of nitrogen—gardeners can plant it with a bean family companion to help deliver this nitrogen. Consider growing it with red clover; oats grow taller quickly, offering structural support for their slow-dancing partner. This herbal duo helps enrich our soil and, as a bonus, we reap three harvests: milky oats, oatstraw, and red clover blossoms.

The grass is sometimes sown in the fall as a cover crop in temperate climates (zone 7 and colder) and "winter killed." You'll reap the benefits of oats as a cover crop—biomass production and reduction of soil erosion—but for those of us in colder climates, fall-sown oats won't yield the medicinal seed heads. In warmer climates (zone 8 and warmer), oats can be fall-sown for a spring milky oats harvest.

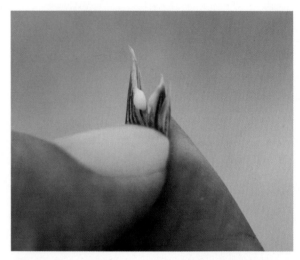

Close-up of oats at the perfect stage for "milky oats"; note the white milk and the seed head taking on a brown tinge as it matures

PROBLEM INSECTS AND DISEASES: Wild turkeys and other birds can eat the seed from the field. The plant is typically free of disease and pest problems in the garden setting but can be susceptible to some rusts and ergot.

HARVESTING: Milky oats are ready to harvest two to three months after planting. The timing of the milky oats harvest can be a little confusing to beginners, but if you understand the plant's reproductive cycle, it becomes clear. The unripe seed heads (milky oats) are harvested from the plant after flowering but before the seeds are fully mature and turn hard. Press a fingernail into the ripening seed, and you'll express a milky substance—this is the marker that it is time to harvest. If you see little yellow structures poking out instead of milk, the plants are still flowering and aren't ready for harvest. If your fingernail meets with a hard seed that doesn't exude milk, it is past its prime. On any given flowering stalk (technically, a panicle), you'll have individual seed heads at varying stages of maturity. You're looking for the narrow window—lasting less than a week—when most of the seed heads are prime for picking. The seed heads should still be green but beginning to take on a tan-yellowish hue.

Harvest when most of the seeds are plump yet immature, pliable, and exuding milk. At this point, strip the milky oats directly from the plants in the field by pulling the seed heads off the stalks into baskets. This goes quickly and is supremely satisfying. If you're stripping a large quantity of tops, you'll want to wear gloves. After stripping the seed heads, you'll be left with the stalks and leaves, which are collectively called "oatstraw." Leave the oatstraw behind to enrich and stabilize the soil, or harvest it with a scythe or long hedge shears.

Process the milky oats into tincture immediately, or dry them in open baskets or screens with good airflow, "schluffling," or tousling daily. Dry the seed thoroughly, or it will spoil upon packaging or jarring. Dry the oatstraw on large screens, and chop into smaller pieces when dry for storage.

## Medicinal Properties

**PART USED/MEDICINAL PREPARATIONS:** *Oat seed:* cooked grain, poultice, soak, and bath. *Oatstraw:* infusion, broth, and vinegar. *Milky oats:* fresh tincture made with alcohol or vinegar

**TINCTURE RATIOS AND DOSAGE:** Fresh milky oat tops (1:2 95%) ½ to 1 teaspoon (3–5 ml) three times a day

**TEA RATIOS AND DOSAGE:**

- Oatstraw: Infusion of 2 teaspoons dried leaves and stem in 1 cup boiling water up to three times a day
- Milky oats: Infusion of 1 tablespoon dried milky tops in 1 cup boiling water three times a day

**VINEGAR DOSAGE:**

- Oatstraw or milky oats, blended: 1 teaspoon (5 ml) up to three times a day

**ACTIONS:**

- Oat seed: Demulcent, emollient, prebiotic, bulk laxative, anti-inflammatory, and cholesterol-lowering
- Oatstraw: Nutritive tonic and mild nervine
- Milky oats: Nervine restorative and antianxiety

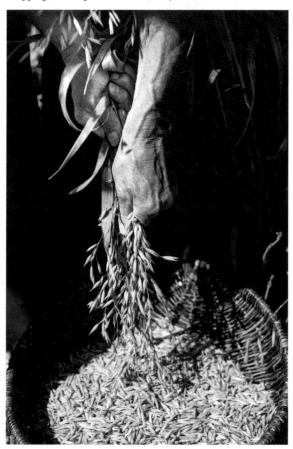

Stripping the unripe seed heads (milky oats) from the stalks

ENERGETICS:

- Oat seed (oatmeal and oat groats) is moistening and slightly warming.
- Oatstraw and milky oats are fairly neutral, energetically.

Milky oats are prepared almost exclusively as a fresh tincture; the unripe seeds are blended with alcohol or vinegar. Use a glass jar blender (not a plastic one) and fully blend to incorporate the milk (technically, liquid endosperm) from the unripe seeds into the solvent. If using alcohol, it will take on an electric lime-green color. Herbalists don't use the dried seed heads for tincturing because they aren't considered to be as potent at that stage. Fresh milky oats vinegar should be refrigerated and used within the year. You'll notice I list higher doses for oats than I use with other medicinals—it's my experience that milky oats are more effective at higher doses.

## Medicinal Uses

Milky oats are beloved among herbalists as a nervine tonic to promote emotional resiliency, easing anxiety, exhaustion, stress, and chronic insomnia. Milky oats are one of the top herbs I recommend, as they're incredibly safe and gentle and deeply nourishing to the spirit. Oatstraw, made from the stem and leaves of the plant, is primarily used as a nutritive tonic. In a similar fashion to milky oats, oatstraw is also a gentle tonic nervine; it can be taken as a remedy to support equanimity, and is especially helpful for people who feel frazzled, jumpy, or easily overwhelmed. However, it's substantially milder in action than milky oats.

### NERVOUS SYSTEM

Most herbal nervines are gentle sedatives, but milky oats act a little differently, being restorative and rejuvenating while simultaneously promoting calmness. For instance, it can be helpful for insomnia that stems from anxiety or depression, but it is taken throughout the day

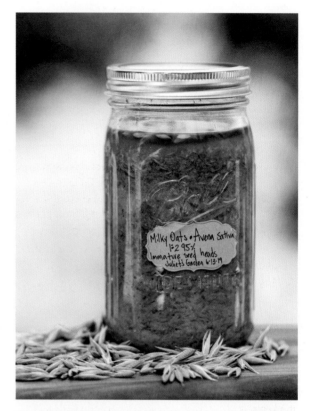

Freshly blended tincture of milky oats

rather than at bedtime. It's not contraindicated to take the herb before sleeping, but the daytime use addresses the underlying emotional issues that are affecting sleep. In a similar capacity, milky oats often find themselves in herbal aphrodisiac formulas. The herb isn't rousing per se; instead, it promotes relaxation and ease. Stress is a buzz killer for the amorous; feeling comfortable and safe fosters intimacy.

I combine milky oats with adaptogens such as tulsi, reishi, and gotu kola to calm stress and anxiety on a deeper level. Antianxiety herbs like motherwort and vervain can also be added to tonic formulas. Vervain and milky oats are helpful remedies for people who easily "lash out" when they're feeling depleted or overwhelmed. Milky oats, along with skullcap, help support people recovering from an addictive relationship with alcohol, tobacco, painkillers, drugs, or other addictive behaviors. The herb bolsters emotional resiliency and dulls the sharpness of withdrawal to an extent. If a person needs to avoid alcohol, as is often the case in recovery, milky oats can be taken as an infusion or as a vinegar-based tincture.

### NUTRITIVE TONIC

Oatstraw is high in minerals—notably iron, calcium, silica, zinc, phosphorus, and magnesium. Infusions and vinegars are the best way to extract the minerals. (See the Resilience Vinegar for Strong Bones and Teeth recipe on page 187.) The flavor of oatstraw tea is pleasant, somewhat like cow's milk. Combine oatstraw with other high-mineral herbs, such as nettles, violet, chickweed, alfalfa, and red clover, for a mineral-rich herbal infusion.

### TOPICAL USES

Oatmeal is a classic home remedy for a number of first aid situations and can be prepared into a poultice, compress, or bath to soothe hot, inflamed skin conditions. It's a classic topical first aid for bug bites, sunburn, and chicken pox.

## Relaxation and Clarity Tea

This tea blend is helpful for promoting relaxation throughout the day, as the herbs aren't sedating and, instead, typically increase alertness.

4 cups water

¼ cup dried milky oats (*Avena sativa*)

2 tablespoons dried tulsi leaf and flower (*Ocimum tenuiflorum*)

1½ tablespoons dried gotu kola leaf (*Centella asiatica*)

1 tablespoon dried lemon balm leaf (*Melissa officinalis*)

In a small pot, bring the water to boil. Add the herbs, turn off the heat, and infuse, covered, for 20 minutes, then strain. Adults, drink one to three cups daily as needed.

## Mineral-Rich Herbal Infusion

This tea is rich in minerals, encouraging strong bones and healthy functioning of the nervous and muscular systems. Add marshmallow for those who have a drier constitution, as it's helpful for offsetting the drying qualities of the stinging nettles.

4 cups water

3 tablespoons dried lemon verbena leaf (*Aloysia citrodora*)

2 tablespoons dried oatstraw leaf and stem (*Avena sativa*)

2 tablespoons dried nettles leaf (*Urtica dioica*)

1 tablespoon dried chickweed leaf (*Stellaria media*)

1 tablespoon dried violet leaf (*Viola sororia* or *V. odorata*)

½ tablespoon dried marshmallow root (*Althaea officinalis*); optional

1 teaspoon dried dandelion leaf (*Taraxacum officinale*)

In a small pot, bring the water to boil. Add the herbs, turn off the heat, and infuse, covered, for 30 minutes, then strain. Adults, drink one to three cups daily as needed.

## Culinary Uses

Being easy to digest, oatmeal, oat groats (the hulled oat kernels), and oat flour are helpful for soothing digestive upsets and the gastrointestinal tract. The soluble fiber in oats escorts extra cholesterol from the body.

> PRECAUTIONS: Although they don't contain gluten, oats do contain the molecule avenin, which is similar in structure and has caused rare reactions in especially sensitive individuals with celiac disease. Some people with celiac disease react to commercial oats because they are often cross-contaminated with wheat and barley. If you can tolerate certified gluten-free oats, then consuming milky oats or oatstraw (especially if grown and processed on an herb farm) likely won't be a problem.

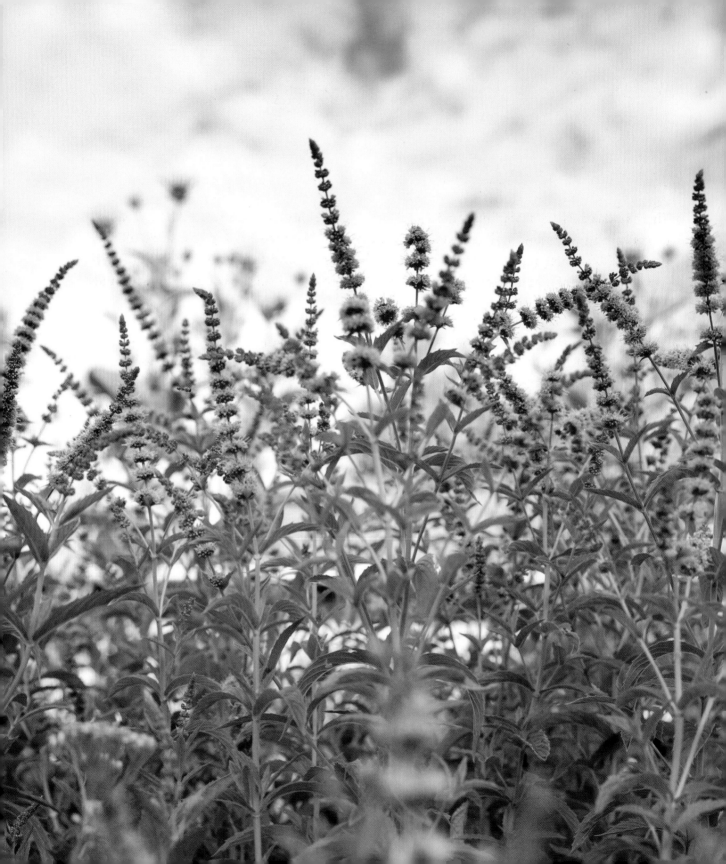

# MINT

## PEPPERMINT, SPEARMINT & OTHER GARDEN MINTS

**SCIENTIFIC NAME:** *Mentha spicata, Mentha* x *piperita, Mentha aquatica, Mentha suaveolens,* and *Mentha* x *gracilis*
**LAMIACEAE,** mint family

There's a dazzling array of mints you might invite into the garden. The species in the *Mentha* genus have been crossed and recrossed for centuries by plant breeders and chance, resulting in over 2,000 named mint varieties. The near-infinite configuration of essential oils has resulted in a cornucopia of scents, likened to apples, ginger, pineapples, lime, coconut, grapefruit, and even chocolate.

The garden mints can all be used medicinally. They are practically interchangeable in their uses, even if they vary in their essential oil content and aroma. Peppermint, spearmint, chocolate mint, lime mint, orange mint, and apple mint are all used similarly for medicine. In contrast, pennyroyal (*Mentha pulegium*) may be in the same genus as the garden mints, but it's in a league of its own: its potent essential oil content makes it a traditional herb for bringing on the menses and repelling insects. However, taken internally, pennyroyal essential oil has proven deadly. Consequently, I am not including pennyroyal in this discussion on mint's medicinal uses. Some of the wild mints have an edge as well, so I won't be generalizing about the entire mint tribe and will only stick to the familiar garden mints mentioned above. Mint has been used throughout the world to sharpen the mind, invigorate the senses, and heighten sexual desire. The herb is also a household remedy for indigestion, headaches, fevers, and sinus congestion.

Mint is an herb to grow and know, even for the brownest of thumbs. Spearmint (*Mentha spicata*) is the most versatile in the bunch as a culinary herb, and its flavor is beloved and familiar. 'Kentucky Colonel' is a common spearmint variety sold by herb growers, and it grows wild throughout the southwestern United States. and Central America. It's one of my personal favorites for herbal iced teas. Apple mint and pineapple mint (*Mentha suaveolens*) are old-timey garden mints—the variegated form with its snow-white leaves makes a bold splash in the landscape.

Peppermint (*Mentha* x *piperita*), a cross between spearmint and water mint (*Mentha aquatica*), has a refreshingly icy flavor. 'Chocolate Mint' is a variety of peppermint with chocolaty undertones. 'Grapefruit Mint' is another peppermint cultivar. Peppermint is especially decongesting and warming, with its high content of menthol, and is a fine mint to have on hand for colds and flu. Water mint, also called bergamot mint, eau de cologne mint, or orange mint, has egg-shaped leaves and rounded tufts of blooms at the tip of its stem. 'Lime Mint' is my darling among the tribe—I adore the confluence of citrusy and minty scents. It originated as a chance seedling at a breeding facility in Oregon and is thought to have mostly genes from *Mentha aquatica*.

Spearmint in bloom (*Mentha spicata*) at the Robison Herb Gardens at the Cornell Plantations

## Cultivation

ZONES: 3–9 (varies by species); full sun to light shade

SOIL: pH 5.5–7.5; moist, fertile, well-drained soil is optimal but will grow in many soils

SIZE: 1–3 feet tall; indefinitely wide

LIFESTYLE: Creeping herbaceous perennial

PROPAGATION: Unless the mint is a wild species, it needs to be propagated asexually by root divisions or stem cuttings. The seeds will not come up true to type, and you'll end up with a mutt-mint of questionable aroma (it won't smell like its parents). Mint is one of the easiest plants to divide and transplant—any piece of the stolon (the running, underground stem) with roots can be divided. Space plants 1 to 2 feet apart.

SITING AND GARDEN CARE: Mint is the best herb for beginner gardeners and a prime suspect for children's gardens. Just know you'll need to curtail the herb's wayfaring tendencies or it will take over the garden. Every spring, we pull back the runners that have invaded neighboring plants and share the waifs with friends. Alternatively, plant mints in large containers or install a rhizome barrier to keep them in check. The flowers beguile an array of pollinators: miniature wasps, flower flies, butterflies, honeybees, solitary bees, and bumblebees.

Curiously, the aroma of garden mints can change with time—after a few years, they might not smell the same as when you initially planted them. This is not due to hybridizing with neighbors, but perhaps is mediated by mycorrhizal relationships or changing soil conditions or pest pressures. If you end up with a smell or flavor not to your liking, you may need to start over with new plants.

PROBLEM INSECTS AND DISEASES: Mints are generally carefree but are susceptible to several fungal diseases, including leaf spot, powdery mildew, rust, wilt, and stem rot. Mulch the plants to prevent soil from splashing up on the leaves. Spider mites, whiteflies, and aphids can also be an issue.

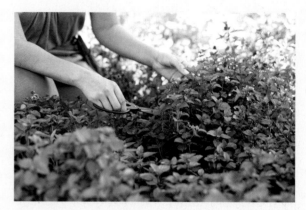

Harvesting mint with the haircut method

HARVESTING: Harvest the flowering stems when the plants are just beginning to bloom, and hang in bundles to dry. This will yield the highest concentration of essential oils and the most potent medicine. For culinary use, the fresh sprigs are the most luscious and often milder in flavor. The aroma and flavor of mints evolve throughout the day and the season; smell them over the months to see which stage you like best. For example, some herbalists prefer the sweeter, milder taste of spring-harvested peppermint to the summer harvest, which is higher in pungent essential oils. If you harvest before flowering, use garden scissors to give the plants a haircut; dry the clippings in baskets or on screens, or use for medicine-making projects as soon as possible, before the plants lose their valuable aromatics.

## Medicinal Properties

PART USED: Primarily the leaves but also the flowering stems

MEDICINAL PREPARATIONS: Infusion, vinegar, honey, oxymel, liniment, compress, poultice, soak, and condiment

TINCTURE RATIOS AND DOSAGE: Fresh (1:2 95%) or dry (1:4 65%); either preparation 1–2 ml up to three times a day

**TEA RATIOS AND DOSAGE:** Infusion of 1 to 2 teaspoons of the dried leaf per 1 cup water up to three times a day

**ACTIONS:** Carminative, nervine, diaphoretic, antimicrobial, decongestant, antiemetic, and anodyne

**ENERGETICS:** Cooling and drying

## Medicinal Uses

Keewaydinoquay Peschel, Anishinaabe herbalist and ethnobotanist, translated her people's name for the herb as "to rise-up or open-up" or "the opener-upper," referring to mint's ability to open up all of a person's senses.

### DIGESTIVE USES

Mint is a classic herb for relieving intestinal gas and bloating, as well as nausea stemming from motion sickness, migraines, or morning sickness. To soothe colicky babies, you can sip on the tea when breastfeeding.

### RESPIRATORY SYSTEM

With decongestant properties, the herb helps clear the sinuses in colds and flu, seasonal allergies, and sinus infections. Peppermint's high menthol content makes it a fine choice here. When drunk as a hot tea, mint is a diaphoretic and can help break a fever. For sore throats, a warm gargle of garden sage and mint is soothing and antimicrobial. Mint, along with thyme and bee balm, makes an excellent steam inhalation for clearing the sinuses and lungs of excess mucus.

### NERVOUS SYSTEM

Mint helps with concentration and focus, especially when combined with rosemary, gotu kola, and tulsi in tea or tincture form. It's also helpful as a mild pain reliever for headaches or menstrual cramps, particularly when the discomfort is accompanied by nausea. Combine it with stronger anodynes like skullcap, vervain, or California poppy.

## Topical Uses

With its anti-inflammatory and antimicrobial qualities, mint is applied as a poultice or compress to inflamed joints and skin afflictions, like insect bites, cuts, and scrapes. It can help quiet itchy conditions. The late herbalist Juliette de Bairacli Levy recommended a vinegar-based liniment for headaches in her *Common Herbs for Natural Health*: Crush fresh mint leaves, heat gently, and then soak overnight in vinegar. Soak a cloth in the cool mint vinegar, and apply to the forehead.

## Culinary Uses

Mint balances spicy dishes with its cooling and refreshing flavor. Worldwide, spearmint is the most popular mint for culinary use, but you might play around with different varieties in your cuisine. I find the citrusy mints to be mild and invigorating and thus bring them into the kitchen as often as spearmint. Minced mint leaves can be added to cucumber salad or sprinkled into yogurt as an accompaniment to lively Indian dishes. Spearmint brightens fruit salads, whipped cream, sorbet, and ice cream. Mint and parsley team up with the likes of lemon, garlic, and olive oil in the Mediterranean herb salad tabbouleh. Mint Chutney is a classic condiment—see the recipe on page 338. Elegant sprigs of flowering mint can adorn and flavor tall glasses of iced herbal teas, mocktails, and cocktails. Combined with other reviving herbs, such as lemon balm, hibiscus, lemon verbena, and hibiscus, mint iced tea cools the body and enlivens the senses on languid summer days. And I would be remiss if I failed to mention the mojito, the Cuban cocktail featuring rum, lime juice, sugar, and spearmint.

> **PRECAUTIONS:** Mint can sometimes aggravate heartburn and irritate ulcers or cause inflammation in the gastrointestinal tract.

# Mint Chutney

YIELD: 1¼ cups

1½ cups (60 grams) packed fresh cilantro leaves and tender stems

1 cup (30 grams) packed fresh mint leaves

½ cup plain yogurt (dairy or plant-based)

½ medium white onion, coarsely chopped

1 tablespoon fresh lime juice

1 small serrano pepper, seeds intact, or substitute jalapeño

¾ teaspoon sea salt

½ teaspoon sugar (optional)

If you're a card-carrying cilantro-hater, you might just turn over a new leaf with this classic Indian condiment. The mint and cilantro perform a culinary duet, their flavors melding into a singular entity. Spearmint is the classic mint in this sauce, but you can use any mint variety; my personal favorite is lime mint. Adjust the serrano pepper to your heat preference.

Enjoy mint chutney as a dip with chips or place alongside hummus in a crudité and charcuterie board. This versatile green sauce can jazz up salads, grilled vegetables, sandwiches, or wraps. And it's no surprise that mint chutney is right at home served alongside traditional Indian dishes, making a fine companion to rich and spicy samosas, sweet and chewy flatbreads, and crispy papadums.

Combine all the ingredients in a food processor and blend until uniform. Store any excess in the refrigerator for up to five days.

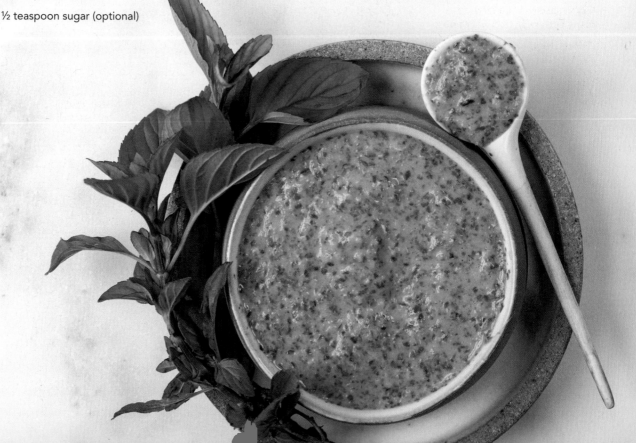

# Minty Sunrise Iced Tea

YIELD: 1 gallon

1½ quarts water

⅓ cup (8 grams) dried hibiscus flower (*Hibiscus sabdariffa*)

¼ cup (4 grams) dried spearmint leaf (*Mentha spicata*)

¼ cup (4 grams) dried lemon verbena leaf (*Aloysia citrodora*)

3 tablespoons (5 grams) dried calendula flower (*Calendula officinalis*)

3 tablespoons (3 grams) dried lemon balm leaf (*Melissa officinalis*)

1 tablespoon (1 gram) dried rose petals or buds (*Rosa* spp.)

Honey, stevia, or sugar, to taste (optional)

1 to 2 quarts ice, for serving

Mint sprigs, for serving

Here is a refreshing minty summertime iced tea with sour undertones from the hibiscus, lemon balm, and lemon verbena. Rose and calendula brighten the mix with a floral touch. This recipe calls for dried herbs, but if you have them growing fresh, you can sub them in, using twice the amount of fresh herbs to dry herbs.

In a large pot, bring the water to a boil, then turn off the heat, add all the herbs, and steep, covered, for 20 minutes. Strain out and discard the herbs. If desired, sweeten the tea with honey, stevia, or sugar. In a pitcher, combine the strained tea with ice and cold water to bring the volume up to about 1 gallon. Serve in ice-filled cups garnished with mint sprigs.

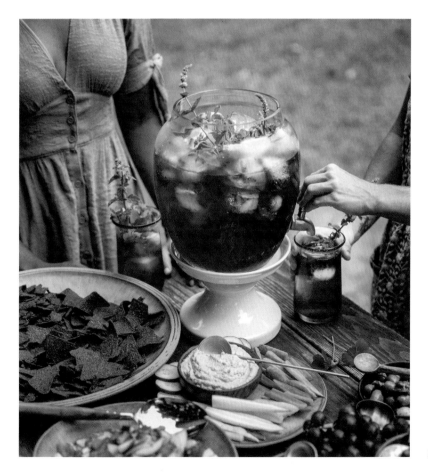

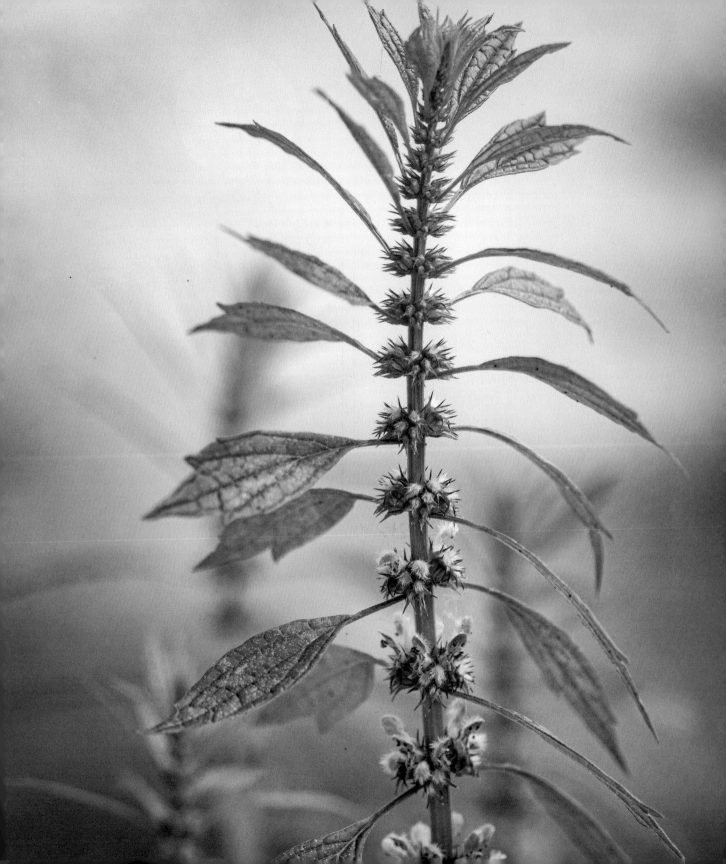

# MOTHERWORT

SCIENTIFIC NAME: *Leonurus cardiaca*
LAMIACEAE, mint family
AKA: lion's ear, lion's tail

With a bitter brew made from prickly parts, motherwort calms prickly personalities. The mint-family herb is a potent remedy for anxiety, stress, ire, and irritability. As an ancient ally for childbirth, postpartum, and menstrual cramps, it has more than earned its illustrious name "herb for mothers." The Chinese use Asian motherwort (*Leonurus japonicus*) similarly; the Pinyin name for the herb is *yi mu cao*, which translates to "benefit mother herb." Motherwort's scientific name, *Leonurus cardiaca*, also has a tale. *Leonurus* signifies "lion's tail" in Greek and refers to the flowering stalk's resemblance to the tufted tip of a lion's tail. (The name *lion's tail* is also used for several species in the *Leonotis* genus that aren't used like motherwort.) The species name *cardiaca* refers to motherwort's calmative effects on the heart.

The plant is a short-lived perennial, native to Eurasia, with extreme garden mettle—even the brownest of thumbs will have good fortune growing motherwort. It produces copious offspring and can easily circulate throughout the landscape if measures aren't taken to check its impishness. Now found throughout the temperate world, the herb grows in fields, along roadsides, in old home sites, and in vacant city lots, forming colonies that can persist for centuries.

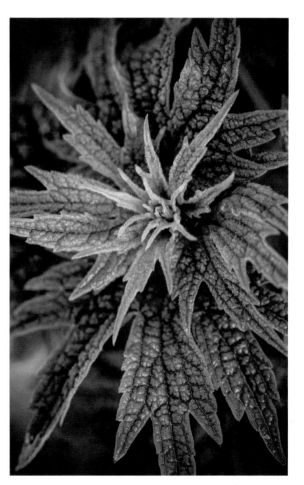

Motherwort's lobed leaves are textured from its rich network of veins

## Cultivation

**ZONES:** 3–8; full sun to partial shade

**SOIL:** pH 6.5–8 (pH 7.5 is ideal); tolerates a wide range of soil types but prefers loose, well-drained, fertile soil that is slightly alkaline

**SIZE:** 2–4 feet tall; 1–2 feet wide

**LIFESTYLE:** Herbaceous perennial

**PROPAGATION:** Stratify the seeds for two weeks before sowing to achieve higher germination rates. Seed germinates in 7 days typically but up to 21 days at 65–70°F. You can make a few divisions from one plant's root system. Volunteers transplant easily. Space 2 feet apart.

**SITING AND GARDEN CARE:** Motherwort is not an especially picky plant and will thrive in a variety of soils. The plants are short-lived perennials, often dying after a few years. If you live in a temperate climate, the herb will replace itself through self-sowing and can become quite weedy. Consider planting it out of the way where it can do its thing without stepping on anyone's toes. Alternatively, harvest the flowers before they form seeds. In colder climates, plant in full sun; in hotter climates, it will appreciate some afternoon cover. In hot climates, plant motherwort in the fall as a winter annual.

**PROBLEM INSECTS AND DISEASES:** Motherwort experiences minimal pressures but can be bothered by spider mites.

**HARVESTING:** Motherwort's long flowering stems are harvested when they're in full bloom; wear leather gloves to avoid the prickles. Bundle to dry. Harvest half of the remaining basal leaves with the "haircut" method, and dry on screens or in loose baskets. As long as you leave some vegetation for the plant to recover, you can obtain two to three harvests from motherwort annually. The second and third harvests will be mostly leaves. When the flowering stalks are dry, strip the leaves and flowers from the stem using gloves, and combine.

## Medicinal Properties

**PART USED:** Leaves and flowering tops

**MEDICINAL PREPARATIONS:** Tincture, infusion, and vinegar (motherwort is quite bitter; most people take it as a tincture or an extract)

**TINCTURE RATIOS AND DOSAGE:** Fresh (1:2 95%) or dry (1:5 60%); either preparation 2–4 ml up to three times a day

**TEA RATIOS AND DOSAGE:** Infusion of 1 teaspoon dried leaves per 1 cup water up to three times a day. The tea is very bitter.

**ACTIONS:** Emmenagogue, parturient, uterine antispasmodic, antianxiety, nervine, anodyne, bitter, diuretic, hypotensive, antioxidant, cardiotonic, and cardioprotective

**ENERGETICS:** Cooling and drying

## Medicinal Uses

Motherwort is a classic remedy for disorders of the nervous, cardiovascular, and reproductive systems.

### NERVOUS SYSTEM

The herb is one of our most potent medicines for anxiety, both tonically and acutely. I frequently combine motherwort with vervain, milky oats, and tulsi as a tonic formula for anxiety and as a remedy for moving through stressful times. The 17th-century herbalist Nicholas Culpeper wrote, "There is no better herb to drive melancholy vapours from the heart, to strengthen it, and make the mind cheerful, blithe, and merry." Indeed, motherwort is specific for anxiety that affects the heart—it quells palpitations and rapid heart rate brought on by panic attacks or acute anxiety. Parents of young children (and teenagers!) find that the herb softens the edginess brought on by sleep deprivation and venturesomeness.

## REPRODUCTIVE SYSTEM

As a birth aid, motherwort helps strengthen and regulate uterine contractions. It was the only herb I used in childbirth, and it gave me great ease. The herb is a traditional remedy to expedite delivery of the placenta when it isn't forthcoming. It can also be used to help with the afterpains of childbirth; combined with vervain and black haw, this medicinal trio helps reduce the pain and intensity of uterine contractions following birth. However, don't use motherwort if there is heavy bleeding after birth, as it can increase uterine bleeding. And because motherwort strengthens contractions, it shouldn't be used during pregnancy until labor has commenced or is impending.

As a remedy for menopausal symptoms, motherwort can help with insomnia, irritability, and mood swings. It can be used with hormone regulators like black cohosh as part of a tonic formula (motherwort won't directly regulate hormones but instead helps mollify menopausal symptoms of hormonal wobbliness).

Motherwort has a curiously dualistic nature, being a uterine stimulant for delayed menses and in childbirth, while also acting as a uterine antispasmodic (relaxant) for heavy menstrual cramps. Motherwort can be combined with other traditional cramp remedies, such as black cohosh, passionflower, black haw, and skullcap; see the recipe below. I find that, in general, menstrual cramps respond better to multiple herbs rather than a single remedy. Motherwort is specific for heavy, dragging cramps with a dark or scanty flow. Be aware that it has the potential to increase menstrual flow and thus should be used cautiously in heavy bleeding. Motherwort, along with feverfew and ginger, can also stimulate the menses when they aren't forthcoming or are sputtering.

## HORMONAL SYSTEM

Motherwort is a specific remedy for hyperthyroidism. However, it doesn't appear to affect thyroid hormones or thyroid function directly; instead, it helps minimize the effects of an overactive thyroid. (Those with hypothyroidism can use motherwort safely.) Motherwort helps lessen the insomnia, anxiety, and cardiac effects that often accompany an overactive thyroid gland. For hyperthyroidism, the herb is traditionally combined with other medicinals that directly support thyroid function, such as bugleweed and lemon balm, under the care of an endocrinologist who can closely monitor hormone levels.

## CARDIOVASCULAR SYSTEM

Motherwort is a traditional remedy for heart palpitations, rapid heart rate, and arrhythmias. Seek the care of a cardiologist when experiencing any new cardiac symptoms, which may be the result of serious heart disease or defect or an underlying noncardiac pathology.

# Menstrual Cramp Tincture Formula

This blend contains medicinals that are traditional pain-relievers and uterine antispasmodics. If the menstrual flow is heavy, omit or decrease the motherwort.

**MAKES 4 OUNCES**

1 ounce motherwort leaf and flower tincture (*Leonurus cardiaca*)

1 ounce passionflower leaf and flower tincture (*Passiflora incarnata*)

½ ounce skullcap leaf and flower tincture (*Scutellaria lateriflora*)

½ ounce black cohosh root tincture (*Actaea racemosa*)

1 ounce black haw or cramp bark root bark tincture (*Viburnum prunifolium* or *V. opulus*)

Use fresh herb or dry herb tinctures. Combine all tinctures and store in a glass dispensing bottle. Dosage is 2–3 ml every few hours up to five times a day.

> **PRECAUTIONS:** Do not use in pregnancy—except during labor—due to its stimulating effect on the uterus. Use caution during heavy menstruation, as it can increase menstrual bleeding. Rare incidence of contact dermatitis has occurred.

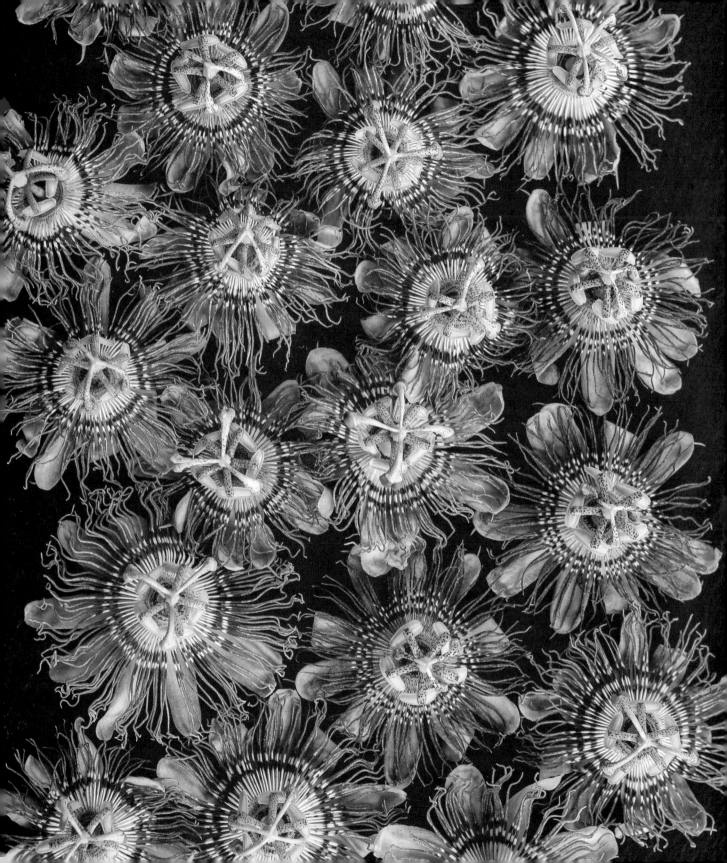

# PASSIONFLOWER

SCIENTIFIC NAME: *Passiflora incarnata*
PASSIFLORACEAE, passionflower family
AKA: maypop, old-field apricot

If ever there was a plant that possessed sufficient charisma to woo the botanically coldhearted, passionflower, with its drop-dead gorgeous flowers and exotic fruits that resemble green dragon eggs, is it. Passionflower is a clambering herbaceous vine—native to the fields and waysides of southeastern North America—that has both medicinal and edible uses. The leaves and flowers are a remedy for insomnia, stress, headaches, and pain. The fruit offers a delectable sour pulp.

Gaze long enough at the vine's evocative blooms, and you'll no doubt notice another admirer: ants. Passionflower beguiles ants with its nectar-producing glands at the base of the leaf and at the base of the flower (pictured in the photo on page 347). The ants return the favor by protecting the plant from insects that would otherwise eat the plant's leaves. Basically, passionflower pays ants in nectar to be their bodyguards.

The *Passiflora* genus is biochemically complex and contains some 500 species, primarily native to the tropics of South America and Southeast Asia. Some species have edible fruit or have medicinal uses, but not all do. Unfortunately, confusion is common on the web and in popular herb books regarding the medicinal uses of various passionflower species. Some authors mistakenly imply that all passionflowers are interchangeable, and many photos are labeled incorrectly. The bottom line: I'm only writing about *Passiflora incarnata* here; please don't extrapolate this information to other species in the genus, as they may not be medicinal and might even be toxic. To grow passionflower for medicine, you'll want to obtain the correct plant or seeds from a seed company or nursery that specializes in medicinals or native plants. If you see a cultivated passionflower vine for sale in a nonspecialist nursery, it's generally not going to be the straight species of *Passiflora incarnata*. It could be a hybrid, but I wouldn't recommend using the hybrids medicinally.

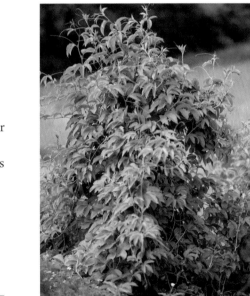

Passionflower needs trellising in the garden or it will overtake surrounding plants

## Cultivation

ZONES: 6–11; full sun to light shade

SOIL: pH 6–7.5; well-drained to average soil

SIZE: 5–15 feet tall depending on support; indefinitely wide as it spreads by underground runners and sprawling vining

LIFESTYLE: Short-lived perennial vine

PROPAGATION: Passionflower is notoriously hard to sprout, but I've had excellent success with the following protocol. First, scarify the seed and then stratify for two to three months. The seed needs warm temperatures to sprout and germinates in one to four weeks, sometimes longer, at 70–80°F. The seeds won't necessarily all come up at once, so hold on to the seed trays after the initial flush of seedlings emerges and wait for stragglers. Softwood to semihardwood 6-inch stem cuttings can be made in the spring to summer with mixed success (plant extra). Dig up runners with as much intact root as possible, cut back the green growth by half, and then transplant to a new location. Plant the starts 3 to 6 feet apart with support for climbing.

To save the seeds from ripe fruit, first, know that both the tan and black seeds are viable as long as they are hard. If the fruits aren't ripe by the first frost, place them in a closed paper bag to mature. Rinse the seeds off as best you can, and ferment the seeds to clean off the pulp, following the directions on page 106.

SITING AND GARDEN CARE: Passionflower is surprisingly easy to grow and, in fact, can be quite rambunctious. The vines will quickly take over the garden if you don't weed out the runners that emerge in inopportune locations. The plant is cold-hardy to zone 6 (zone 5 in sheltered locales) and needs a trellis, wall, fence, or plant to climb up. For those of you in colder climates, it's worth it to find local vines to propagate, as they will have genes for cold-hardiness. In colder climates with regular hard freezes, the plant survives the winter with only its subterranean root system (new shoots emerge from the earth in the spring). In warmer climates, it's evergreen or loses leaves in cold snaps but keeps its green stems.

Passionflower often goes hog wild in the garden for several years—sending up new shoots far from the parent vine with its copious runners—and then the whole colony will up and die one winter. It appears to be a short-lived perennial, or perhaps very sensitive to mean looks. The vines prefer full sun and are relatively drought tolerant but will flower in partial shade, albeit more demurely. Train passionflower up a pergola, tipi bamboo trellis, or arbor, and undersow with shade-loving herbs such as gotu kola and jiaogulan.

PROBLEM INSECTS AND DISEASES: The most common "pests" you'll likely encounter are the caterpillars of beautiful native butterflies, especially if you live in North America. Passionflower leaves are the only food source for gulf fritillary caterpillars, but other butterfly larvae also feed on their leaves. If caterpillars are a big problem in your garden, you could always relocate them in a faraway passionflower patch or create a larval relocation patch in an out-of-the-way spot.

HARVESTING: Harvest the long vines when they're beginning to flower and haven't yet set much fruit. Let the vines sit in the shade for an hour to give the insects time to crawl off and inspect the vines for caterpillars. Hang to dry or prepare immediately as medicine. Passionflower has a lot of water weight and can dry slowly, especially in humid climates. It has a propensity to turn an unsavory yellow if it dries slowly, so speed the drying process by using a fan and heat, or place in a dehydrator or in an air-conditioned room.

---

*Clockwise from top left:* A developing passionfruit (the remnants of the flower are still visible); a honeybee gathering passionfruit pollen; the pithy shell of a developing passionfruit surrounds the juicy seed mass; an ant feeding on an extrafloral nectary

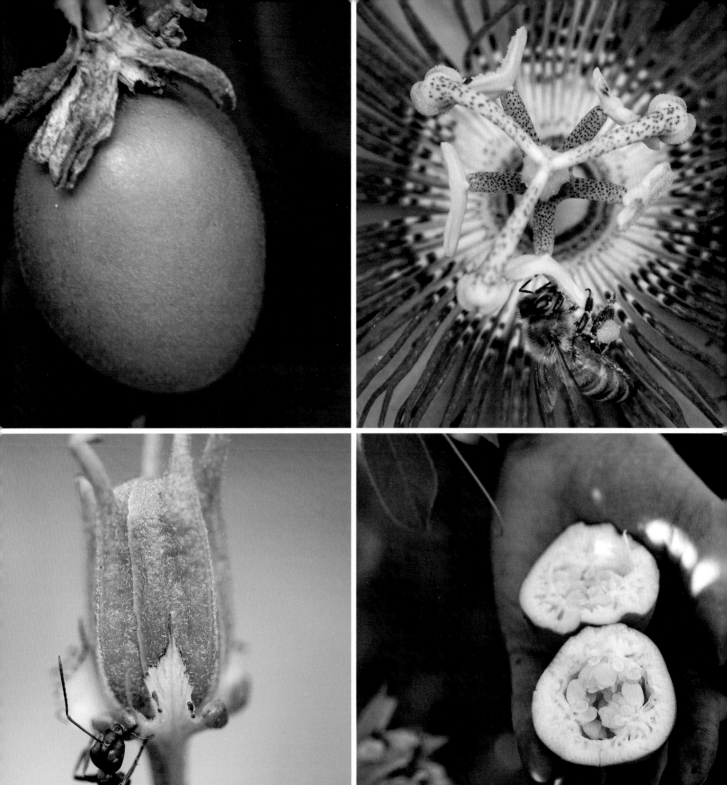

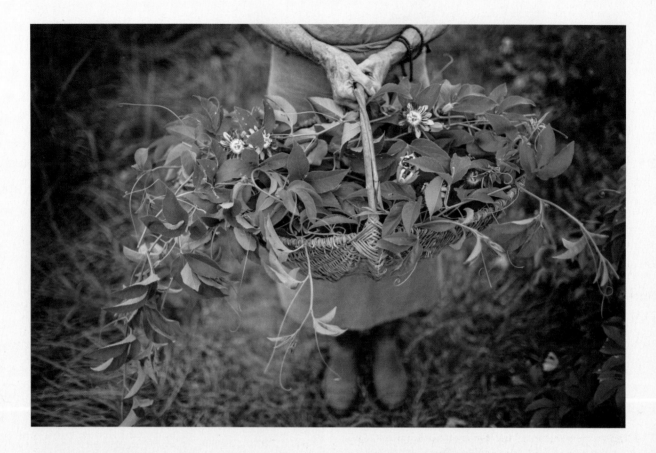

## Medicinal Properties

PART USED: Leaf and flower

MEDICINAL PREPARATIONS: Infusion, tincture, poultice, and compress

TINCTURE RATIOS AND DOSAGE: Fresh (1:2 95%) or dry (1:5 60%); either preparation 1–5 ml up to three times a day.

TEA RATIOS AND DOSAGE: Infusion of 2 teaspoons dried leaf and flower per 1 cup water up to three times a day

ACTIONS: Anodyne, hypnotic, hypotensive, nervine, antidepressant, antianxiety, and antispasmodic

ENERGETICS: Fairly neutral

## Medicinal Uses

The contemporary use of the herb stems from Native American uses of the medicine, although the modern applications are actually quite different from early recorded uses. Contemporary herbalists primarily use the leaves, stems, and flowers, whereas the ethnobotanical literature cites medicinal use of the roots.

### NERVOUS SYSTEM

Passionflower is one of the most beloved nervine remedies, finding its way into formulas for insomnia, menstrual cramps, headaches, musculoskeletal pain, stress, shingles, anxiety, and pain from injury. The herb is helpful for insomnia with circular thinking, such as when you're lying in bed mulling over an unpleasant situation or some silly thing you said and you just can't let it go. Passionflower offers relief from anxiety and stress, especially when accompanied by pain. The herb can be used internally to take the edge off teething and to help children relax when they are climbing up the walls. Passionflower helps promote sound sleep, and many parents give it to their little ones who frequently wake throughout the night. As one of our safer antianxiety herbs, it's helpful in calming children's chronic anxiety and also helps little ones deal with traumatic or stressful situations.

### REPRODUCTIVE SYSTEM

Passionflower is one of the herbs I favor for menstrual cramps, often in combination with motherwort and black cohosh. Many people find the herb brings them relief from cranky premenstrual moments and moodiness in menopause. Contemporary herbalists and midwives use passionflower to help with pain and insomnia in pregnancy.

### MUSCULOSKELETAL SYSTEM

Passionflower is one of my trusted remedies for acute musculoskeletal pain. I use it in combination with meadowsweet, black birch, and skullcap for muscle strains, sprains, and joint inflammation in general.

### RESPIRATORY SYSTEM

As a respiratory antispasmodic, it can be added to formulas for hacking or spasmodic coughing and asthma, especially if the asthma presents with hacking nighttime coughing.

### CARDIOVASCULAR SYSTEM

Passionflower helps lower blood pressure, especially when stress is involved. Of course, if you have high blood pressure, you'll want to monitor blood pressure levels and seek the care of a cardiologist or, in pregnancy, a midwife or obstetrician. High blood pressure that isn't managed properly can have serious consequences, including stroke and preterm labor.

## Rest Easy Tincture Formula

This blend is helpful for insomnia: both for difficulty falling asleep and for wakefulness that disturbs prolonged sleep. Because some individuals react to valerian with stimulation, it is prudent to take a little of this formula in the middle of the day and see how you react. If you are sensitive to valerian, omit the valerian and keep the remaining proportions.

MAKES 5 OUNCES

2 ounces passionflower leaf and flower tincture (*Passiflora incarnata*)

1 ounce skullcap leaf and flower tincture (*Scutellaria lateriflora*)

1 ounce valerian root tincture (*Valeriana officinalis*)

1 ounce lavender flower tincture (*Lavandula angustifolia*)

Use fresh tinctures if possible, but you can substitute dried tinctures or use different preparations for each tincture. Combine all tinctures and store in a glass dispensing bottle. Dosage is 2–5 ml as needed. For short-term relief of pain lasting no more than two days, you can take 3 ml up to six times a day.

## Culinary Uses

Passionfruits wrinkle and turn yellow when ripe. They have a spongy, foam-like wall, which houses the edible flesh surrounding the seeds. Pop open the ripe fruit—ignoring the inedible rind—and slurp up the seedy flesh, seeds and all. The part you eat resembles a bullfrog egg mass. I prefer to chew up the crunchy edible seeds, but some folks opt to spit them out. The taste is sour and sweet, with the unripe fruits being decidedly more sour.

> PRECAUTIONS: Use with caution in individuals with low blood pressure and slow heart rate (bradycardia). Use cautiously in individuals with a known latex allergy; an allergic reaction is extremely rare. Avoid high doses in pregnancy.

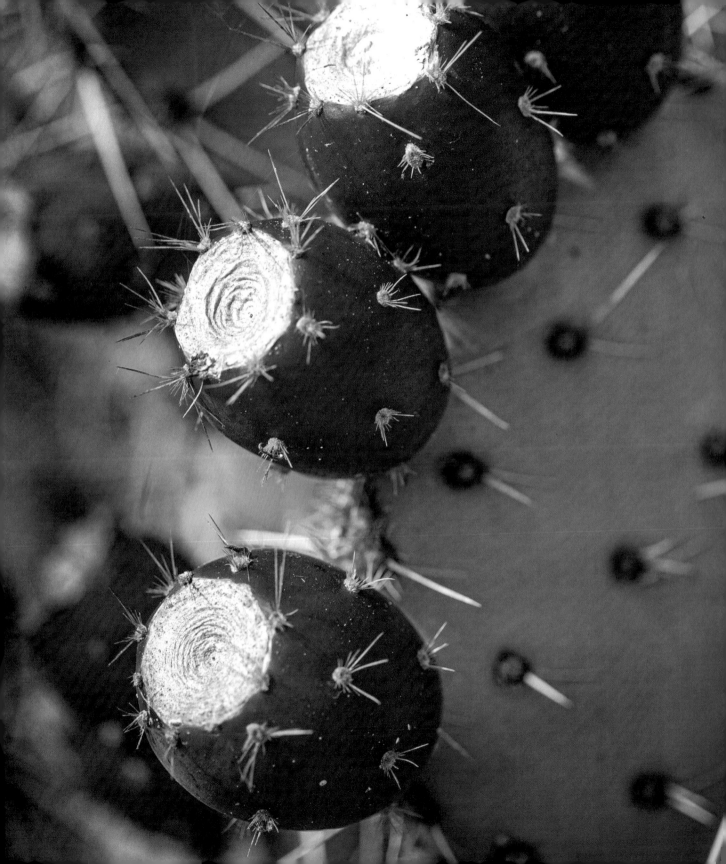

# PRICKLY PEAR

**SCIENTIFIC NAME:** *Opuntia*, various species
**CACTACEAE**, cactus family
**AKA:** Indian fig, Barbary fig, cactus pear; pads: *nopales* (Mexico); fruit: *tunas* (Mexico), *fichindindia* (Italy), *sabur* or *sabra* (Middle East)

Perhaps you think prickly pears have no place in an herb gardening book for temperate climates, but I promise you *can* grow this cactus, and its bounty is worth its bedevil. Native to the Americas, prickly pears are a large group of species in the *Opuntia* genus. These cacti have been a central food, medicine, and dye plant for Indigenous peoples for millennia. The edible cactus pads, or *nopales,* once disarmed, can be batter-fried, pickled, and added to salsas and scrambled eggs. The egg-shaped fruit is eaten fresh after peeling, and the juice is prepared into jam, lemonade, sauces, margaritas, and syrup. Nopales (*nopal,* singular) are a folk remedy for several ailments, including burns, diabetes, infections, and hangovers. The name *nopal* is rooted in the Aztec word *nōpalli,* and the fruit's name, *tuna,* originates with the Taino languages of the Caribbean.

The Barbary fig (*Opuntia ficus-indica*)—a type of prickly pear thought to have originated from a wild prickly pear in Mexico—is the most widely grown and consumed cactus in the world. It's cultivated in northern Africa, Italy, and Mexico for its fruit, which comes in an array of colors from tomatillo-green to peach and crimson. The Barbary fig is often spineless and can grow quite tall. There are a number of strains, with varying degrees of cold-hardiness, but most are suited for warmer climates. In the Sonoran Desert, *Opuntia engelmannii*—with its fantastically fuchsia fruits—is harvested for food and medicine.

Various species of prickly pear (primarily *Opuntia stricta*) have been cultivated throughout the world for their myriad uses. In addition to their edible pads and fruit, they are fodder for cattle, sheep, and goats and are grown for the natural dye, carmine, which is made from cochineal, an insect that feeds off the cactus stems. Prickly pears are now seriously invasive in South Africa, parts of northern Africa and the Mediterranean, and in Australia, and Hawai'i. The plants differ in their tenderness and taste—some varieties have larger or tastier fruits, and others bear succulent pads. The species are plentiful and freely hybridize, making identification of species sometimes challenging. As long as you know you have a prickly pear in the *Opuntia* genus, you can see if you enjoy the flavor of a particular variety's pads or fruit.

Prickly pears are doubly armed: first, with the conspicuous, needle-like spines and, second, with practically invisible spiny hairs called *glochids*. These persnickety hairs grow from the pads, fruit, and base of the flower. Glochids annoyingly lodge their hooked ends into the skin, tongue, and throat alike and can be felt for days if not gingerly removed with tweezers. Some friendlier varieties have fewer glochids and no spines. (See page 353 for how to remove the spines and glochids.)

Wild prickly pear fruit

## Cultivation

**ZONES:** Varies by species but some are cold-hardy to zone 4; full sun

**SOIL:** pH 6–8; well-drained soil

**SIZE:** Varies by species and climate, ranging from knee-high to 20 feet tall

**LIFESTYLE:** Perennial succulent

**PROPAGATION:** It's easiest to propagate the plant by rooting the pads. If you have a strain with distinct traits, like a spineless variety or one with double blooms, this is the only way to maintain its characteristics. Wearing thick leather gloves, cut full-grown pads free from the plant with a sharp knife, taking care to leave the parent pad unscathed. Using tongs, place the pads on a plate in a dark area for several days—the cut area will harden, or form a callus, which protects the cactus from rot. Plant the pad, cut-end down, in a few inches of well-drained, premoistened soil, and prop it up with small rocks if necessary. If you live in an arid climate, you can plant your pad directly in the ground in its ultimate site. Otherwise, plant the pad in a small pot, keep in dappled or indirect light in a warm location, and water when the soil dries out. Tug the transplant gently with tongs after a month to check if rooting has occurred—if you sense resistance, the roots have formed, and the cactus is ready for full sun and can be transplanted into a larger pot or the earth.

Germinating prickly pear is not for the faint of heart. First, ferment the fruit to clean germination inhibitors from the seed. Then, scarify the seed. Finally, there is a grueling stratification regime, which may take one to two years before germination. Sow the fresh seeds shallowly directly in the garden or in outdoor trays. Cover only with a thin layer of sand. Keep the "cactuslings" protected from the full sun for the first few months.

**SITING AND GARDEN CARE:** There's a prickly pear for just about any climate. Look for plants that are adapted to your region by checking with local nurseries or gardeners. Mail-order cactus companies can also be a good source. I recommend growing a spineless variety, which has obvious advantages when it comes to cultivating, harvesting, and processing. Unfortunately, the spineless strains aren't especially cold-hardy, but you can still grow them in temperate climates with some finagling. Before the first frost, harvest a handful of pads to overwinter. Save the cactus pads in a basket, placed in an out-of-the-way dark spot that doesn't freeze—they're amazingly tenacious and can survive for months without any care or water. Come spring, root the pads in a pot and keep indoors. After the threat of frost has passed, plant the rooted cactus pads out in the garden, where they'll grow throughout the season, producing fresh pads for harvest. Before the first kiss of frost, harvest a fresh cache of pads to overwinter once again. I also grow my spineless prickly pear in pots as an edible houseplant that spends its summers outdoors.

There are cold-hardy species with thorns you can grow outdoors as a perennial, but you'll need to spend more time and take more care when harvesting and processing. An advantage to growing spiny varieties in cold climates is their ability to set fruit. Again, it's best to source your plants from local nurseries or growers who can let you know if their cultivar fruits in your region. If you live in a climate that doesn't freeze or has light frosts, you can skip all this and smugly grow the cactus outdoors year-round. As you can imagine, the plant prefers full sun and well-drained soil. Here in North Carolina, where we have clayey soils, I grow my prickly pear in my garden's "Mediterranean" section—an area amended with copious amounts of coarse sand. The ample blossoms resemble roses and entice several species of bees, including solitary bees, leafcutter bees, and sunflower bees.

**PROBLEM INSECTS AND DISEASES:** Prickly pear can be affected by prickly pear cactus bugs, cactus moth borers, and cochineal, which produces fluffy white patches on the pads (read more about cochineal above). If you're growing prickly pear outside its native range, insect pressure is less intense. The plants are also affected by various fungal pathogens, causing rot.

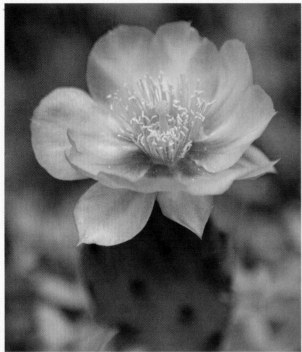

Prickly pear in flower

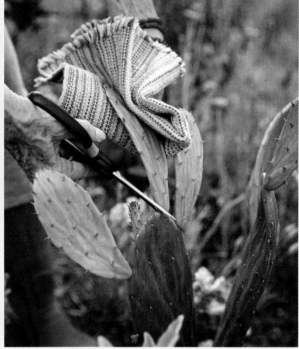

Harvesting garden-grown spineless prickly pear

HARVESTING AND PROCESSING PRICKLY PEAR: Young pads sprout rubbery green nubs, resembling teddy-bear-like spines (these are actually the leaves of the cactus, which fall off as the pad ages). If a pad has filled out but is still a lighter green color with some tender nubs, it's at the best stage to harvest. Cultivated plants have softer pads than their wild counterparts—pick their nopales when they are still pliable but have reached the size of a large hand. Collect wild, thorny species earlier in their development, when the nopales are about 6 or 7 inches long.

Wearing leather gloves, grasp the pad with a tong and, with the other hand, cut it free from the plant with a knife. Place your harvest in a bowl or bucket. If you have a spineless variety, it will still have glochids. These are easily scrubbed free with a vegetable brush and liberal rinsing. If you have a spiny pad, place it sideways on a cutting board, and, wearing dishwashing gloves, scrape off the spiny nubbins with a knife. Turn over the pad and repeat. Slice off the thick base and outer edge of the nopal. Then give the pads a final scrub and rinse to be sure all the glochids are washed free. Alternatively, spines can be singed off by roasting over a fire on a grill. Store-bought nopales are often ready to eat; sometimes, you'll find them despined and sliced into little pieces, called *nopalitos*. They're also sold "as is," in which case, you'll need to remove the prickles at home, as described above. Once you've disarmed the pads, you can proceed with any nopales recipe or prepare them into a slurry by blending the pad with a little water, as described below.

To pick the fruit (tunas), which often doesn't bear spines but are nonetheless armed with glochids, forager Pascal Bauder shares a tip he learned from an Indigenous elder: using fallen branches, fashion a small bundle and vigorously brush the fruits with it. The idea is to remove most of the glochids before you collect the fruit. Give them a spray-down with a hose or kitchen sprayer to remove the first round of hairs. You'll need to then peel the fruits or process them to remove the remaining prickles. To peel the tunas: wearing dishwashing gloves, cut the two edges off the fruit and make a longitudinal slit; remove the peel. Eat raw or prepare into a sauce or syrup. Alternatively, place the fruits—peel and glochids intact—in a blender or food processor with a little water and lightly pulse until it reaches a slurry consistency but the seeds are mostly intact. Strain the mash through a colander lined with a straining cloth so the juice and pulp pass through but the glochids, seeds, and peels remain. Press the slurry with a spoon to express all the liquid. The juice can then be enjoyed fresh, frozen for later, or prepared into syrup, jam, sauce, or fruit leathers. Too much of the raw juice can be problematic for some people—see more in the Precautions section on page 355.

## Medicinal Properties

**PART USED:** Pads and fruit

**MEDICINAL PREPARATIONS:** Fruit: chutney, juice, jam, syrup, lemonade, cocktails, and vinegar. Pads: slurry, capsules, juice, pickles, salsa, poultice, and various foods.

**TINCTURE:** Not recommended, as it doesn't extract the soluble fiber

**SLURRY RATIOS AND DOSAGE:** Blend two small pads with enough water to form a slurry. Drink one-third of the slurry with each meal throughout the day.

**ACTIONS:** Pads: Demulcent, cholesterol-lowering, hypoglycemic, diuretic, and vulnerary. Fruit: antioxidant, antirheumatic, anti-inflammatory, nutritive tonic, and cardiotonic.

**ENERGETICS:** Cooling and moistening

## Medicinal Uses

The pads are high in soluble fiber, which helps remove excess cholesterol from the body. Studies have demonstrated the pads' ability to lower LDL-cholesterol and triglyceride levels. Another benefit of fiber is that it contributes to the sensation of being full without adding calories, which explains the herb's tradition as a weight-loss remedy.

### ENDOCRINE SYSTEM

Prickly pear is one of the most popular folk remedies for type 2 diabetes in Mexico and the southwestern United States. It has demonstrated hypoglycemic effects, possibly through increasing insulin sensitivity at the level of cellular membranes. The pads appear to be more active in moderating blood sugar levels as a food, either broiled or consumed as slurry, than in the form of capsules. The blood-sugar-lowering effect peaks at 2 to 3 hours after consumption and may last up to 6 hours. It is recommended to consume 1 to 2 pads (150 to 300 grams) of prickly pear throughout the day in divided doses. The pads can be prepared into food or consumed before meals as a slurry or juice. (See the notes in the Culinary Uses section below.) Prickly pear doesn't affect blood sugar in those with healthy glucose levels. Be sure to monitor blood sugar levels and work with an endocrinologist when managing diabetes.

### TOPICAL USES

The gloop of prickly pear is used throughout the world as a soothing topical remedy, much like aloe vera gel. The pad can be sliced down its length and the flesh scooped from the center. Apply the gel as a fresh poultice to soothe sunburns, burns, chafed skin, insect bites, bruises, sores, and inflamed joints. Store the excess in the refrigerator for up to a week.

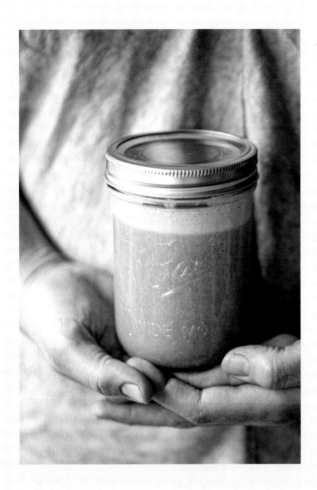

### NUTRITIVE TONIC

The fruit is remarkably high in vitamin C and magnesium and also contains a fair amount of fiber. Varieties with fuchsia flesh contain high levels of betalains, pigments that are highly antioxidant, anti-inflammatory, anticancer, and hepatoprotective (protecting the liver). Given the levels of fiber and antioxidants in the fruit, it is an excellent food for nourishing the cardiovascular system and protecting the body against free radical stress, thus lowering the risk for inflammatory disease and cancer or cancer recurrence. The pads are high in vitamins A and C and contain moderate amounts of minerals, including magnesium, iron, manganese, and calcium. As discussed, they also provide a substantial amount of soluble fiber.

## Culinary Uses

The pads are tangy and mucilaginous, like a muddle of okra, lemon, and green beans. After disarming them, slice nopales into ½-inch pieces. These can be parboiled or roasted with a little oil and salt and added to salsas, casseroles, or scrambled eggs. I find nopales delightful in salsas, as the punch of the other ingredients distracts from the gooeyness. (See my recipe on page 356.) Likewise, mix them into a pot of beans or layer them into a casserole, and their texture melds with the other ingredients.

You can also consume the raw blended nopales as a slurry, but be forewarned: it's gloopy! As a daily dose, blend two small nopales with a little water. Adding lime juice and a touch of cayenne helps counteract the viscousness. Also, consider adding celery juice or cucumber juice. People who do not have diabetes may want to add a little pineapple juice. Drink in divided doses with meals to manage cholesterol levels or blood sugar in diabetes. Go slow at first, as high doses can cause gastric upset and nausea. You can prepare bigger batches to save time and refrigerate the blended nopales for up to four days.

I prefer to consume the melon-flavored fruit in small amounts as a juice concentrate: an ounce or two diluted with water, lemonade, cocktails, or vegetable or fruit juice. If you have one of the carmine-colored varieties, the juice is an electrifying fuchsia. It audaciously wakes up salad dressings, chilled summer soups, herbal teas, pancakes, and margaritas. You can buy the juice bottled without preservatives. Freeze any excess in ice cube trays, and pop out the cubes into freezer storage bags to store.

> PRECAUTIONS: Use caution and consult your medical practitioner if you are taking pharmaceutical hypoglycemic agents, as prickly pear may dangerously compound blood-sugar-lowering effects. High doses of the pads may cause gastric distress—bloating and nausea—in some individuals. Some people react to raw prickly pear flesh or the juice with chills, nausea, and body aches. Start with small doses and increase slowly.

# Rainbow Nopales Salsa

YIELD: 3 cups

1 ear sweet corn, or substitute ¾ cup frozen sweet corn

3 cups water

¾ cup (80 grams) diced nopal pads (about 3 small pads or 1 large store-bought pad)

1½ cups (215 grams) diced tomatoes

⅓ cup finely diced white onion

¼ cup finely minced cilantro leaves

1½ tablespoons fresh lime juice

1 small fresh jalapeño pepper, finely minced, or to taste (optional)

2 garlic cloves, finely minced

10 fresh calendula flowers (*Calendula officinalis*), yellow rays removed from the tough green base

Sea salt, to taste

Fresh, seasonal salsa says *festive*, especially when it's prepared with edible flowers and nopales in the mix. Use store-bought nopales (typically these are already despined), or gather the tender young pads and prepare them yourself, using the directions found on page 353. You can substitute other seasonal edible flowers; visit page 178 for inspiration.

1. Steam or boil the sweet corn, let cool, and slice the kernels from the ear; set aside.

2. In a small pot, bring 3 cups of water to boil, add the diced nopal pads, and simmer, uncovered, for about 2 minutes. Strain immediately, briefly rinse with cold water, and let cool completely.

3. In a large bowl, combine the corn, nopales, tomatoes, onion, cilantro, lime juice, jalapeño, and garlic. Add the calendula flowers and season with salt just before serving.

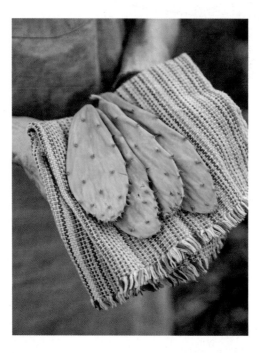

Prickly pear pads at the perfect stage for harvesting

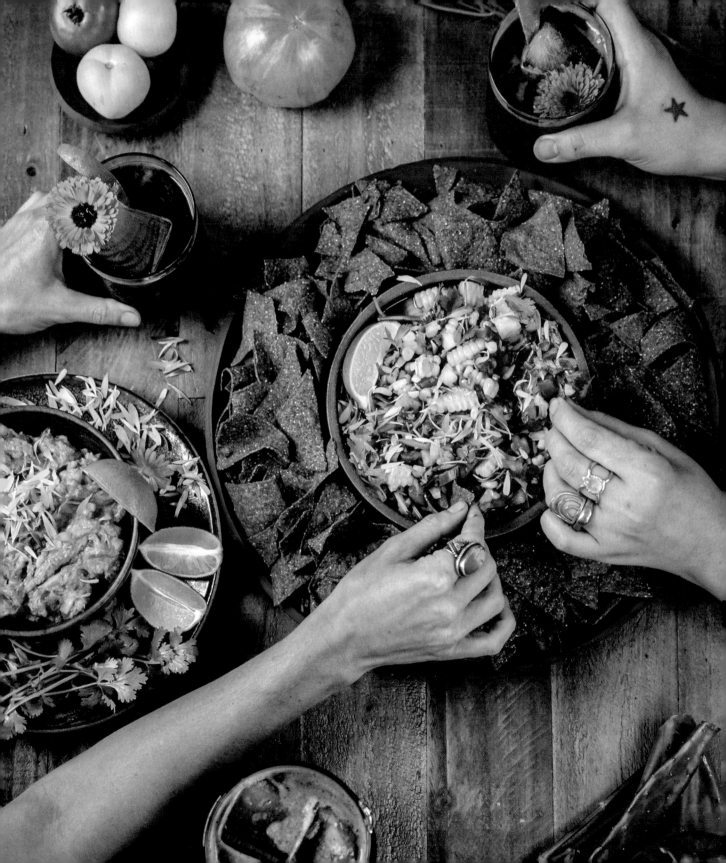

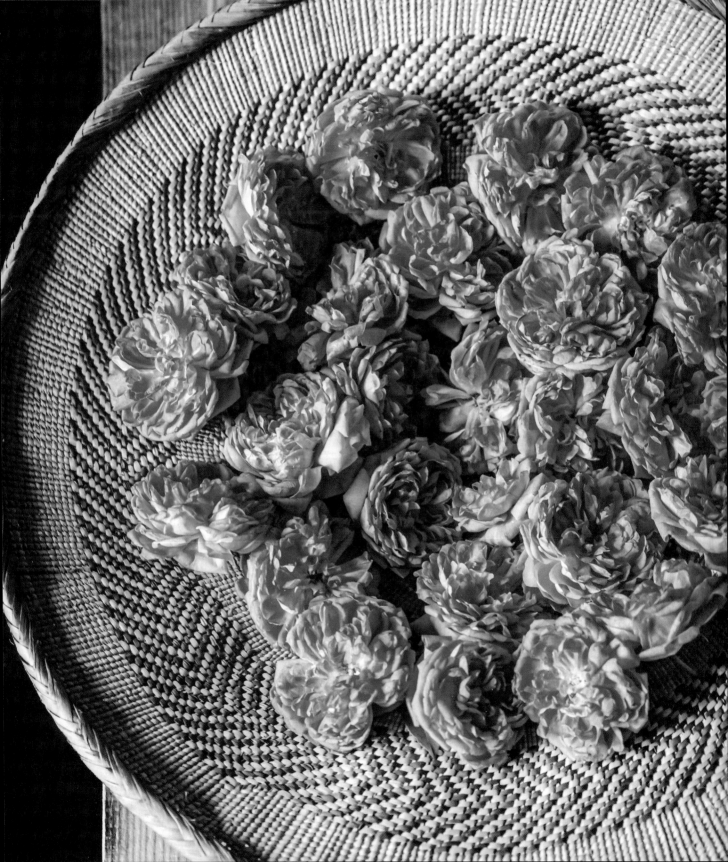

# ROSE

SCIENTIFIC NAME: *Rosa* spp.
ROSACEAE, rose family
AKA: sweetbriar, briar rose

Cultivated for millennia, rose has long been a beloved medicine, food, and botanical fragrance throughout many cultures, including those of India, Greece, Egypt, North America, China, and the Middle East. There are over 300 species and thousands of cultivars; all species are edible and medicinal, but they vary widely in their aroma, hue, and astringency. Roses are woody shrubs with prickles and can be compact or vining with arching or trailing stems. Wild species have five petals and a profusion of stamens. Roses are native to Eurasia, North America, and North Africa, with a concentration of species clustered in Asia.

Velvety and puckery, rose petals are edible and can add a fragrant flourish to salads, butters, jams, and frosting. Once fertilized, the blooms give rise to rosehips—a plentiful food medicine that is rich in antioxidants and bioflavonoids and one of the most concentrated sources of vitamin C in the world. Tragically, some roses have been bred solely for their visual charm and do not produce rosehips, as their blooms are too packed with petals to allow pollinators access to their tenderest parts.

When selecting a rose, choose a variety suited to your climate and soil. You'll also want to know if it sets fruit or has fragrant blooms. If possible, partake of the fragrance before buying: many of the modern hybrids have traded in their aromatic allure for a prolonged blooming season. The most fragrant and long-cherished varieties include the cabbage rose (*Rosa centifolia*), musk rose (*Rosa moschata*), and the Damask rose (*Rosa x damascena*), a cultivated hybrid. Consider growing a rose native to your bioregion, which is the best way to support biodiversity in the landscape and will attract birds to their bright rosehips in the fall. There are more than 35 species native to North America to choose from—consult a native plant nursery in your area to see what's available.

Another strategy is to befriend the invasive, non-native wild roses growing in your midst. Learning how to identify these species and use them medicinally is an innovative strategy for curbing their growth *and* filling your pantry. Ramanas rose (*Rosa rugosa*)—also known as Japanese rose or beach rose—and multiflora rose (*Rosa multiflora*) are both native to Asia and have naturalized elsewhere. Multiflora rose is a standard rootstock of ornamental roses and is highly opportunistic in central and eastern North America. Its creamy white floral clusters and tart hips can both be used medicinally.

Ramanas rose has spread throughout much of the world, especially coastal areas. It covers the dunes along the coastline of New England and proliferates along European shores. It's easy to grow, is especially disease resistant, and makes enormous orange-red rosehips. Shrubby and thicket-forming by nature, *Rosa rugosa* is a lovely choice for an edible hedge or protective border where it isn't invasive. Despite its merits, the plants can be invasive in some areas, especially coastal regions. If it grows abundantly in your area, I recommend wild harvesting it and not bringing it into the landscape, as it easily displaces native plants and may be difficult to control.

## Cultivation

ZONES: 3–9; full sun (hardiness varies by species)

SOIL: pH 5.5–7 (6.5 is ideal); well-watered, fertile soils with good drainage

SIZE: Varies by species, from 2 feet to 20 feet tall

LIFESTYLE: Woody shrubs and clambering woody vines (depending on the variety)

PROPAGATION: It's easiest to make new roses through cuttings or layering, as the seeds take a long time to germinate and also don't come true to type. If you have a named variety, you'll want to make clones to keep the desired traits. Semi-ripe softwood cuttings are the easiest way to propagate the plants (see page 103). Hardwood cuttings are taken in the fall or early winter and root more slowly than semi-ripe cuttings. Vining or clambering species can be propagated through layering (see page 103). Seed can take 18 months to germinate. Scoop the seeds from fresh rosehips and wash off the pulp. Scarify the seeds and plant them directly in the garden or in an outdoor seed tray. Alternatively, stratify the seeds using the plastic bag method once they've been washed and scarified; they require three months of warm, moist stratification followed by three months of cold, moist stratification before sowing.

SITING AND GARDEN CARE: Roses do best in full sun, preferably in an area that receives good airflow. They are notoriously thirsty and hungry, preferring moist, fertile, yet well-drained soil. Be prepared to fertilize them annually, and give them an additional monthly shot of compost tea or organic liquid fertilizer. Water the plants at their base during dry weather instead of overhead, which can promote fungal diseases. Depending on your variety, you may need to prune the plant to encourage flower production and vigorous growth—research your particular strain and its pruning requirements. In general, the old-fashioned garden roses and clambering varieties need little pruning apart from cutting away dead growth or controlling their spread. Contemporary varieties like hybrid tea, floribunda, and grandiflora roses produce

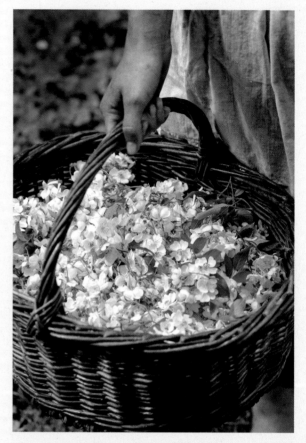

A harvest of multiflora rose (*Rosa multiflora*)

flowers on new growth and are thus cut back hard in the early spring to thin the bushes and galvanize new growth and a gorgeous display of blooms later in the season.

PROBLEM INSECTS AND DISEASES: Roses, in general, are susceptible to fungal diseases like black spot and powdery mildew. Prune diseased growth, and remove fallen damaged leaves to minimize spread. Look for disease-resistant varieties or hearty heirloom strains from local sources. Japanese beetles, thrips, leafhoppers, and slugs are also potential pests.

HARVESTING: Collect the flowers in the morning, soon after they've opened, on a dry, sunny day, and quickly move the harvest into the shade or drying location. Dry on screens or loose-weave baskets. If you're making medicine with the fresh flowers, harvest when you're ready to prepare your remedy, so you capture most of the aromatic compounds. If you're collecting wild roses, be sure of your identification, and make sure the plants aren't sprayed. Don't use roses from the florist, as they have been grown with chemicals.

If you'd like to harvest rosehips, leave some of the flowers intact; the hips develop from the flowers. Collect rosehips when they are red and fleshy and the seed is hard inside. If you live in a climate that freezes and the rosehips are developing close to the first frost, wait to harvest until after the first frost; the cold will sweeten the flesh. Prepare the fresh hips into medicine as soon as possible. Or dry on screens or baskets, and cut open a sample hip to make sure it's dry in the middle. Larger hips need to be split open to dry or the inside will mold. If you'll be preparing the rosehips into a food that won't be strained, remove the seeds first as they have irritating hairs that get caught in the throat.

## Medicinal Properties

**PART USED:** Flowers, flower buds, rosehips, and leaves

**MEDICINAL PREPARATIONS:** Infusion, tincture, honey, syrup, oxymel, vinegar, butter, hydrosol, oil, salves, compress, poultice, and soak

**TINCTURE RATIOS AND DOSAGE:** Flowers and buds: Fresh (1:2 95%) or dry (1:4 60%); either preparation 1–4 ml up to three times a day. Tincture of rosehips not recommended.

**TEA RATIOS AND DOSAGE:** Infusion of 1 to 2 teaspoons dried flowers, flower buds, rosehips, or leaves per 1 cup boiling water up to three times a day

**ACTIONS:** Flowers and flower buds: Nervine, astringent, anti-inflammatory, cardiotonic, antimicrobial, diuretic, anticatarrhal, antianxiety, and aphrodisiac. Rosehips: Astringent, antimicrobial, blood tonic, and nutritive

**ENERGETICS:** Cooling and drying

## Medicinal Uses

To understand rose as a medicine, first know that it is supremely cooling and tightening. Those qualities are helpful for hot and inflamed sinuses from colds and the common flu and equally soothing for hot and irritated digestive conditions.

### NERVOUS SYSTEM

Rose petals and rosebuds are an ally for heavy hearts—for those suffering from grief, despair, and loss. I find the uplifting scents of citrusy herbs like lemon balm and lemon verbena complementary to rose's sweet and calming nature. The romantic associations with rose—petals strewn upon the bed or a dozen red roses gifted to a beloved—are consistent with the flower's soothing and aphrodisiacal nature. Rose's signature aroma stirs romance and passion in many hearts. Likewise, it encourages relaxation in intimacy, especially when one has experienced sexual trauma.

### NUTRITIVE TONIC

Rosehips are high in vitamins and bioflavonoids and are a supreme herbal blood-builder and antioxidant. Read more about their uses in the Culinary section.

### TOPICAL USES

Rose flowers are cooling and tightening to the skin and can be prepared as a poultice, wash, or soak to assuage burns, sunburns, insect bites, bruises, and weeping skin conditions. The leaves of rose are highly astringent and antimicrobial and can be combined with the flowers. Rosehip seed oil is pressed from the seeds and is a classic serum for restoring tired, aged skin and soothing acne. See my recipe for Floral Serum: Rose-Calendula-Elder Oil on page 364—it contains both rosehip seed oil and infused rose petals. Rose hydrosol is a light and fresh astringent that can be spritzed on the face as a toner or sprayed on the body as a cooling and refreshing after-bath anointment.

### ROSE AROMATHERAPY

Pure rose essential oil, known as *rose otto,* is extremely precious. The flowers are picked by hand, and 50 blooms are needed to produce one drop of the oil, which explains why it's one of the most expensive botanical fragrances in the world. Thankfully, a small amount goes a long way. Rose otto can be diluted in a massage oil to help one feel sensual and relaxed. It's also helpful for softening and dispelling heavy emotions like jealousy, rage, and resentment.

## Sensual Tea

Sweet and spicy, this tea blend can help ignite a romantic spark and set the mood for intimacy.

4 cups water

2 tablespoons dried rose buds or petals (*Rosa* spp.)

1 tablespoon dried damiana leaf (*Turnera diffusa*)

½ teaspoon cinnamon bark chips (*Cinnamomum verum*)

¼ teaspoon hulled cardamom seeds (*Elettaria cardamomum*)

Honey or maple syrup (optional)

In a small pot, bring the water to a boil. Turn off the heat, add all the herbs, cover, and infuse for 20 minutes. Strain and sweeten with honey or maple syrup if desired. Drink a cup or two and enjoy!

## Culinary Uses

All true roses (*Rosa* spp.) have edible petals and hips as long as they haven't been sprayed. The petals of pink and red varieties contain an array of antioxidant compounds—including bioflavonoids, carotenoids, and anthocyanins—imbuing roses with the ability to neutralize free radicals as adeptly as green tea. Pluck the petals and layer them into salsas and fruit salads. They can be stirred into frosting, smoothies, soft cheeses, ice cream, and sorbet. Rose petals and butter are one of the most exquisite floral duets—try my Spiced Rose Butter on page 167. I add the petals to berries when making jam; for a cheater version, add the minced petals to store-bought jam. In the summertime, I combine the beautiful fresh blooms with hibiscus and mint to make a cooling and refreshing herbal iced tea. The petals can likewise be steeped in wine, brandy, or other liquors. And rose is delectable infused into herbal vinegars and honeys.

Rosehips are more astringent than the blooms, and depending on the variety, they are often delightfully sour. They are high in vitamins A, B, C, and E, along with bioflavonoids. Take care before popping whole hips in your mouth—inside the flesh of many species are small hairs that can be irritating to the throat. In which case, you'll need to slice each one open to scrape out the seeds. Rosehips can be added to sweeter fruit or fruit juice and prepared into fruity jams, compotes, chutney, and syrups.

> PRECAUTIONS: Rose is drying and can aggravate dry constitutions if taken regularly. Roses from florists are heavily sprayed and should not be used for medicine or food. Avoid high doses in pregnancy. Note that there are many plants with "rose" in their name that are not related to the true roses (*Rosa* spp.) and are thus not used as medicine or as food in similar fashion (some are poisonous!). These include Lenten rose (*Helleborus* spp.), rock-rose (*Cistus* spp.), rose mallow (*Lavatera* spp.), and others. Many ornamental flowering bushes superficially resemble roses—be more than positive in your identification!

*Clockwise from top left:* Ramanas rose (*Rosa rugosa*); Ramanas rose (*Rosa rugosa*) has large rosehips; rosehips add color to the garden throughout the fall and winter; rosehips grow sweeter after the frost (*Rosa* sp.)

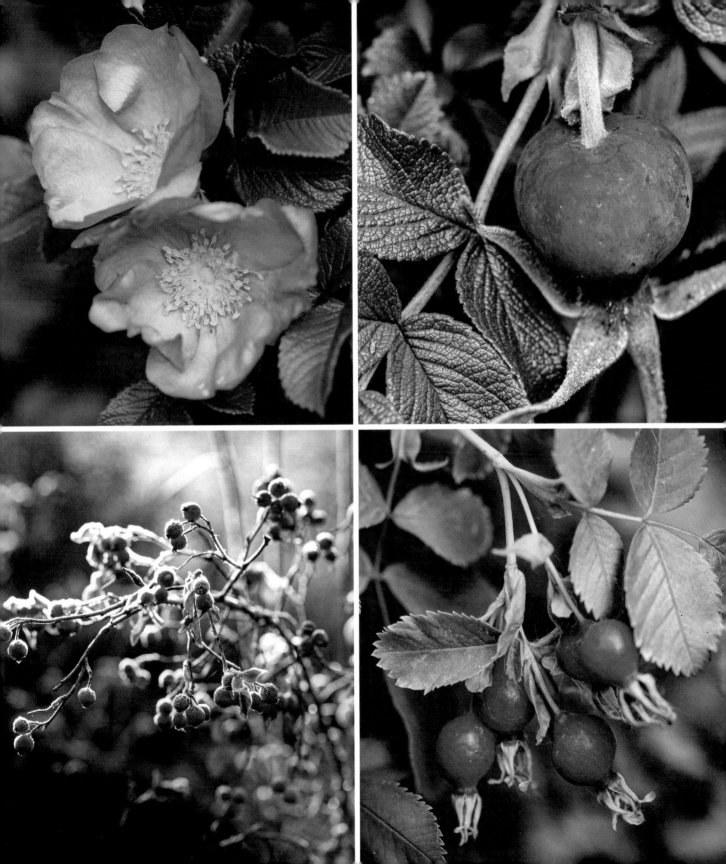

# Floral Serum: Rose-Calendula-Elder Oil

YIELD: About 1½ cups (4 ounces)
PREP + COOK TIME: 20 minutes plus 5 hours infusion

¼ cup (4 grams) packed dried rose petals or buds (*Rosa* spp.)

¼ cup (7 grams) tightly packed dried whole calendula flower (*Calendula officinalis*)

¼ cup (5 grams) packed dried elderflower (*Sambucus nigra*)

½ cup (4 fluid ounces) unrefined cold-pressed jojoba oil

2 tablespoons (1 fluid ounce) unrefined cold-pressed rosehip seed oil

12 drops geranium essential oil (*Pelargonium graveolens*; optional)

3 drops sweet orange essential oil (*Citrus sinensis*; optional)

9 drops lavender essential oil (*Lavandula angustifolia*; optional)

Facial serums are a balm against the meanness of gravity and the vagaries of life. In this version, rose, elder, and calendula are infused into jojoba oil, imparting their aroma, astringency, and anti-inflammatory qualities. Jojoba—a golden oil hailing from the desert—is renowned for its permeability, and rosehip seed oil is a premier oil for skin regeneration. Lavender, geranium, and sweet orange essential oils have restorative qualities, particularly for mature, tired, or compromised skin. You can leave them out if you prefer; the serum will still be decadently therapeutic. Apply the oil to scars, stretch marks, and sun-damaged skin. It will breathe new life into listless areas. A little goes a long way with this potent concoction—add wee dollops to areas that need love and attention, and follow up with your usual moisturizer or lotion.

1. INFUSE THE HERBS IN JOJOBA OIL: Chop the dried herbs finely or grind them to a powder in a spice grinder or clean coffee grinder. Combine the dried herbs and jojoba oil in a small canning jar and stir, making sure the oil covers the herbs; you may need to press them down. Place a lid on loosely (**do not screw tight, to let air escape**). Place the jar in a small pot filled with water, using canning jar rings to elevate the jar from the bottom of the pot. Heat on the lowest stovetop setting for 5 hours. Take care that the oil's temperature doesn't go above 120°F by periodically testing with a kitchen thermometer. Depending on your stovetop settings, you may need to intermittently take the pot off the heat to let the oil cool.

2. After the infusion is complete, remove the jar from the water bath, take off the lid, and let the oil cool until comfortable to touch yet still warm. Strain the oil through a cloth, and press and wring thoroughly, like you really mean it. (Despite your best efforts, you'll lose some of the oil. That's okay.)

3. Add the rosehip seed oil and essential oils (if using) to the infused jojoba oil and stir. A small glass serum bottle is handy for dispensing minute amounts of the precious infusion. Try a small amount on your wrist first to determine if you react to the essential oils. The serum will keep for 1 year unrefrigerated and up to 2 years in refrigeration.

# Raspberry-Rose-Lime Bubbly

YIELD: 4 drinks

PREP TIME: 5 minutes

---

4 cups sparkling water

⅓ cup Raspberry-Rose-Lime Simple Syrup (page 189)

¼ cup fresh lime juice (from 2 to 3 limes)

1 teaspoon Dandy-Orange Bitters (page 264)

4 cups crushed ice, for serving

Lime wedges, for serving

This ruby refreshment is a delectable herbal version of sparkly punch, perfect for lakeside picnics or pool parties. The drink is only slightly sweet, and the addition of the bitters gives it a cocktail feel without the addition of alcohol. Transform the rose bubbly into a happy-hour libation by adding 1 ounce of vodka to each drink.

---

Combine the sparkling water, raspberry-rose syrup, lime juice, and bitters in a large jar and stir vigorously. Distribute equally into 4 large cocktail glasses filled with ice, and garnish with lime wedges.

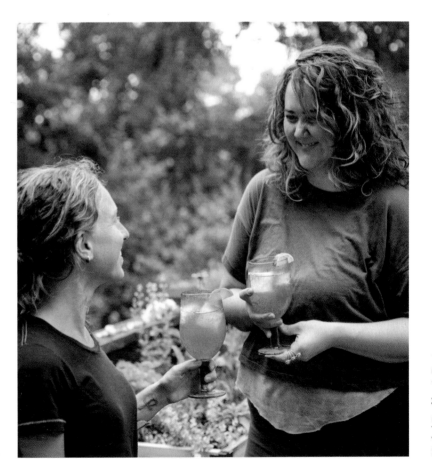

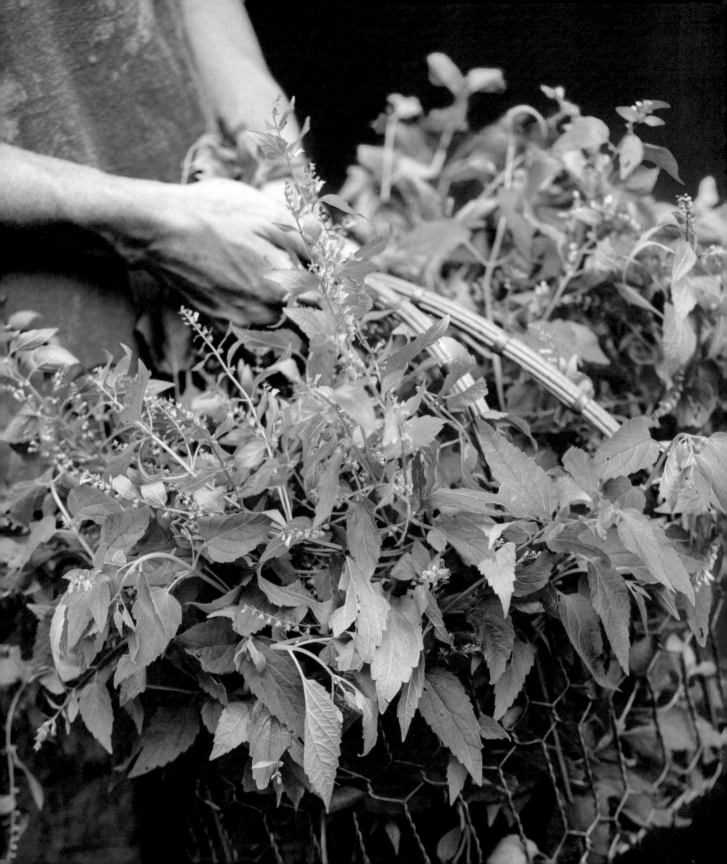

# SKULLCAP

**SCIENTIFIC NAME:** *Scutellaria lateriflora*
**LAMIACEAE,** mint family
**AKA:** mad-dog skullcap, blue skullcap, hoodwort, and scullcap

I first befriended skullcap when living in the Berkshire Mountains on a community farm. Every morning, I would set out from our woodland longhouse with my morning jar of nettles tea to seek out my secret sunlit perch—a fallen tree next to an active beaver pond—to see how the landscape was changing. Blue vervain, boneset, and skullcap grew among the sedges and grasses in the cool soil next to the water's edge. As a fresh-faced herb devotee with a fascination for beavers, that roost was my version of heaven on earth. I've since brought the herb into my garden and have tended a skullcap patch no matter where I've lived. Today, my skullcap is planted alongside boneset and blue vervain, a living homage to that beaver pond. As a garden herb, skullcap grows quite contentedly—spreading by runners into a small colony—as long as it has rich soil with ample moisture and a spot of shade in the brightest time of day.

The flower has an unusual trait—its calyx is crested, or hooded, like a tiny cap fit for a damselfly—inspiring the name *skullcap*. The herb is native to the northern reaches of the United States and southern Canada, growing in wet meadows and nearby streams, rivers, and lakes. Truth be told, you might step right over skullcap without even noticing the plant. With small scalloped-edged leaves smaller than a beaver's paw and tiny bluish-purple flowers the size of a robin's beak, the plant's diminutive traits don't exactly make it a garden showstopper. Nonetheless, the herb is a potent remedy for insomnia, anxiety, pain, and restlessness. I keep a bottle of skullcap on my nightstand in case I wake in the middle of the night, and the bottle accompanies me whenever I travel.

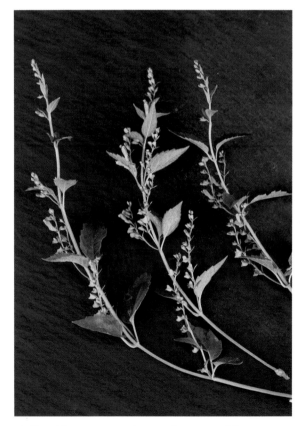

Skullcaps' flowers point in the same direction, and their calyx (green flower part under the petals) has a distinctive protuberance, or "skull cap"

## Cultivation

ZONES: 3–8; partial shade to full sun (if the soil is sufficiently moist)

SOIL: pH 6–8 (pH 6.2–7 optimal); moist, rich soil

SIZE: 1–2 feet tall; indefinitely wide

LIFESTYLE: Herbaceous perennial

PROPAGATION: Skullcap easily divides from the underground running stem. Be sure each division has rootlets and a bud or two, and you're good to go. Stratify the seeds for 60 days before starting in trays, or sow directly in the soil in the fall. Space the plants 1 foot apart.

SITING AND GARDEN CARE: Skullcap is glad to grow alongside a stream, pond, river, or lake as long as it's not in full shade, preferring dappled light. If you haven't such a spot, it will also do just fine in regular garden soil, especially if you add generous amounts of organic matter and compost and mulch well. The herb will grow in full sun if there's enough moisture and the climate isn't too hot. You'll need to keep its feet wet during droughty periods, and if you live in an arid or sweltering climate, shade in the heat of the day is essential. When I lived in hot and humid Florida, I grew skullcap as a winter annual. The herb may die back during the summer, going dormant, and reemerge in the fall as long as the soil is moist and kept mulched. In arid climates, skullcap can be grown in large, wide containers like the one shown opposite, which hold in moisture. Water frequently, and place the container in dappled light or afternoon shade.

There are more than 300 *Scutellaria* species worldwide, many of which are medicinal. However, the species are not all interchangeable. More than a few times, I've seen showier species of skullcap—mislabeled as *Scutelleria lateriflora*—for sale at herb nurseries. Accordingly, it's imperative you know and trust your sources if you're buying the potted plant. *S. lateriflora* has paired blossoms that are just over a ¼ inch in length, growing in one-sided racemes; the bluish flowers emerge from one side of the stem, pointing in the same direction. This characteristic is unique among the North American skullcaps and is the origin of the herb's species name, which means "side-flower."

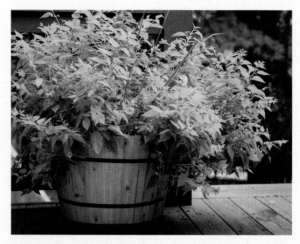

Skullcap thrives in containers; water frequently and use a large vessel to help hold in moisture

PROBLEM INSECTS AND DISEASES: Powdery mildew is sometimes a problem. I've had my patches ravished overnight by rabbits—perhaps they were having trouble sleeping that night! Various species of caterpillars can also munch the leaves.

HARVESTING: Harvest the flowering stalks of the herb when it's beginning to flower, leaving about 8 inches of the growth intact for the plants to regenerate; hang in loose bunches. The plant is quite succulent, so it will take longer to dry than other herbs. Strip the leaves and flowers from the stem after drying.

## Medicinal Properties

PART USED: Leaves and flowering tops

MEDICINAL PREPARATIONS: Tincture, infusion, and vinegar

TINCTURE RATIOS AND DOSAGE: Fresh (1:2 95%) or dry (1:5 60%); either preparation 2–5 ml up to three times a day

TEA RATIOS AND DOSAGE: Infusion of 1 to 2 teaspoons dried leaf and flower per 1 cup water up to three times a day

ACTIONS: Nervine tonic, antianxiety, hypnotic, anodyne, and antispasmodic

ENERGETICS: Slightly cooling and drying

## Medicinal Uses

Indigenous peoples from North America use various species of skullcap as herbal remedies for a variety of situations, including menstrual and digestive disorders and in childbirth. Eurasian species of skullcap are also used medicinally, but the part used and the therapeutic applications do not always overlap.

### NERVOUS SYSTEM

Skullcap is one of our most beloved hypnotic remedies, encouraging deep, restful sleep. Stronger than the gentle sedatives lemon balm and chamomile, skullcap is in the same league as sleep aids like passionflower, hops, and valerian; yet it is not overly sedating, and many people use the herb throughout the day to allay anxiety, restlessness, or pain. As a pain remedy, it can be combined with California poppy, passionflower, and vervain to assuage headaches, menstrual cramps, musculoskeletal aches, and pain from injuries or surgery. (See the recipe in the next column.) These herbal pain relievers are, in all honesty, generally less effective than pharmaceutical pain relievers, but they're still useful when pain isn't severe or in between doses of pharmaceutical pain relievers (to lessen the needed dose and decrease the frequency of dosages).

To calm anxiety and reduce stress, skullcap can be called on during acute situations or taken tonically. It's helpful for folks who hold on too tight—to their plan, to their lists, to their misgivings. As a tonic remedy for stress, it can be combined with milky oats and adaptogens such as tulsi, gotu kola, or reishi mushrooms.

### MUSCULOSKELETAL SYSTEM

Skullcap relieves muscle cramps and can be used to lessen tension in the jaw and to reduce teeth grinding and clenching at night. The herb is also helpful for back pain, tension headaches, sore and tight muscles, and twitching muscles.

## Pain-Relieving Formula

This blend is helpful for lessening the pain from headaches, toothaches, menstrual cramps, sore muscles, and pain due to injury or surgery. Avoid in pregnancy.

MAKES 4 OUNCES

1½ ounces skullcap leaf and flower tincture (*Scutellaria lateriflora*)

1 ounce California poppy leaf and flower tincture (*Eschscholzia californica*)

½ ounce passionflower leaf and flower tincture (*Passiflora incarnata*)

½ ounce vervain leaf and flower tincture (*Verbena hastata* or *V. officinalis*)

½ ounce rose bud or petal tincture (*Rosa* spp.)

Use fresh tinctures if possible, but you can substitute dried tinctures or use different preparations for each tincture. Combine all tinctures and store in a glass dispensing bottle. Dosage is 2–4 ml up to three times a day. For short-term relief of pain lasting no more than two days, you can take 3 ml up to six times a day.

> PRECAUTIONS: Germander (*Teucrium* spp.) looks similar to skullcap and for many years has been used as a skullcap adulterant (substitute) by herbal merchants. Unfortunately, at least one species of germander (*T. chamaedrys*) possesses compounds that are toxic to the liver. Be sure that any skullcap products you purchase come from a reliable source (companies can test for adulteration), as substitution may still be a concern.

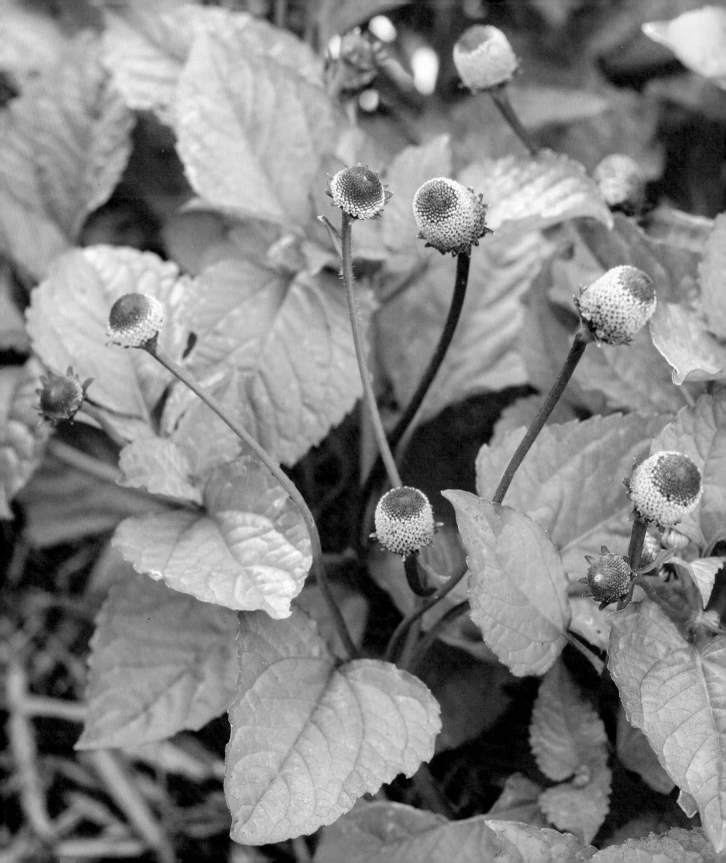

# SPILANTHES

SCIENTIFIC NAME: *Acmella oleracea*; formerly *Spilanthes oleracea*
ASTERACEAE, aster family
AKA: toothache plant, eyeball plant, para-cress, jambu (Brazil), Szechuan buttons, buzz buttons, electric buttons (New York City), electric daisies (Las Vegas), brede mafane (French-speaking countries), and peek-a-boo plant (silly seed companies)

Spilanthes is a tropical herb with globular golden blooms marked by a crimson center, earning the plant one of its many aliases, *eyeball plant*. Its flower and leaf have a potent effect on the salivary glands; even the tiniest nibble will set your mouth to shimmer and drool, culminating in a tingly numbing sensation. Wow! The name "toothache plant" is a nod to the dulling sensation the herb affords to toothache pain.

Spilanthes is a short-lived perennial in the tropics. Elsewhere, the frost-sensitive plant is grown as an annual. It has gained recent acclaim as an ornamental bedding plant and also as a culinary herb. The herb has a host of medicinal uses and yields a substantial amount of medicine in one season: one to two plants will yield over a quart of tincture. Spilanthes has been one of my closest garden companions for over two decades and is one of the primary medicines I turn to in my apothecary year after year. The herb is native to South America, most likely Brazil, but has been cultivated as a medicinal and culinary herb for so long that its native range is unclear. In fact, spilanthes is no longer known in the wild and only exists in the gardens of humans or escaped nearby (we call such plants *cultigens*). Spilanthes is now grown in India, China, and South and Central America.

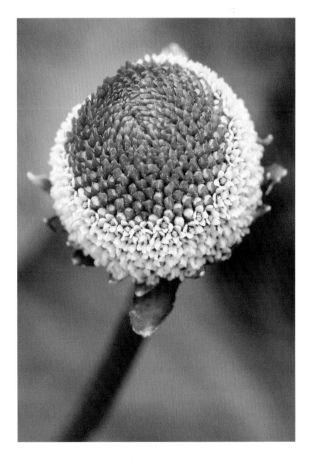

Spilanthes is a medicinal groundcover with succulent leaves. The inflorescences grow singly and consist of only ray florets, giving the flower heads the appearance of button-like "buds" when, in fact, they are fully mature, bearing hundreds of fertile little flowers.

## Cultivation

ZONES: Perennial in zones 10 and warmer; grown as a frost-tender annual in all other zones; full sun to light shade

SOIL: pH 6–7; average to moist fertile soil

SIZE: 1 foot tall; 1–2 feet wide

LIFESTYLE: Frost-tender perennial but commonly grown as an annual

PROPAGATION: Sow the tiny seeds on the surface of the soil, and lightly tamp in. The seed germinates in 5 to 10 days at 70–85°F. It's easy to divide spilanthes roots: sever a rooted side shoot, cut back half of the vegetation, and replant. Or take cuttings from vegetative stems and cut each leaf in half before placing in the cutting medium. Plant 1 foot apart after the danger of frost has passed.

SITING AND GARDEN CARE: Spilanthes is grown as a frost-tender annual unless you live in the tropics. Plant it in average to rich soil after the danger of frost has passed. Water during dry spells, as it relishes water more than many other medicinals. It will let you know when it's thirsty; spilanthes is one of the first plants to wilt in my herb garden during droughty conditions. When I lived in Florida, I planted the herb in the dappled shade under tangerine trees and mulched the plants heavily to hold in the moisture. If you live in an arid climate or have well-drained soil, plant it in soil amended with extra organic matter or add clay to aid with water retention.

Spilanthes easily transplants and self-sows if you don't mulch too heavily, but the volunteer sprouts take their time coming up—I don't usually see them until mid-June, so you may want to start the seeds fresh every year to get a head start on the season. Spilanthes happily sprawls as a dense groundcover under taller herbs or vegetables, such as tomatoes, peppers, hibiscus, basil, tulsi, and calendula. Spilanthes with all-yellow flowers, sometimes called "lemon drops," can be used medicinally the same as the ones with red centers. (This yellow-bloomed spilanthes is perhaps *Acmella alba*, or it may be a cultivar of *A. oleracea*. The taxonomy is unclear.) Spilanthes does well in containers and can be interplanted with other ornamental medicinals, such as lemongrass, purple basil, and artichoke.

PROBLEM INSECTS AND DISEASES: Slugs relish spilanthes. One solution is to plant the herb in a hanging basket, which elevates the plants far from the reach of even the most adventurous gastropods. Aphids and spider mites can sometimes be a problem.

HARVESTING: It's possible to harvest the plants two to three times during the growing season. Cut the plants back to 6 inches, and if there's still time before the frost, the plants will regrow nicely and give you another harvest. Dry the herb on screens or in loose-weave baskets.

## Medicinal Properties

PART USED: Leaves and flowers

MEDICINAL PREPARATIONS: Tincture, tea, poultice, compress, tooth powder, nibble, and cocktail fancier

TINCTURE RATIOS AND DOSAGE: Fresh (1:2 95%); 2–4 ml three times a day; more frequent dosages (up to five times a day for two to three days) can be used for virulent infections. Dried tincture not recommended.

TEA RATIOS AND DOSAGE: Infusion of 1 to 2 teaspoons of dried leaf and flower per 1 cup water up to three times a day

ACTIONS: Sialagogue (salivary stimulant), oral anodyne, immunostimulant, diuretic, antioxidant, anti-inflammatory, antibacterial, antifungal, and anthelmintic

ENERGETICS: Stimulating and dispersing, slightly warming; mildly drying owing to its diuretic actions

## Medicinal Uses

Spilanthes has been one of my top ten herbal allies for the past two decades. I first learned about it from a

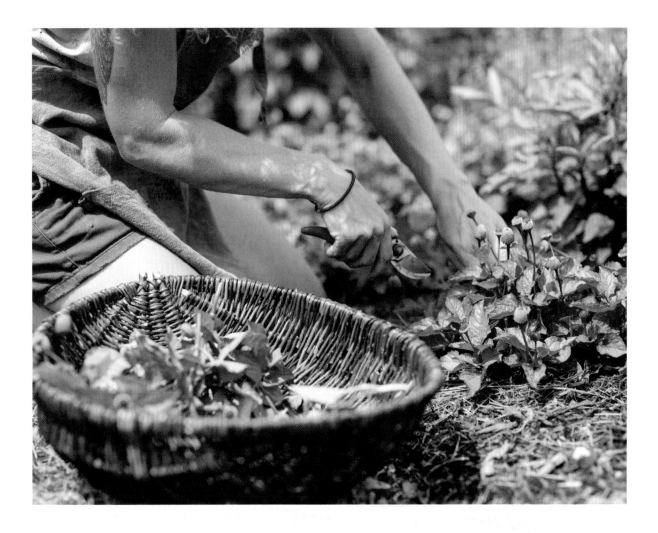

former apprentice of herbalist Deb Soule, who has long favored it as a garden medicinal and writes about it in her book, *The Roots of Healing: A Woman's Book of Herbs*. I became a spilanthes devotee the first year I began growing it and using it for medicine. The herb's unmistakable salivary sparkle—and immune-stimulating quality—is brought about by constituents named *alkamides,* also known as *alkylamides*. *Spilanthol* is the most abundant isobutylamide (class of alkamides) in the spilanthes plant. The presence of prickly alkamides is shared with a number of medicinal and culinary plants, including purple coneflower, prickly ash, and Sichuan pepper, or Szechuan peppercorns—a Chinese spice that is derived from the fruits of several trees in the *Zanthoxylum* genus.

All the aboveground parts are medicinal and can be chewed fresh in moderation or made into a tincture. The flowers are the most tingle-inducing part, possessing the highest concentration of alkamides, but the leaves and stem are a close second in terms of tingle and medicine. The plant can be dried and used medicinally, but it is more bioactive and potent when fresh. Be sure the dried plant is tingly when you nibble on it—this is a good indicator of its strength. When the plant is in season, it can be used fresh as a poultice, tea, nibble, or chew.

### IMMUNE SYSTEM

One of the most common ways I use spilanthes is as an immune stimulant to augment the body's internal defenses against the common cold and flu. Immune stimulants are helpful to ward off infection after potential exposure, like flying on an airplane or caring for a sick family member. This class of herbs can also be called on to stimulate immune activity throughout infectious illness, which ultimately helps a person get over the sickness more quickly. I combine spilanthes with other antimicrobial herbs, such as usnea, goldenseal, and honeysuckle, when combating infectious illness. (See the recipe on page 291.) Spilanthes can be called upon to help the body fight many infectious diseases, including sinus infections, urinary tract infections, ear infections, cold sores, colds, and influenza. The herb is used around the globe as a digestive remedy against intestinal infections and parasites.

### ORAL USES

Toothache plant truly lives up to its name, as it can temporarily numb the mouth during tooth infections and abscesses. It can be combined with licorice root for this purpose while one waits for the relief of a needed dental procedure. In India and Southeast Asia, spilanthes is a traditional toothache remedy and is also used to strengthen teeth and prevent tooth decay. The herb helps maintain healthy gums by increasing salivation and blood flow. The dried flowers can be added to tooth powders to address periodontal disease. Alternatively, after brushing with toothpaste, add the powdered flowers to a wetted toothbrush and brush the gums and tongue. Add goldenseal powder (cultivated only) to increase the antimicrobial and astringent qualities. If you have fresh plants on hand, chewing on a bit of the flower head is a fine substitute for the above methods. When spilanthes-grazing, I find that the buzz of the plant is not limited to my mouth—I feel mentally refreshed and vitalized after ingesting even a tiny bit of the plant.

### TOPICAL USES

Deb Soule recommends diluting the tincture of spilanthes, along with echinacea and usnea tinctures, with calendula tea as a douche for bacterial vaginosis. I've used the diluted tincture of spilanthes topically as a compress or soak on various insect bites and stings, including spider bites. It seems to take away the sting and swelling. Topically, it's used to fight infections and heal burns.

## Culinary Uses

Spilanthes' sparkly, palate-numbing properties make for a unique gustatory sensation. The "buds" can be found adorning specialty cocktails; the flower heads are pressed firmly into the rim of a glass to fully release the bling. One enterprising bartender concocted a cocktail known as the *Electriquila,* prepared from tequila, sake, and citrus and served in a glass with a salted spilanthes rim. The herb can be used in lieu of Sichuan pepper to season a number of traditional Chinese, Nepali, and Tibetan dishes. South Americans flavor stir-fries and sauces with the tingly floral heads. In Brazil, jambu (their name for spilanthes) is used to flavor meat and prepare a zingy soup, along with chili peppers, garlic, and cassava.

> **PRECAUTIONS:** Immune-stimulating herbs like spilanthes have a potential to increase autoimmunity and have caused flare-ups in people with autoimmune conditions, although this is more the exception than the rule. As spilanthes is in the aster family, it has the remote potential to cause a reaction with people who are highly sensitive to plants like ragweed and chamomile; however, there are no documented adverse allergic reactions, despite its widespread international use. Take care not to squirt the tincture on the back of your throat or chew too large a wad of spilanthes, as the throat may take offense and clamp down.

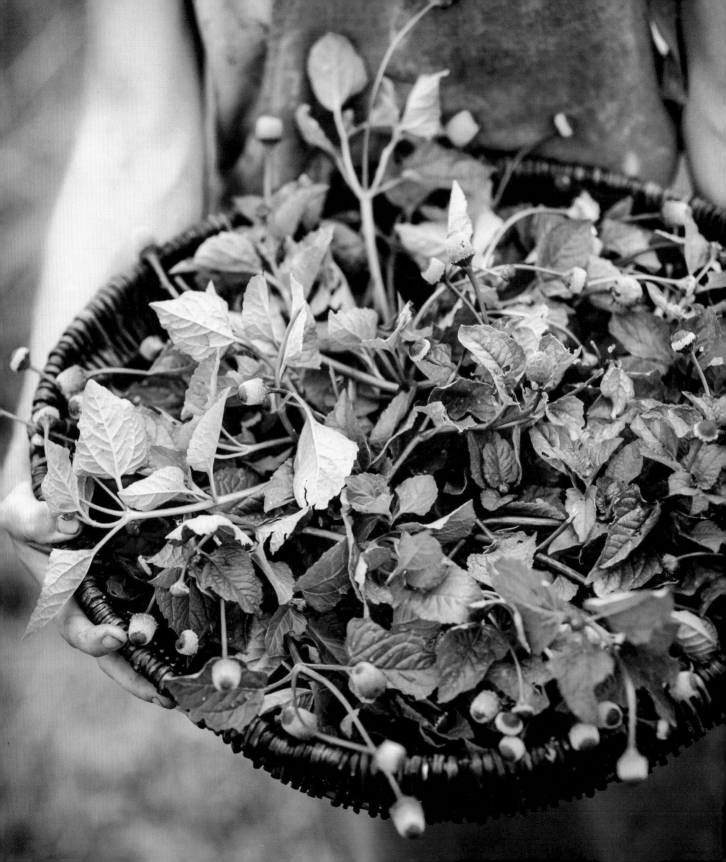

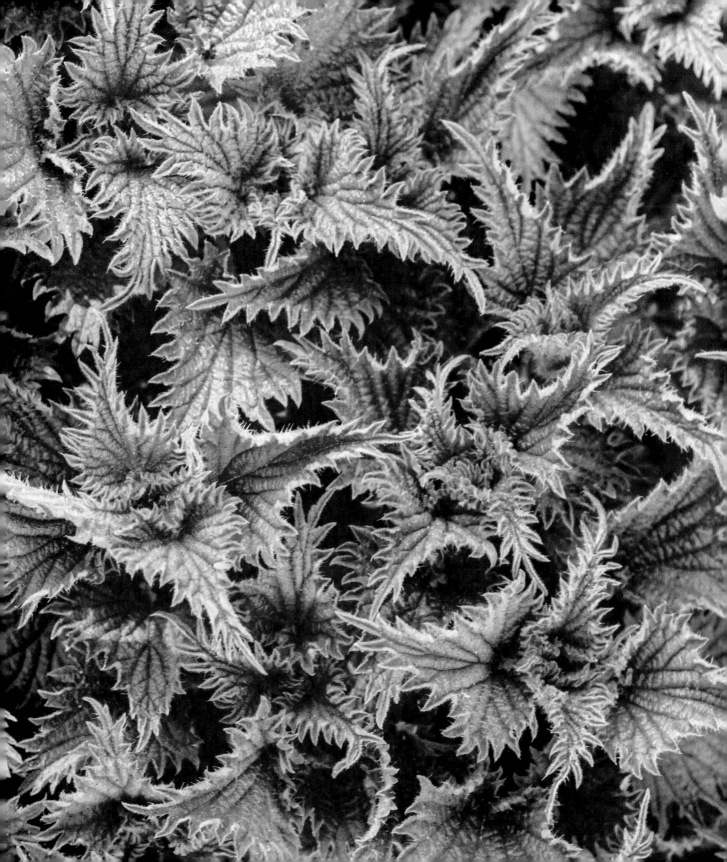

# STINGING NETTLES

SCIENTIFIC NAME: *Urtica dioica*
URTICACEAE, nettles family
AKA: nettles, nettle

The emerald nettles queen reigns over the herbal realms with vim and vigor. She is not to be trifled with. Nettle wears a crown of nearly invisible silver prickles, primed to sting any who might dare to trespass. The leaves of this legendary herb are packed with vitamins, minerals, and chlorophyll, and this vitality infuses into nutritive herbal teas, vinegars, and medicinal foods. The sting of nettles is disarmed when the leaves are dried or cooked. The plant forms dense colonies through spreading rhizomes. It is native to Eurasia, northern Africa, and North America but is now widely cultivated and naturalized throughout the temperate world.

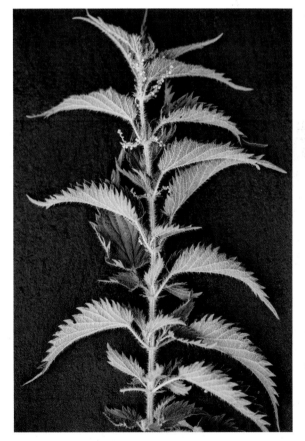

A nettle stalk in flower midsummer

The sting of nettles is orchestrated by trigger-happy hairs (trichomes) that inject a slew of inflammatory compounds, including histamine, serotonin, oxalic acid, and acetylcholine. These chemicals cause an electrifying tingle. Your skin might bloom with miniature welts and swelling, both of which dissipate within 24 hours. Nerve sensation can be altered, making bathing a novel sensory experience. Interestingly, the juice of nettles is a traditional antidote to the sting, as are poultices of the leaves of yellow dock and jewelweed. I find these remedies to be underwhelming, but they do assuage the emotional upset of being one-upped by a plant in the most nettlesome fashion. The prickle of nettles is oddly therapeutic for arthritic joints. Self-flagellation with nettles, called *urtication*, helps to relieve pain and inflammation temporarily. The reprieve varies, but for some brave souls, the effect lasts a few weeks. (If you want to try this at home, seek the guidance of an experienced herbalist, as the skin irritation and inflammation can be quite uncomfortable.)

## Cultivation

ZONES: 2–9; full sun to partial shade

SOIL: pH 5.5–7.8; rich, moist soil with a high nutrient content

SIZE: 3–5 feet tall; indefinitely wide

LIFESTYLE: Herbaceous perennial

PROPAGATION: Root division (technically, rhizome division) in the fall or spring is the easiest way to propagate the plant. Dig shallow furrows, spaced every 10 inches, and lay the rhizomes along the entire length of the furrows. This dense spacing will give you a solid bed of nettles in one year. Obtain the rhizomes from clean wild patches or neighboring herb growers. To start from seed, stratify seeds for one to two months or direct-seed in the fall. Don't cover the seeds when planting. Seedlings emerge in 7 to 14 days at 65–70°F. Space the plants every 9 inches.

SITING AND GARDEN CARE: Planting nettles into the garden requires foresight and planning, as the plant can spread by seeds and runners alike and become a troublesome and painful weed. But with strategic placement and management, it is a valuable asset in the landscape: nettles are a perennial food crop, medicinal herb, and garden amendment. If you already have nettles growing nearby in a pristine locale, perhaps you don't need to invite it closer. I've found, however, that our family consumes more nettles when we have easy access. Throughout the spring and summer, my partner's morning ritual consists of clipping a few shoots from the nettle patch for his herbal infusions, and I'm apt to run out the back door to harvest the greens for dinner.

To avoid encounters with unsuspecting humans, plant nettles out of the way in a wet meadow, at a damp wood's edge, or near an old compost or manure pile. If you haven't such a spot, you can plant them as a perennial garden herb. But consider well. Nettle might be the most tenacious herb you plant, persisting for decades or longer, and will require your vigilance to curb its colonizing tendencies. The stakes are high, considering the potential for bare feet and hands to encounter nettle's stinging hairs. If you do decide to grow it, enrich the soil with abundant organic matter, and mulch heavily the first year; nettles will soon fill the entire bed, excluding most weeds. Mulch the pathways heavily with wood chips, or mow to discourage spreading nettle shoots. Alternatively, plant nettles in a raised bed with wood sides, or install a semi-buried barrier around plantings. In many locales, the plant will spread by seed, making containment even more challenging. Dispose of the fruiting branches before they can release their seeds. In a warm or arid climate, the plants appreciate afternoon shade and irrigation. In drier regions, plant nettles in a retired bathtub, trough, or pond liner.

Nettle plants are in hog heaven growing in aged manure and compost piles. Otherwise, feed nettles annually with aged compost or manure, and they'll reward you generously with exuberant growth. Nettle is a *dynamic accumulator*—a term used to describe plants with the ability to mine nutrients (such as nitrogen, potassium, phosphorus, and calcium) from deep in the soil and concentrate the nutrients in their leaves. These stored nutrients are released into the upper layers of the soil when the plants die or lose their leaves, making the surrounding neighborhood more hospitable for other plants. Gardeners can capitalize on this process by adding the nutrient-dense leaves to the compost pile or using them as a fertile mulch. Or prepare a fermented compost tea out of nettles following the directions on page 52.

PROBLEM INSECTS AND DISEASES: Aphids relish the tender greens and can pose a real problem in spring, resulting in stunted growth and disfigured young leaves. Grasshoppers can also be a nuisance. The larvae (caterpillars) of many native butterflies and moths feed off nettles, which can sometimes result in marked defoliation.

IDENTIFICATION AND HARVESTING: Nettles have an unmistakable trait: the ability to needle humans with its microscopic burning hairs. Even though its sting is remarkable, other plants have a similar defense mechanism, so it's essential to look at all the characteristics below.

> **NETTLE'S IDENTIFYING TRAITS**
>
> - Opposite, stinging leaves with large teeth and distinct veins, giving the leaf a "quilted" texture. The shape of the leaf varies, depending on the strain, and can be triangular to loosely heart shaped, or elongated, two to three times as long as it is wide.
>
> - The green stem is never woody and is loosely four-sided with four grooves; it has stinging hairs. The plant has four little strap-shaped stipules (leaf-like appendages) at the node (leaf-stem junction).
>
> - Nettles grow in colonies close to humans and waterways—floodplains, forest edges, ditches, hedgerows, trailsides, and old farms, especially in barnyards.
>
> - Green, demure flowers grow from the leaf-stem junction. The plant can be dioecious, with separate female and male individuals, or monoecious, with male and female flowers on the same plant. Its species name—*dioica*—refers to its dioecious form.

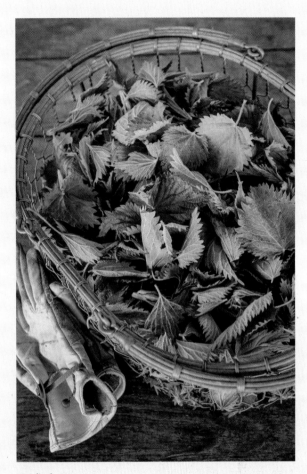

Nettles harvest

The wood nettle (*Laportea canadensis*) is a close relative of stinging nettle found growing near shaded streams and trailsides in central and eastern North America. It has alternate stinging leaves, whereas stinging nettle (*Urtica dioica*) bears opposite leaves. Wood nettle has edible leaves, but the leaves are not used medicinally like stinging nettle. There are other species of stinging nettle used as medicine or as food; consult a local wild foods expert or herbalist to learn about regional varieties. Note that a few unrelated plants are also called *nettles* because of a similar ability to sting. These meddlesome plants aren't used in the same way as *Urtica* species. An example is bull nettle (*Cnidoscolus stimulosus*), a stinging plant in the spurge family. Two North American species of plants—false nettle (*Boehmeria cylindrica*) and nettle-leafed vervain (*Verbena urticifolia*)—closely resemble stinging nettle but lack the characteristic stinging hairs.

When harvesting nettles, wear thick clothing that covers arms and ankles, and use leather gardening gloves, preferably ones that cover the forearms, such as leather rose gloves. Use a scythe or similar tool for large-scale harvesting and pruners or kitchen scissors for smaller yields. The shoots emerge in the earliest spring and can be harvested weekly. When you pick the greens repeatedly, you'll be rewarded with tender new regrowth throughout the spring. When harvesting for food, take only the tender upper leaves; pinch off the tips or strip the upper leaves from the stem. Later in the summer, the leaves become too chewy to eat. For medicinal uses, harvest the plants when they are knee-high but have not yet flowered. Don't crush the leaves. If you pile up the shoots in a harvest basket, the bruised leaves oxidize to

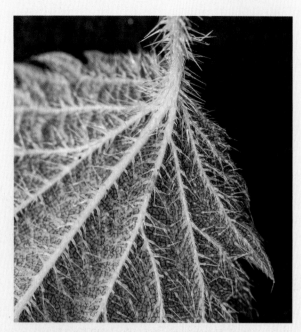

Close-up of nettle's stinging hairs, or trichomes, on the underside of a leaf

an unsavory black color, diminishing the herb's vitality. I learned this the hard way one spring. After hiking a few miles to a lush, pristine nettle patch, I eagerly stuffed a large duffel bag full of shoots, only to discover the crop ruined when I returned home.

Come midsummer, nettles tire, raggedy from the heat. The plants are sometimes besieged by ravenous caterpillars. Cut the plants back after the caterpillars have metamorphosed and moved on, and fall's cooler temperatures will rouse nettles back to life. Many traditional herbalists caution against harvesting nettles after the plants have begun to flower because older nettle leaves can irritate the kidneys. Other herbalists dismiss this precaution. I tend to heed the warnings of those with more experience, and I'm conservative when it comes to other people's health. In any case, the plant doesn't look especially perky by the time it's flowering, so I harvest the leaves earlier in the season when it still looks vital. If you're harvesting the plant from the wild, be sure your location is pristine, as it can bioaccumulate toxins.

## Medicinal Properties

**PART USED:** Leaves, seeds, and roots (rhizomes)

**MEDICINAL PREPARATIONS:** Infusion, tincture, vinegar, pesto, cooked greens, juice, broth, powder, capsules, and finishing salts

**TINCTURE RATIOS AND DOSAGE:** Fresh (1:2 95%) or dry (1:4 60%) leaves; either preparation 2–4 ml three times a day

**TEA RATIOS AND DOSAGE:** Infusion of 2 teaspoons to 2 tablespoons dried leaves per 1 cup water up to three times a day

**ACTIONS:** Alterative, antirheumatic, anti-inflammatory, galactagogue, astringent, diuretic, and nutritive tonic

**ENERGETICS:** Cooling and drying

## Medicinal Uses

Nettle is a supreme blood builder and nourishing tonic. If you're hankering for the minerals in nettles, take the herb as an infusion, broth, or vinegar, or enjoy it as a food. (Alcohol-based tincture won't deliver the minerals.) Because it's a food plant, nettle can be consumed frequently, with less attention to dosage as compared with other herbs. However, the herb can be drying, resulting in dry skin and sinus membranes. To counter this effect, take nettles with demulcent herbs like marshmallow, linden, or chia seeds. The herb may still prove too drying for everyday use if you run dry.

### NUTRITIVE TONIC

With its high iron content, nettle is highly useful as an infusion, vinegar, or broth for iron-deficiency anemia. It can be consumed during pregnancy and the postpartum to help with the extra nutritional demands of childbirth and breastfeeding. The herb can be part of a nutritional and herbal strategy for rebuilding iron levels after heavy bleeding from childbirth or menstruation. Nettle is a traditional tonic for promoting breast milk production, especially for those with lower nutritional reserves. (See my Mineral-Rich Herbal Infusion recipe, which includes nettles, on page 333.)

### SKIN TONIC

Nettle is a traditional spring tonic and blood cleanser, and it's an excellent herbal ally during fasting and cleansing. The herb is prepared into teas, along with red clover and burdock, to assuage eczema, psoriasis, and acne. Nettles will perk you up when you feel tired or depleted and can help build reserves after a long or intense illness. I often add the herb to milky oats and tulsi to support people undergoing challenging transitions and periods of extra workload.

### URINARY SYSTEM

The leaves and seeds of nettles are a diuretic and kidney tonic. Combine it with uva-ursi, goldenrod, and corn silk to prepare a tea for addressing urinary tract infections. The root is an ingredient in many herbal formulas used to address benign prostatic hyperplasia (BPH). Nettle leaf enhances the excretion of uric acid, making it useful in the treatment of gout. It is also a traditional remedy for dissolving kidney stones. The seeds are the primary part of the plant used to support kidney function, but the leaves are also a kidney tonic.

### ALLERGIES

Freeze-dried nettle, in capsule form, is used as a tonic antihistamine for allergies. In one study, 58 percent of hay fever sufferers reported freeze-dried nettles as moderately to highly effective at alleviating allergy symptoms. There is a good bit of controversy in the herbal community as to whether preparations other than the freeze-dried capsules are equally effective. Some herbalists swear that the freeze-dried nettles are more efficacious, and some practitioners use concentrated tinctures and infusions instead with good results. I recommend beginning with the freeze-dried nettles and seeing how effective they are before experimenting with other methods. Start the nettles 3 months before seasonal allergies typically begin, continuing throughout the duration of allergy season. Nettle is also helpful for dander or dust allergies, in which case the regimen can be started at any time.

## Culinary Uses

Nettle is a nutritious spring green eaten steamed or added to soups and stir-fries. The sting disappears when the leaves are cooked or dried. The cooked greens and tea of nettles are high in chlorophyll, vitamins, and minerals, including vitamins A and C, calcium, potassium, magnesium, and iron. Use nettle greens anywhere you might use spinach or kale. Add them to quiche, omelets, or soup. Nettle greens are a tad fibrous, but you can mask their texture by sneaking them into creamy soups or blending them into pesto or pâté. Make a large batch of nettles pesto (page 172) or pâté (page 384) and freeze it in smaller portions to use throughout the winter months. Rehydrate the dried leaves in soups and stews, but make sure you cook them until they're tender, as they can be a bit chewy otherwise. Nettle, along with its sister-wife, seaweed, finds its way into my wintertime broths, including my Herbal Immunity Broth Concentrate on page 174. Another way to enjoy the herb's rich store of minerals is to prepare an herbal vinegar from the dried leaves. (See the recipe for Resilience Vinegar on page 187.)

> **PRECAUTIONS:** Nettles can be drying when ingested daily; use in moderation for those with dry skin and dry mucous membranes. Additionally, its diuretic effects may compound pharmaceuticals with the same action. The herb may alter blood sugar levels—people with diabetes should consult a medical practitioner and monitor blood sugar levels. Wild-harvest the plants from clean locales only, as they are adept at concentrating heavy metals and other toxins.

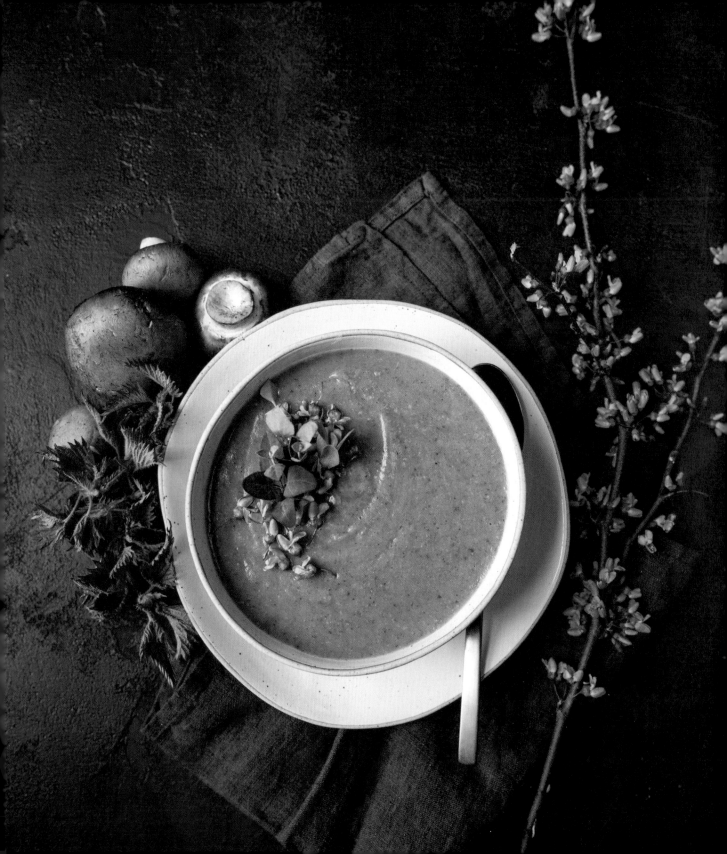

# Creamy Nettles Potato Soup

YIELD: 3 quarts if using fresh nettles; 2½ quarts if using dried nettles

5 large (about 3 pounds) russet potatoes, cubed

2 quarts vegetable or chicken stock or Herbal Immunity Broth (page 174)

4 strips bacon (turkey, tempeh, or pork)

2 quarts (115 grams) fresh nettles (to substitute dried, see the note below)

1 tablespoon butter or extra-virgin olive oil, or more to taste

1 medium leek, trimmed, well washed, and sliced

10 medium (310 grams) cremini mushrooms, chopped

Sea salt, to taste

½ teaspoon freshly ground black pepper, to taste

¼ teaspoon red pepper flakes, to taste

Sprigs of chickweed or microgreens, for garnish

Note: If using dried nettles, use 1 cup (20 grams) dried nettles plus 4 cups finely chopped seasonal greens such as kale, spinach, lamb's-quarter, or Swiss chard (2 to 3 bunches)

This hearty emerald soup sneaks mineral-packed nettles and immunomodulating mushrooms into a classic and comforting dish. If nettles aren't in season or you don't have access to fresh nettles, you can use dried nettles plus fresh cooking greens. This soup tastes much like a baked potato; try it with a garnish of fresh minced chives and sour cream, or add a generous drizzle of grass-fed heavy cream to each bowl. For a punch of umami, throw some crumbled blue cheese or feta into the mix. Whatever garnishes you choose, this soup is as welcoming as it is nourishing.

1. In a large pot, bring the potatoes and stock to a boil. Turn the heat down to simmer.

2. In a skillet, fry up the bacon. While the bacon is frying, wash the fresh nettles thoroughly (it may require several washings). Strip the leaves from the fibrous stems using leather garden gloves. When bacon is fried, place on a paper towel to drain; set aside.

3. In the same skillet, heat the butter or oil. Sauté the leek and cremini mushrooms until tender.

4. Coarsely chop the cooked bacon. Add the bacon, nettles, and sautéed leek and mushrooms to the pot with the potatoes and stock. Continue cooking over medium heat until the nettles are green and tender and the potatoes are thoroughly cooked, about 10 minutes. Turn off the heat. Using an immersion blender, puree the soup until completely smooth and creamy. Or let the soup cool slightly and then blend it in a food processor or blender; transfer it back to the pot to reheat.

5. Add the salt, pepper, and red pepper flakes, to taste. Add more butter or extra-virgin olive oil if desired for a richer flavor. Serve in wide bowls to showcase the color, and garnish with sprigs of chickweed or microgreens.

# Nettles Pâté

YIELD: 4 cups with fresh nettles; 4½ cups with dried nettles

---

15 to 20 (60 grams) small to medium sun-dried tomatoes (about ½ cup)

4 quarts (225 grams) loosely packed fresh nettles, or substitute 2½ cups dried nettles (55 grams)

1 cup (105 grams) walnut halves

10 medium (100 grams) shiitake mushroom caps, chopped

½ cup extra-virgin olive oil, plus a little more for sautéing the mushrooms

3 garlic cloves, peeled

½ cup (70 grams) whole pitted Kalamata olives

½ cup (115 grams) feta cheese

⅓ cup (70 grams) grated Parmesan cheese

Nettles pâté is pesto's voluptuous cousin, thicker and earthier by nature. Smother it on pasta, bake it into lasagna, or spread it on pizza or focaccia. Serve as a dip with crudités or crackers. You can enjoy this dish year-round by following the directions below for dried nettles. If you avoid dairy, substitute extra olives for the feta and Parmesan cheese. Or, use a coconut- or nut-based cheese alternative, tasting for saltiness as needed.

---

1. Pour just enough hot water over the sun-dried tomatoes to cover, and let sit for 3 hours. If you don't have the time to presoak, soaking them in hot water while you prepare the other ingredients is sufficient. You can also substitute jarred sun-dried tomatoes in olive oil. Strain the soaked tomatoes after hydrating.

2. Prep your nettles:

IF USING DRIED NETTLES: Bring 1⅔ cups water to a boil in a small saucepan. Turn off the heat, add the dried nettles, and stir every 5 minutes as the nettles rehydrate. Set aside (you won't be straining the rehydrated nettles).

IF USING FRESH NETTLES: Strip the nettle leaves from the fibrous stem using leather garden gloves. Wash the leaves thoroughly (it may require several washings). Steam until the nettles are tender yet still vibrantly green. Let the nettles cool with the lid off.

3. Toast the walnut halves in a dry, preheated skillet over medium heat, stirring continuously, until their aroma permeates the kitchen and they are slightly browned, about 1 to 2 minutes. Do not leave unattended, as they can quickly burn. Place the toasted walnuts on a plate to cool. In a small skillet, sauté the mushrooms in a little extra-virgin olive oil over medium heat until tender, about 5 minutes.

4. When the nettles and mushrooms are cool enough to handle, combine all the ingredients in a blender or food processor, and blend until the pâté reaches an even consistency. Add more olive oil and salt, if necessary. Refrigerate for up to 5 days or freeze in small portions.

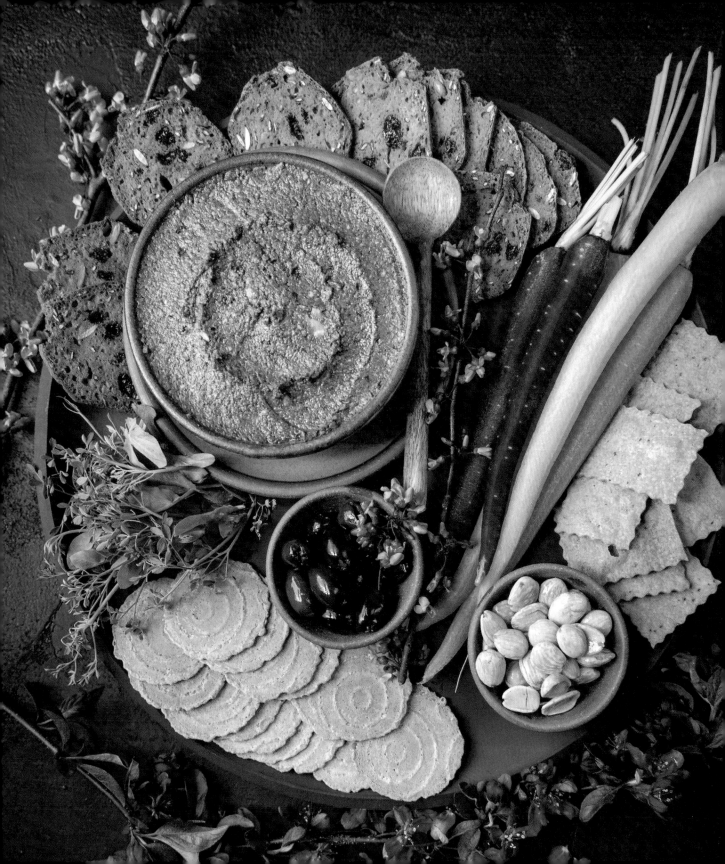

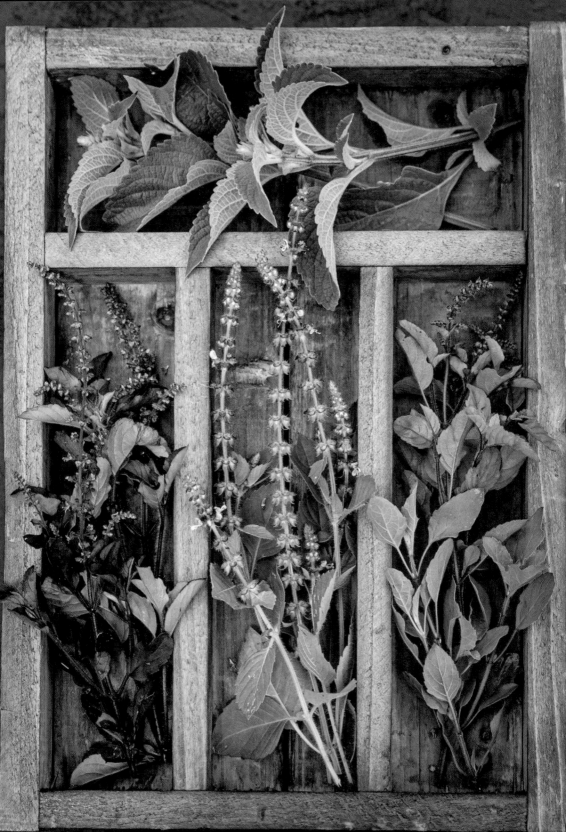

# TULSI

SCIENTIFIC NAME: *Ocimum tenuiflorum*, formerly *Ocimum sanctum*, and other *Ocimum* species and crosses
LAMIACEAE, mint family
AKA: holy basil, sacred basil, *tulasi* (Sanskrit), *kaphrao* or *kha phrao* (Thai)

Tulsi truly is one of the most versatile medicinals you can grow in your garden and bring into your apothecary. It has long been a sacred plant in India, prized for its myriad medicinal uses and calming, uplifting nature. In the past decade, it has gained herbal superstardom status in the West as a tasty beverage tea and panacea—the leaves and flowers are a remedy for colds, flu, sinus infections, anxiety, depression, allergies, asthma, coughs, cardiovascular disease, poor memory, and lack of concentration. The tender shoots are used in cooking throughout southern Asia as a spicier variation of its affable culinary and botanical cousin, Genovese basil (page 217). In the tropics, it is a semiwoody small shrub, reaching hip-high or taller. Elsewhere, it is grown as a frost-tender annual. Tulsi is native to the tropics and subtropics of Asia and has spread from cultivation in the Caribbean, parts of Africa, and the Pacific Islands.

## Tulsi Varieties

Depending on the cultivar, tulsi's size and the appearance of its leaves and flowers vary. Each variety is nuanced in flavor, medicinal use, and aroma owing to its unique essential oil profile. The botanical classification of the basil genus (*Ocimum*) is in flux, and there's confusion regarding the scientific naming of the various tulsi varieties, perhaps due in part to its long history of cultivation. If you live in the temperate world, you'll find the highest yield with 'Kapoor' (*Ocimum* sp.), also called 'Temperate Holy Basil', as it's the easiest to germinate and grow in cooler climates. If you purchase tulsi seeds from a North American seed company or buy the plant from an herb nursery, it will usually be 'Kapoor', even if it isn't labeled as such. It is milder in flavor than the other cultivars, which I find preferable for pesto.

'Rama' (*O. tenuiflorum*) has a purplish stem and smallish green leaves; it is the most common variety grown in India. 'Krishna' (*O. tenuiflorum*) is a pungent variety with striking purplish leaves and stems; it is especially helpful for clearing the sinuses and enlivening the senses. 'Vana' tulsi (*Ocimum* sp.) goes by many names, including wild tulsi, African basil, wild basil, clove tulsi, forest-type, or van tulsi (which is perhaps a separate species, but its classification is unclear). 'Vana' tulsi is covered with velvety gray hairs, has pale lavender blooms, and looks markedly different from the other tulsi strains. It has a clove-like aroma from its high content of eugenol. It is native to Africa and southern Asia and has naturalized in Central America, Hawai'i, South America, and Polynesia.

*Top:* 'Vana' tulsi; **bottom left to right:** 'Krishna', 'Temperate', 'Amrita'

# Cultivation

ZONES: Perennial in zones 10 and warmer; grown as a frost-sensitive annual elsewhere; plant in full sun

SOIL: pH 5.5–7.5 (6–7 optimal); fertile, well-drained soil with consistent moisture

SIZE: Varies by cultivar and location. As an annual, most varieties are 18 inches tall and 12 to 18 inches wide; 'Vana' tulsi grows 5 feet tall and 3 feet wide; tulsi is much larger in the tropics

LIFESTYLE: Most varieties are woody perennials in the tropics but grown as annuals in temperate zones

PROPAGATION: The seed is small and should be planted shallowly; barely cover the seeds. Bottom heat will significantly increase germination. Sprouts in 5 to 21 days at 70–85°F. 'Kapoor' typically germinates the quickest of the tulsi varieties. When the soil and air temperatures are cool, the plant is slow to grow; when the days grow longer and the nighttime temperatures warm, it will take off! Tulsi is frost tender; transplant or direct-seed after the danger of frost has passed. You can also propagate it through semiripe softwood cuttings. In the temperate world, space plants 12 inches apart, except for 'Vana' tulsi, which should be spaced 2 feet apart. In the tropics, you'll need to space the plants farther apart.

SITING AND GARDEN CARE: Tulsi enjoys full sun in temperate regions but doesn't mind a little afternoon shade in warmer climates. It will grow in almost any garden soil, but it's lusher with good fertility and consistent moisture. If you live in a cool, damp, cloudy climate, you may have more success growing it in a greenhouse or hoop house. Tulsi thrives in containers placed in full sun. I've successfully grown most varieties of tulsi in pots.

As with culinary basil, pinching back the shoots and early flowers encourages the plant to bush out and promotes more vegetative growth. Tulsi truly is an early bloomer, sometimes flowering when it is only a few inches high. Pinching off those early flowers helps it develop into a well-rounded plant. I pinch tulsi back a couple of times a week for the first month the plants are in the ground. These aromatic herbal pinchings are a lovely ingredient in herbal-infused water with slices of lemon or lime.

PROBLEM INSECTS AND DISEASES: Slugs and aphids can be a problem. Container-grown plants may become infested with spider mites, aphids, or whiteflies. Seedlings are susceptible to damping-off.

HARVESTING: Harvest in the morning after the dew has evaporated, and quickly move the harvest to the shade or to its drying location. Take care not to pile up the plants, as tulsi easily oxidizes and, if bruised, will turn an unsavory black color. Several harvests can be obtained each year: simply cut back the mature plant to 8 inches, and it will regrow quickly. This keeps the plants frisky and producing flushes of tender foliage. If the plant is allowed to flower and fully set seed, growth slows dramatically. Harvest the flowers along with the leaves, as both are medicinal. Late in the season, the harvest will be more floral. Dry in bundles or on large screens. Tulsi is quite succulent, so it can take longer to dry than other leafy medicinals. After the plants are dry, strip the leaves and flowers from the stems and jar together.

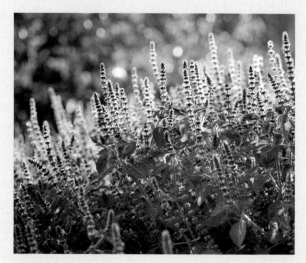

The popular 'Temperate' variety of tulsi

## Medicinal Properties

PART USED: **Leaves and flowers**

MEDICINAL PREPARATIONS: **Infusion, tincture, pesto, medicated ghee, infused oil, infused vinegar, compress, and poultice**

TINCTURE RATIOS AND DOSAGE: **Fresh (1:2 95%) or dry (1:4 60%); either preparation 2–4 ml up to three times a day**

TEA RATIOS AND DOSAGE: **Infusion of 2 teaspoons dried leaf and flower per 1 cup water up to three times a day**

VINEGAR: **1 teaspoon (5 ml) one to three times a day**

ACTIONS: **Adaptogen, antioxidant, antidepressant, antianxiety, antibacterial, antifungal, antiprotozoal, antiviral, carminative, diuretic, expectorant, galactagogue, anticatarrhal, immunomodulator, anti-inflammatory, hypotensive, antimutagenic, hypoglycemic, and hypocholesterolemic**

ENERGETICS: **Slightly warming and slightly drying**

## Medicinal Uses

Tulsi is one of those amazingly versatile herbs that might be characterized by which medicinal actions it does *not* possess rather than which it does. It's no wonder that the herb is highly revered as a sacred plant and highly valued as a home remedy in many cultures throughout southern Asia and northern Africa.

In India, tulsi is considered a sacred plant and is planted outside homes and temples to purify and bless the surroundings. Many Indians drink the tea daily to increase compassion, sharpen awareness, and promote focus in meditation. The leaves are used in worship, and the woody stem is made into prayer beads, which are worn or prayed over to cultivate the higher emotions of compassion, devotion, and love. Tulsi is a folk remedy in India for respiratory infections, digestive upset, and colic in babies. In Thailand it is a home remedy for gas, indigestion, peptic ulcers, coughs, sinusitis, and headaches. Ayurvedic doctors use the herb in the treatment of type 2 diabetes, and it has demonstrated favorable effects on blood sugar levels and lipid metabolism.

### CARDIOVASCULAR SYSTEM

Tulsi is a traditional heart tonic herb thanks to its antioxidant qualities (helping to prevent the free radical damage and inflammation that precipitate atherosclerosis) and aid in lowering blood pressure and reducing excess cholesterol.

### RESPIRATORY SYSTEM

Tulsi is a folk remedy in India for asthma, bronchitis, chest colds, sinus infections, allergies, and cold and flu. Benefiting the respiratory tract through several channels, tulsi reduces excess mucus through its expectorant, anti-inflammatory, and anticatarrhal qualities, and it supports the immune system through its antimicrobial and immunomodulating qualities.

### NERVOUS SYSTEM

Tulsi helps increase focus and clarity, making it especially useful for elders with declining cognitive abilities, children and adults with attention deficit/hyperactivity disorder (ADHD), and students who are simply wishing to increase their ability to assimilate and retain new material. It can be combined with gotu kola, milky oats, peppermint, calamus, and rosemary in formulas to increase concentration and cognition (see the recipe for the Focus and Clarity Tea Blend on page 296). Tulsi is a fine ally for people who are naturally scattered or distracted, as it is both calming and "centering." (See the Relaxation and Clarity Tea recipe on page 333.)

An adaptogenic herb, tulsi fosters resiliency when going through big life changes, such as moving or starting a new job or relationship. I find tulsi helpful for depression and anxiety, and I frequently add it to formulas as the "backbone" adaptogenic herb along with classic nervines that are used for those ailments. It pairs well with vervain and motherwort for anxiety and stress. For depression, I often combine tulsi with lemon balm, lavender, St. John's wort, and mimosa.

## Rejuvenation & Equanimity Formula

This blend helps alleviate stress and overwhelm and is especially helpful for folks who are feeling "bottomed out" from overwork.

MAKES 6 OUNCES

2 ounces tulsi leaf and flower tincture (*Ocimum tenuiflorum*)

2 ounces milky oats tincture (*Avena sativa*)

1 ounce skullcap leaf and flower tincture (*Scutellaria lateriflora*)

1 ounce motherwort leaf and flower tincture (*Leonurus cardiaca*)

Use fresh tinctures if possible (1:2 95%), or you can substitute dried tinctures or use different preparations for each tincture. Combine all tinctures and store in a glass dispensing bottle. Dosage is 4 ml (⅘ teaspoon) up to three times a day.

## Hope Tea Blend

Helpful for assuaging grief, these herbs are traditional remedies for despair and despondency. This blend is inspired by the work of herbalist David Winston. If you're unable to obtain the mimosa, substitute a teaspoon of lavender flowers.

1 tablespoon cinnamon bark chips (*Cinnamomum verum*)

2 teaspoons dried angelica root (*Angelica archangelica*)

4 cups water

1 tablespoon dried tulsi leaf and flower (*Ocimum tenuiflorum*)

1 tablespoon dried mimosa flower (*Albizia julibrissin*)

1 teaspoon dried hawthorn berries or flowers (*Crataegus* spp.)

1 teaspoon dried rose petals or buds (*Rosa* spp.)

In a small pot, combine the cinnamon and the angelica with the water. Bring to a boil, covered, and turn the heat down to simmer for 20 minutes. Turn off the heat, and add the tulsi, mimosa, hawthorn, and rose. Infuse, covered, for 20 minutes, and strain. Adults, drink up to three cups a day.

## Culinary Uses

Tulsi can be enjoyed as a culinary herb, tasting like a pungent version of Genovese basil. I like to combine the tender tips with milder forms of basil (lemon or lime basil and Genovese basil) in pesto and freeze it for year-round enjoyment. (See my recipe for Basilicious Benediction Pesto on page 391.) Tulsi's enlivening flavor complements quiches, marinara sauce, and pasta dishes. There are plenty of other ways to enjoy the flavor and medicinal qualities of tulsi year-round: blend the leaves with a little olive oil and freeze in ice cubes; dry the leaves and use them as a seasoning; prepare a compound butter and freeze in rolls; or use as an ingredient in an herbal finishing salt. In Thailand, tulsi is known as *kaphrao*; it's used as a culinary herb in stir-fry dishes with rice and meat or seafood.

> PRECAUTIONS: Avoid during pregnancy or if trying to conceive. There is some controversy around the use of tulsi in pregnancy, but it has been used traditionally as an abortifacient and antifertility herb in some cultures. Tulsi may modify blood sugar regulation—people with diabetes should monitor blood sugar closely and talk to their physician prior to use. Several studies on male animals have shown a decrease in fertility and sexual behavior with extremely high doses of tulsi. It's not clear whether this has any bearing on human physiology with moderate consumption of tulsi.

# Basilicious Benediction Pesto

YIELD: 2½ cups

1½ cups (55 grams) walnut halves

4 cups (80 grams) loosely packed fresh Genovese basil leaves

3 cups (55 grams) loosely packed fresh tulsi leaves

1¼ cups extra-virgin olive oil, or more if needed

1 cup (90 grams) grated Parmesan cheese

7 medium garlic cloves, peeled but left whole, or more to taste

2 teaspoons fresh lemon juice

Freshly ground black pepper, to taste

Sea salt, to taste

With the first spoonful of this aromatic pesto, you'll know deep in your core that the herbal deities have blessed you a thousand times over. This pesto makes a delicious pasta topping or a base for white pizza, and it's a scrumptious spread on sandwiches, wraps, or sourdough toast. You can even pull out some crackers and start dipping.

Toast the walnuts in a preheated dry (non-oiled) skillet over medium heat, stirring frequently, for 1 to 2 minutes, until they are brown and aromatic. Do not leave unattended, as the walnuts can burn quickly. Set aside on a plate to cool. Combine all the ingredients in a food processor and blend until combined. Add more olive oil if the pesto is too thick. Taste, and add more garlic, freshly ground black pepper, or sea salt, if desired.

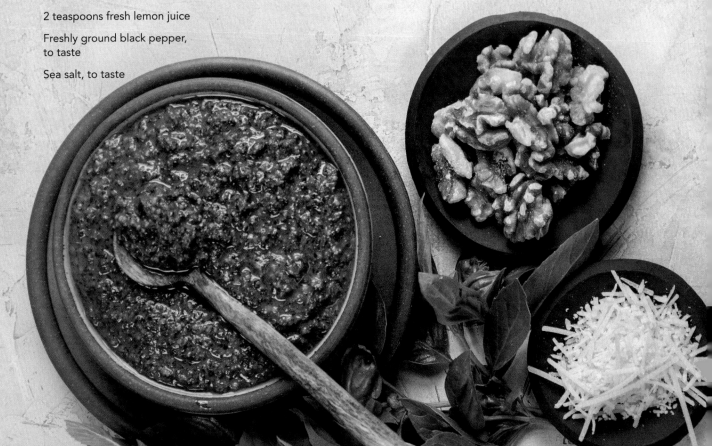

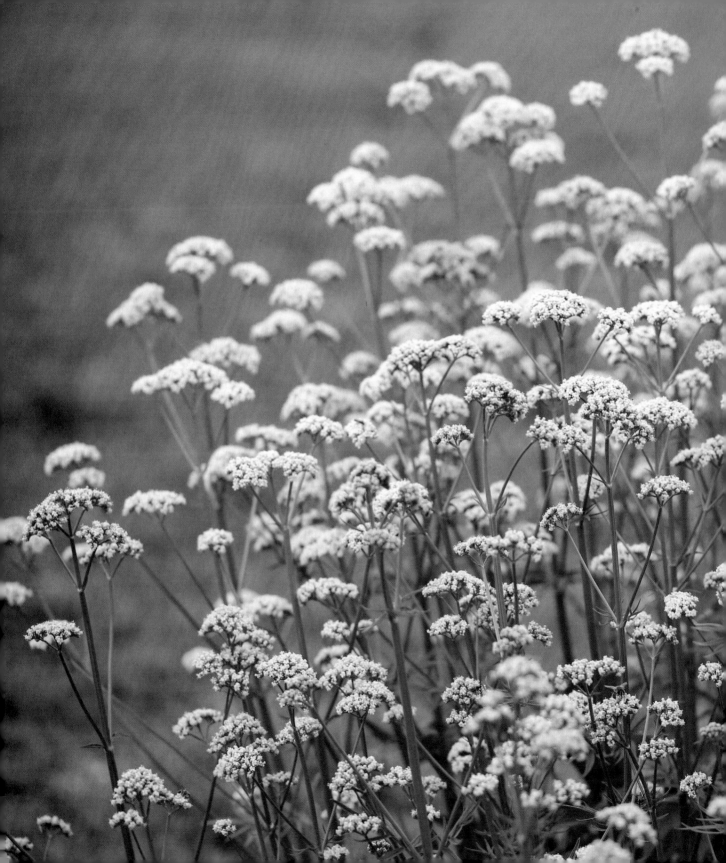

# VALERIAN

SCIENTIFIC NAME: *Valeriana officinalis*
CAPRIFOLIACEAE, honeysuckle family (formerly placed in the Valerianaceae)
AKA: garden heliotrope, all-heal, cat's love, moon root

Valerian imparts a folksy flair to the garden—its creamy blooms and ferny leaves are especially charming against a stone wall or white picket fence. The roots are a trusted remedy for insomnia, anxiety, and pain and have been a mainstay in household medicine chests for over 2,000 years. Its name is a testament to its popularity as a medicinal, originating from the Latin *valere*, "to be well" or "to be strong." The plant is native to Eurasia and has naturalized in many parts of the temperate world. It can now be found feral in fields, home sites, and waysides throughout much of North America. Kitties go wild for valerian, similar to their affection for catnip. Interestingly, rats are equally fascinated by the herb, lending a botanical twist to the tale of the Pied Piper, who is rumored to have lured the rats out of Hamelin with valerian in his pocket.

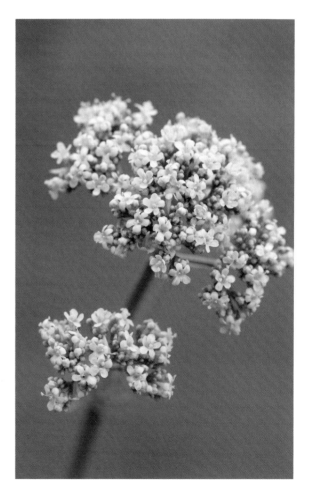

## Cultivation

**ZONES:** 3–9; full sun to partial shade

**SOIL:** pH 6–7; average to rich, moist garden soil

**SIZE:** 3–6 feet tall, 1–2 feet wide

**LIFESTYLE:** Herbaceous perennial

**PROPAGATION:** Valerian is a light-dependent germinator; surface-sow seeds. Germination takes place in 7 to 21 days at 65–70°F. Seeds are short-lived, lasting one year, and low germination rates are common: sow heavily. The easiest method of propagation is root division. Space plants 1½ to 2 feet apart.

**SITING AND GARDEN CARE:** Valerian is a notorious garden wanderer, prone to taking up residence throughout the garden and adjoining countryside. To quench its wanderlust, clip the flower heads soon after blooming, before they can produce seeds. Valerian does well in regular garden soil in full sun, especially if the soil is kept moist through mulching and the plants are watered during drought. Plant it in part shade if you live in an arid or warm climate. It will still flower in partial shade, especially if it receives some sun during midday. If you have a wet meadow, pond, or sunny stream or riverside, valerian will be quite content and reward you with a whole colony of cheery grandchildren.

**PROBLEM PESTS AND DISEASES:** Valerian is notoriously carefree in the garden, but it is susceptible to powdery mildew and downy mildew. As noted above, felines have been known to love valerian to death.

**HARVESTING:** Dig the roots in the spring or fall but wait until the fall of the second year after planting for your first harvest, which allows the roots to reach sizable proportions. The smellier, the better, as the aroma is an indicator of medicinal strength. Valerian's roots are often packed with dirt and will need a bit of pruning and cutting prior to washing to get in all the crevices. After washing, while the root is still fresh, chop in small pieces and dry on screens or open-weaved baskets. The dried roots maintain their potency for a long time, up to three years. In fact, my herbal teacher, Michael Moore, remarked that he had observed dried herbarium specimens 100 years old that were still aromatic!

## Medicinal Properties

**PART USED:** Root and rhizome

**MEDICINAL PREPARATIONS:** Decoction, tincture, powder

**TINCTURE RATIOS AND DOSAGE:** Fresh (1:2 95%) or dry (1:5 70%); either preparation 1–4 ml up to three times a day

**TEA RATIOS AND DOSAGE:** Decoction of 1 to 2 teaspoons dried root per 1 cup water, one to three times a day

**ACTIONS:** Hypnotic, sedative, nervine, anodyne, anxiolytic, carminative, hypotensive, and skeletal and smooth muscle relaxant

**ENERGETICS:** Warming and drying

## Medicinal Uses

Across the European continent, valerian has a long tradition of easing insomnia, anxiety, pain, and muscle tightness. It was so treasured by early North American colonial settlers that they brought the roots with them across the sea, transplanting them into their new gardens. Being a warming herb, valerian is most helpful for those with a cool constitution, demonstrated by paleness and a tendency to feel cold, especially in the extremities. Paradoxically, valerian is stimulating for a small portion of the population—exacerbating the tension and agitation one is hoping to soothe. This wired state can be quite vexing and confusing to the unaware. One evening, a dear friend called me up in distress after giving her wound-up toddler valerian in preparation for bedtime. Her daughter had gone off the deep end in a terrifying fanfare of puppy-level jitters. We quickly ascertained that her daughter was one of the few who has an unusual response to the root. Unfortunately, there's no easy way to determine who will have an atypical reaction. Try a small amount of the herb in the middle of the day to see how it affects you.

## NERVOUS SYSTEM

Valerian is famously known as a sleep remedy and can be combined with passionflower and skullcap to create a safe and effective hypnotic herbal blend. Dosages vary; for some folks, a few drops are adequate, whereas others may need up to a teaspoon of the tincture. Start with a small amount and increase the dosage as needed. Valerian isn't habit-forming. A number of clinical studies have demonstrated the effectiveness of the root as a sleep aid, the hypnotic action attributed to the presence of volatile oils and valepotriates. In one double-blind study, valerian significantly decreased sleep latency (the time it takes to fall asleep) as compared with a placebo. Additional clinical studies have shown that an infusion of valerian root considerably increases sleep quality in those who experience poor and irregular sleep.

Valerian's aromatic roots are also used as a gentle sedative, pain reliever, and muscle relaxer for anxiety, tension headaches, injury, menstrual cramps, and tight muscles. My herbal teacher, 7Song, uses valerian as a first aid remedy for calming the agitation that can accompany painful injuries.

## DIGESTIVE SYSTEM

A carminative and smooth muscle relaxant, valerian offers digestive support for intestinal gas, irritable bowel syndrome (IBS), and Crohn's disease.

## MENSTRUAL SYSTEM

Along that same vein, valerian relaxes the uterus, relieving the pain and force of menstrual cramping. I combine valerian with skullcap, black haw, and motherwort to alleviate menstrual cramps.

> **PRECAUTIONS:** Avoid concurrent use of valerian with barbiturates or benzodiazepines, such as Valium and Xanax.

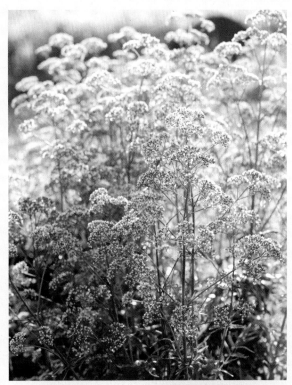

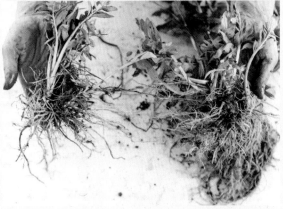

Valerian is easy to propagate through root division

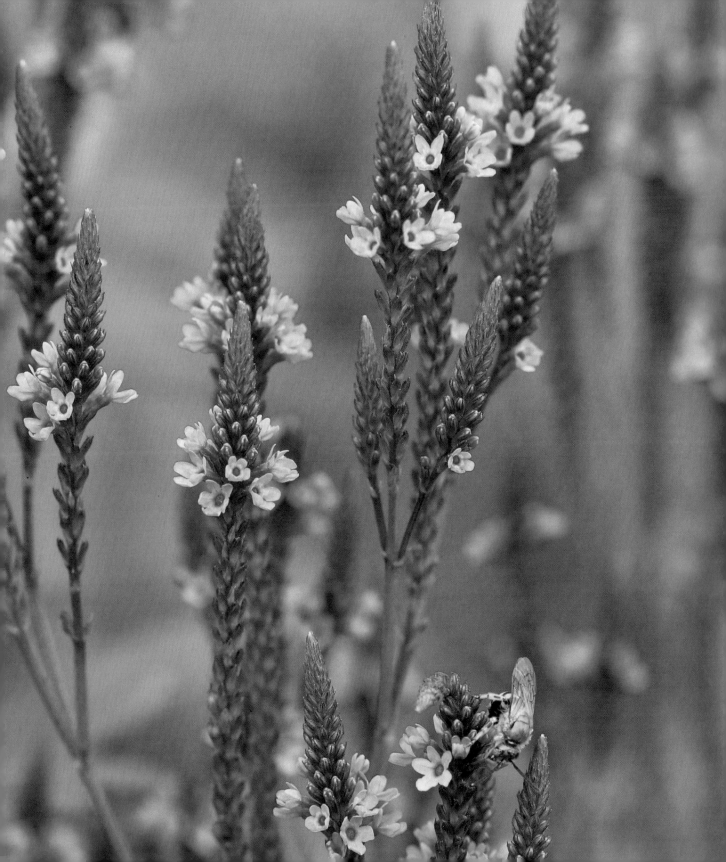

# VERVAIN

SCIENTIFIC NAME: *Verbena hastata* (blue vervain); *Verbena officinalis* (European vervain)
VERBENACEAE, vervain family
AKA: simpler's joy, holy herb, herb of grace, herb of the cross, herbe sacrée (French), wild hyssop, devil's bane, and common verbena

With names like "herb of grace," "holy herb," and "devil's bane," you can easily guess that vervain is a plant steeped in ancient and rich folklore. Indeed, European vervain was a highly sacred herb to the Druids and Romans. Classical Roman and Greek priests used flowering vervain branches to anoint and "sweep" the altar. The Druids have long worn it as a talisman to protect against venomous bites and to promote good fortune. Christian folklore shares that the vervain growing at the foot of the cross on Mount Calvary was used to stanch Christ's wounds, hence the name "herb of the cross." In Germany, brides wore vervain to bless their union in long-lasting amicability, and mothers hung the herb around their children's necks for protection against sickness and evil.

Blue vervain (*Verbena hastata*) is native to much of the temperate United States and Canada, growing in wet ditches and open wetlands and alongside streams, ponds, and lakes. Native peoples have a long relationship with the herb as a remedy for coughs, fevers, and digestive and urinary complaints.

European vervain (*Verbena officinalis*) is native to Eurasia and North Africa but has spread as a weed in much of the world, including Polynesia, Australia, New Zealand, Africa, and the Americas. It grows wild in fields, waysides, ditches, farmland, and open woods with sandy soils. The herb was a prominent folk remedy for many complaints, including edema, sore eyes, and poorly healing sores. The Chinese use *V. officinalis* similarly to the traditional European uses.

Contemporary use of both vervain plants is inspired by both traditional European folklore and North American Indigenous uses. British herbalists employ vervain for a wider degree of maladies than their American contemporaries. Much of what I know about vervain comes from British-trained herbalists such as Amanda McQuade Crawford and Anne McIntyre. Most modern herbalists use vervain plants interchangeably, but I feel they are distinct remedies with some overlapping uses. I tend to use blue vervain (*V. hastata*) more for fevers, colds, and flu, and European vervain (*V. officinalis*) more for its nervine qualities, as I feel it's a stronger anodyne, hypnotic, and antianxiety remedy. I invite you to experiment with the two species and see for yourself. Even though the two species' medicinal qualities are similar, their range, preferred habitat, and cultivation requirements are quite different.

Blue vervain (*Verbena hastata*)

## Cultivation

**EUROPEAN VERVAIN**
(*Verbena officinalis*)

ZONES: 4–11; full sun to light shade

SOIL: pH 5.5–7.8; average to well-drained soil

SIZE: 1½–3 feet tall; 1–1½ feet wide

LIFESTYLE: Herbaceous perennial

**BLUE VERVAIN (*Verbena hastata*)**

ZONES: 3–8; sun to part shade

SOIL: pH 5.5–7; fertile garden soil to rich, moist soil

SIZE: 2–4 feet tall; 1–2 feet wide

LIFESTYLE: Herbaceous perennial

PROPAGATION: For either species, stratify the seeds for two weeks to a month and then plant on the surface of the soil. The seeds are tiny, as are the sprouts; water with a mister to avoid dislodging or disturbing either. Alternatively, broadcast the seeds directly in the garden in early spring and lightly tousle into the surface. Blue vervain roots can be divided, yielding a few divisions per plant.

SITING AND GARDEN CARE: Blue vervain (*V. hastata*) prefers moist, rich soil but will tolerate regular garden soil. It grows companionably with boneset, skullcap, and marshmallow. In warmer climates, it will benefit from partial shade—consider planting it under an elderberry bush. European vervain (*V. officinalis*) has sparse growth and looks a little scrappy in the garden. Its casual appearance belies the medicinal potency of its leaves and flowers. It does well in regular garden soil and appreciates not being overwatered. In colder climates, European vervain will often appear as an annual; in warmer climates, it will survive as a short-lived herbaceous perennial.

PROBLEM INSECTS AND DISEASES: Generally, very few, but caterpillars can be a problem, especially on younger plants.

HARVESTING: Harvest the top two-thirds of the plant when in full flower, and hang in bunches to dry or prepare as medicine. Strip the leaves and flowers from the stem after the leaves are crumbly, and store.

## Medicinal Properties

PART USED: Leaves and flowers

MEDICINAL PREPARATIONS: Infusion, tincture, poultice, compress, and wash

TINCTURE RATIOS AND DOSAGE: Fresh (1:2 95%) or dry (1:5 60%); either preparation, up to 2–3 ml three times a day

TEA RATIOS AND DOSAGE: Infusion of 1 teaspoon dried leaf and flower per 1 cup water up to three times a day

ACTIONS: Bitter, cholagogue, anti-inflammatory, nervine, antianxiety, antidepressant, hypnotic, anodyne, diaphoretic, diuretic, hypotensive, emmenagogue, galactagogue, and emetic (in high doses)

ENERGETICS: Cooling and drying

## Medicinal Uses

European vervain is a traditional relaxing tonic for the nervous system to assuage pain and insomnia. Topically, its use is legendary for relieving inflammation, stopping bleeding, and healing wounds. The Chinese use *V. officinalis* (*ma bian cao*) to promote the menses in amenorrhea (absence of periods) and painful menstrual cramps with scanty flow. It is also used as a diuretic to lessen edema, and for malarial disorders. Many Indigenous peoples use blue vervain for fevers, stomach cramps, diarrhea, and edema.

## DIGESTIVE SYSTEM

Vervain is a bitter digestive remedy with an affinity for the liver and the gallbladder. A few drops of the tincture or vinegar can be taken before meals to stimulate digestion.

## NERVOUS SYSTEM

Vervain assuages anxiety and depression, nourishes deep sleep, and reduces pain. I find the herb to be especially suited for those who are hotheaded, quick to anger, and display aggression or overly "alpha" tendencies. Vervain helps nurture the receptive side of one's nature, allowing one to ease into vulnerability in safe relationships, especially after suffering trauma.

## REPRODUCTIVE SYSTEM

Vervain is both a tonic and an acute remedy for many reproductive issues. As a bitter remedy that stimulates bile production, it helps balance estrogen and progesterone indirectly by encouraging healthy intestinal flora and supporting the liver in removing excess hormones via the bile. I add vervain to tonic formulas with more overt hormone balancers, like black cohosh and chaste tree, to address menstrual cramps, menopausal symptoms, uterine fibroids, amenorrhea, and premenstrual headaches or moodiness. (See page 369 for my recipe.) In menopause, it offers relief through cooling hot flashes and lessening night sweats.

Vervain is a helpful herb for many postpartum maladies. It increases breast milk production, especially if one is feeling stressed or overwhelmed. Combine it with fenugreek for this purpose. Vervain is also helpful for postpartum depression, especially when paired with motherwort and passionflower. (It is not a replacement for mental health care—consult with your medical practitioner if you are experiencing postpartum depression.) Along with black haw and skullcap, vervain can help reduce the intensity of afterbirth pains following childbirth.

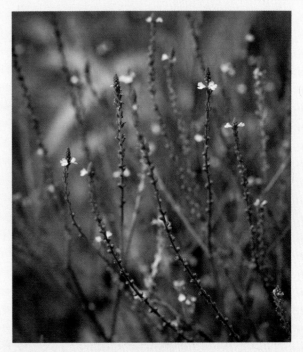

European vervain (*Verbena officinalis*)

## IMMUNE SYSTEM

Blue vervain promotes sweating, which helps to break fevers. I combine it with yarrow and elder to prepare a bitter brew that must be drunk hot to augment its diaphoretic qualities. (See page 417.)

> **PRECAUTIONS:** Do not use in pregnancy; it has been used traditionally as an abortifacient and stimulates the menses. Coadministration of vervain and iron supplements reduces absorption of the iron. High doses may cause abdominal pain, diarrhea, nausea, vomiting, and headache. Rare incidences of transient hepatotoxicity have occurred.

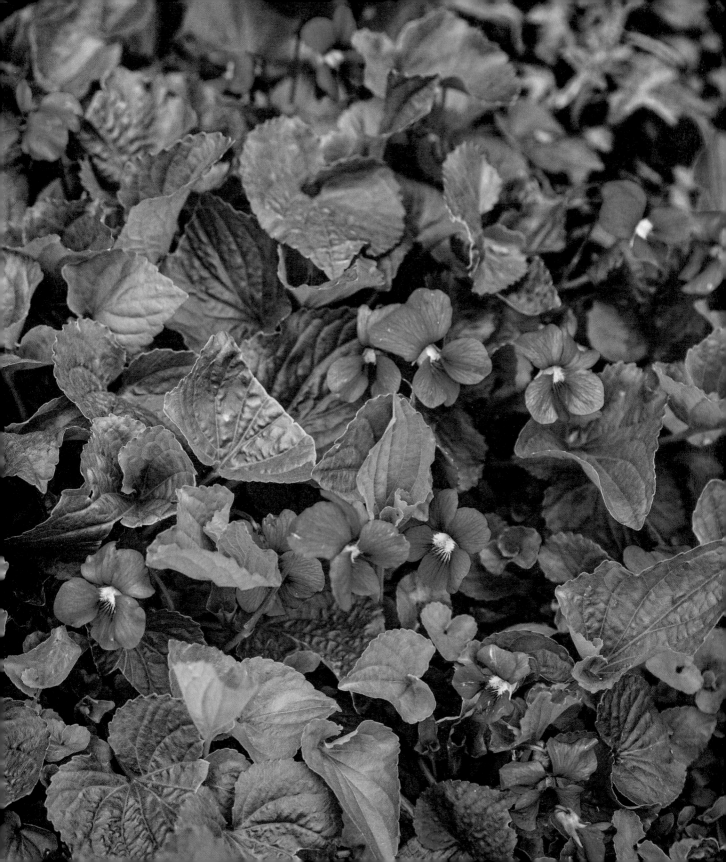

# VIOLET
## SWEET & COMMON

SCIENTIFIC NAME: *Viola sororia, Viola odorata,* and *Viola tricolor*
VIOLACEAE, violet family

Violets are welcome "weeds" in my garden. These springtime charmers are more than congenial wildflowers; they are nutritious wild edibles and medicinal herbs with a long history of use. Think twice before weeding out violet; it may be one of the most valuable plants in your garden, even if you didn't put it there. The sweet violet has been cultivated for its aroma since 400 BCE. Violet growers brought the fragrant blooms to market in Athens; in Rome, they made violet-infused wine from the blooms. In the late 1800s, sweet violet was widely grown in Europe for its cut flowers and for perfumery. Sadly, many scented varieties bred in the violet heyday have since been lost due to the advent of synthetic violet-scented compounds. A few native butterflies, such as the great spangled and meadow fritillaries, are wholly dependent on violets: their caterpillars feed exclusively on *Viola* leaves. Sweat bees and mason bees nectar on the early blooms, and grouse, mourning doves, and juncos feed on the seeds. Violets produce two types of blooms: the familiar aboveground flower, pollinated by insects, and then a colorless flower that's self-fertile and subterranean. These *cleistogamous* flowers never open for pollinators or breezes yet produce viable seeds.

The violet tribe, or *Viola* genus, contains close to 500 species, most of which hail from the temperate climates of the world. They can be challenging to identify, and they readily hybridize. Since this is a large group of plants and they aren't all interchangeable, I'll avoid generalizing about their uses, especially considering some violets are rare forest wildflowers and should not be harvested. Instead, I'll feature a few abundant species I know and love. There's a good chance you already have one of these growing in your garden.

Common blue violet (*Viola sororia*; formerly *V. papilionacea*) is the most ubiquitous violet species growing in central and eastern North America and in California. It grows in lawns, gardens, sidewalk cracks, and along trailsides, which naturally gives one the impression it's a "weed." It's actually native to North America and just happens to capitalize on human disturbance. The leaves and flowers are edible and medicinal and are used similarly to the sweet violet. Cherokee healers use this species internally as a spring tonic and as a remedy for coughs and diarrhea, as well as to externally treat headaches and boils. The "Confederate violet" is a cultivar of *Viola sororia*—it has white flowers with blue streaks and is a common inhabitant of lawns in the southeastern United States. There's also a variety with pink blooms. Both are used in the same way as the blue variety.

Common blue violet (*Viola sororia*)

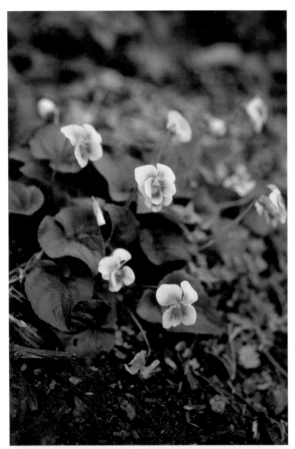

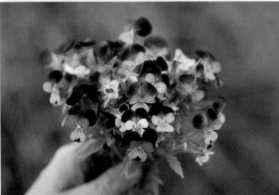

Common blue violet 'Confederate violet'; heart's-ease (*Viola tricolor*)

The sweet violet, or English violet (*Viola odorata*), is the principal medicinal and culinary species used in Europe and Asia. Cultivated for over 2,000 years for its fragrance and medicine, it has escaped from the garden in many locales, including throughout North America and Australia. This perennial herb grows in hedgerows, fields, gardens, and the edges of woodlands. Much of the contemporary use of violet in the United States is rooted in the European herbal traditions of the sweet violet. Interestingly, most violet species in North America lack the signature aroma of the sweet violet.

Heart's-ease, also known as Johnny jump-ups or wild pansy (*Viola tricolor*), is native to temperate Europe and has escaped cultivation in many locales. It's an old-fashioned bedding plant, resembling a miniature pansy, with many cultivars still being sold today. Use the scientific name when shopping for the plant, as other violets also go by "Johnny jump-ups." When my daughter Ruby was a toddler, heart's-ease, with its colorful edible blooms, was her favorite garden herb. Crouching on our stone walkway, she would find the heart's-ease growing in the cracks, pick them with her chubby fingers, and gleefully stuff her mouth. Years later, as her first foray into entrepreneurship, she grew Johnny jump-ups in our herbal nursery and sold them in our booth at the farmers' market. (A little parental reality check: Ruby's now a teenager with zero hearts for heart's-ease.)

Pansies are hybrids, crosses originating with *Viola tricolor* and other *Viola* species. They have edible flowers, but most commercial bedding plants are grown with chemicals, so be sure they haven't been sprayed. Try looking for pansy starts from your local organic herb nursery or grow your own. Because they are of unknown parentage and are novel hybrids, they aren't used medicinally. However, the flowers contain high levels of flavonoids and related antioxidant compounds.

The African violet (*Saintpaulia* spp.) is not related to *Viola* species and isn't used similarly.

## Cultivation

ZONES: *Viola sororia* 3–9; *Viola odorata* 6–9; *Viola tricolor* 6–9; all species full sun to partial shade

SOIL: Fertile, moist, well-drained soils

SIZE: On average, 6–12 inches tall; 1 foot wide (varies by species)

LIFESTYLE: Primarily herbaceous perennials

PROPAGATION: Sow the seeds of sweet and common violet directly on the surface of the soil in the fall, or stratify for two months and then surface-sow the seed in flats. Roots can be divided in the early spring or fall. Sweet violet is known for its low germination rates: sow heavily. Germination can be sporadic and take up to a year. In the early spring, plant heart's-ease seeds on the surface of the soil, and lightly tamp in, directly in the garden or in flats.

SITING AND GARDEN CARE: Some of you may turn your nose up at the idea of planting violet, especially if it's a rampant weed in your area, but I find the plant to be one of the most useful and productive herbs in my garden. That said, the herb will likely spread throughout your entire landscape, and you'll be corralling it for years to come, weeding it out of areas where it's crowding other plants. Try planting violet under shrubs or fruit trees, where it can do its thing without outcompeting its neighbors. Sweet and common violet prefer the dappled sun of open woodland with rich, moist soil but can grow in the sun if the soil is fertile and moist. In warmer climates, partial shade will keep the plants perkier during the summer. Because sweet violet can spread throughout the landscape, consider planting the common blue violet instead, if it's native to your region. Violet often makes a comeback in the fall, with a flush of tender new growth. Leave the dying growth intact at the end of the season, as fritillary caterpillars overwinter under the insulation of leaf litter. Johnny jump-ups are annuals to short-lived perennials who don't shirk from cool weather; plant them in full sun to light shade and they'll generally self-sow. Once you have a patch established, it's common not to have to replant as long as you don't mulch too heavily.

PROBLEM INSECTS AND DISEASES: Sometimes affected by thrips, spider mites, powdery mildew, and slugs and snails.

IDENTIFICATION AND HARVESTING: Violets are quite tricky to identify when they aren't in flower, as there are several low-growing plants with similarly shaped leaves, some of which are poisonous. Therefore, you'll only want to harvest violet when it's in flower, and even then, there are still look-alikes. Use a local field guide to determine which violets you have growing in your garden, and only harvest if you're absolutely certain of your identification. The leaves and flowers can be harvested with scissors in a "haircut" style. Violet can be harvested multiple times throughout the early spring until the leaves become too fibrous for eating. At this point, you can collect the tough leaves for medicine. Violet often puts forth a fresh flush of growth in the fall, giving us a second season to harvest for culinary uses. Dry the leaves and flowers on screens or in open-weaved baskets.

## Medicinal Properties

PART USED: Leaves and flowers

MEDICINAL PREPARATIONS: Infusion, vinegar, honey, syrup, oxymel, pesto, salad, poultice, compress, infused oil, and salve

TINCTURE RATIOS AND DOSAGE: Not recommended (see page 404)

TEA RATIOS AND DOSAGE: Infusion of 2 teaspoons dried leaves and flowers per 1 cup boiling water three times a day

ACTIONS: Alterative, demulcent, diuretic, anti-inflammatory, and lymphagogue

ENERGETICS: Cooling and moistening

## Medicinal Uses

Alcohol-based tinctures aren't the best way to prepare violet because the mucilage and minerals aren't extracted by alcohol. Instead, consume the herb as a food or prepare it as an infusion, honey, or syrup. The following information is a general overview of the traditional therapeutic uses of the common blue and the sweet violets. I'll lump the two together and simply call them *violet*. Violet is one of our more cooling and moistening herbs and is used internally as a blood cleanser, respiratory remedy, and lymphatic stimulant. It is taken as a tea or syrup and can also be eaten for its medicine. As a gentle food herb, violet is generally safe for elders and youngsters. Like chickweed, violet is a slow and steady medicine, dependable but not heroic. It truly shines for nurturing wellness and supporting the eliminative channels of the body. For acute scenarios like urinary or respiratory infections, combine it with other, more potent, medicinals.

### RESPIRATORY SYSTEM

Violet has a rich tradition in Europe as a soothing remedy for dry, hacking cough. The tea or syrup of violet, along with marshmallow and licorice root, soothes coughing from the common cold, bronchitis, and whooping cough.

### IMMUNE SYSTEM

Violet, along with calendula and cleavers, is a tonic remedy for chronically swollen lymph nodes.

### NUTRITIVE TONIC

The leaves are high in vitamin C, beta-carotene, and rutin, a glycoside with antioxidant, anti-inflammatory, and venotonic (increases tone in veins) qualities.

### URINARY SYSTEM

With its cooling, moistening, diuretic, and anti-inflammatory qualities, violet soothes the urinary tract and

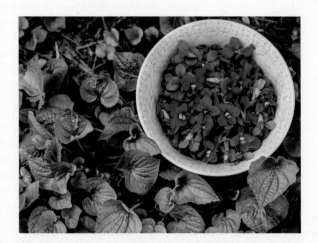

remedies painful urination. Violet, along with urinary antimicrobials, such as uva-ursi or cranberry, is a medicine for urinary tract infections.

### DIGESTIVE SYSTEM

Violet leaves soothe the mucus membranes of the digestive tract, and their soluble fiber content makes them a gentle laxative. Like oatmeal or barley, which are also high in soluble fiber, violet leaves help lower cholesterol levels.

### TOPICAL USES

Topically, violet is applied as a poultice, compress, infused oil, or salve in the treatment of dry or chafed skin, abrasions, insect bites, eczema, varicose veins, and hemorrhoids. It's cooling, soothing, and anti-inflammatory to the skin.

Heart's-ease (*Viola tricolor*) has the same medicinal uses as common and sweet violets, with additional cardiovascular applications. The leaves and flowers of heart's-ease are a folk remedy for the heart. With its high levels of flavonoids, especially in the flowers, the plant is highly antioxidant and has a number of anti-inflammatory and blood vessel–strengthening applications. Heart's-ease contains salicylates and has been used internally as a musculoskeletal anti-inflammatory.

## Soothing Respiratory Tea

This formula is helpful for dry, hacking coughs that are unproductive and to soothe sore throats and quiet coughs that start in the throat. The demulcent qualities of the violet, marshmallow, and licorice help to coat the throat and lessen respiratory inflammation. See the safety warnings for licorice on page 58.

4 cups water

1 tablespoon dried marshmallow root (*Althaea officinalis*)

2 teaspoons dried licorice root (*Glycyrrhiza glabra* or *G. uralensis*)

3 tablespoons dried violet leaf (*Viola sororia* or *V. odorata*)

2 tablespoons dried mullein leaf (*Verbascum thapsus*)

2 teaspoons dried wild cherry bark (*Prunus serotina* or *P. virginiana*)

In a small pot, combine the water, marshmallow root, and licorice root. Bring the water to a boil and turn down the heat to medium-low. Simmer for 20 minutes, turn off the heat, and add the violet, mullein, and wild cherry. Infuse, covered, for 20 minutes, then strain through a cloth to avoid ingesting the irritating hairs from mullein. Adults, drink up to 3 cups a day.

## Culinary Uses

Tender raw violet leaves and flowers can be added to salads, prepared into pesto, and nestled inside sandwiches and wraps. Violet is delicious in hummus; see my recipe for violet hummus on page 410. One of my favorite springtime breakfasts, pictured here, is a toasted whole-grain bagel, with an olive oil and raw garlic spread, topped off with chickweed and violet greens. Violet leaves can also be sautéed or steamed and stirred into soups and stews—the leaves act as a nutrient-dense thickener. To prepare a mineral-rich springtime fairy vinegar, add the leaves and flowers to other spring edibles,

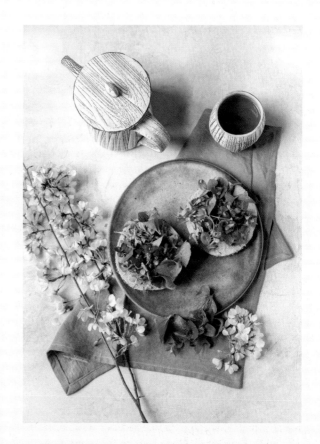

such as chickweed, dandelion, and nettles, and follow the directions on page 185 for herbal vinegars. The flowers are a delightful garnish: sprinkle them on salads or confections like cakes, muffins, cupcakes, and pancakes. Violet blooms are dazzling when candied or frozen into ice cubes. The crown jewel of *Viola* concoctions is violet syrup—see my recipe on page 406.

> PRECAUTIONS: Some species contain salicylates and should be avoided if you have salicylate sensitivity. Avoid internal use with individuals who have the rare inherited disorder G6PD deficiency. The roots of most violet species can cause nausea, vomiting, and diarrhea and should not be eaten. Violet has many poisonous look-alikes—be sure of your identification before harvesting.

# Regal Violet Simple Syrup

YIELD: 1½ cups (12 ounces)

1 cup water

2 cups (22 grams) loosely packed purple violet flowers, green sepals removed (see note below)

About 1½ cups organic white sugar (the whiter the better, if you want the brilliant purple)

About 10 drops lemon juice

Note: Harvest 2 heaping cups (43 grams) of purple violet flowers and give them a brief rinse. Remove the sepals and receptacle (the green floral parts underneath the purple petals), retaining the violet petals for the recipe.

Purple violet flowers possess a profusion of flavonoids—natural pigments that act as antioxidants. Add violet flowers to sugar water to concoct a ravishing syrup, primed for sweetening and flavoring drinks and confections. For a regal violet syrup, you'll need to remove the green undersides of the violet flowers, a fiddly affair. Now, before you start thinking about skipping this step, I'll let you know I tried the same shortcut. (Did you fancy me an idler?) When I left the green floral parts on the flowers, I was rewarded with the saddest of syrups, lilac-gray in hue. Picture a Victorian-era pillow, once lavender, stained with two lifetimes of tears and mildew, and you get the gist. Do you really want to be the evil queen who transforms the hope of springtime violets into disconsolate woe?

I thought not! You want to be revered for your cocktail benevolence. Use this syrup to make Orange Viola Mocktails (page 408), Grapefruit Violas (page 408), and Viola-ritas (page 409). Add a dash of violet syrup to sparkling water, lemonade, orange juice and vodka, or a violet margarita.

1. In a small pot, bring the water to a boil. Turn off the heat, add the violet petals, and stir until all the flowers are submerged. Cover and let sit until the liquid has cooled to room temperature. Pour the flower and water mixture into a jar, cover, and let it sit in the refrigerator for 12 hours.

2. Strain the infusion as described on page 137. Measure the volume of the violet infusion, and use twice the volume of sugar. For example, if your strained violet infusion, comes out to ¾ cup, add 1½ cups of sugar. Add the sugar and violet water to a small pot and heat on low, stirring a few times, until the sugar is dissolved. Take care not to heat too quickly, or you may destroy the color.

3. Remove from the heat and add the lemon juice 1 drop at a time. The lemon juice will transform the syrup from blue-purple to lavender.

4. Jar the syrup and store in the refrigerator for up to 6 months, watching for signs of spoilage.

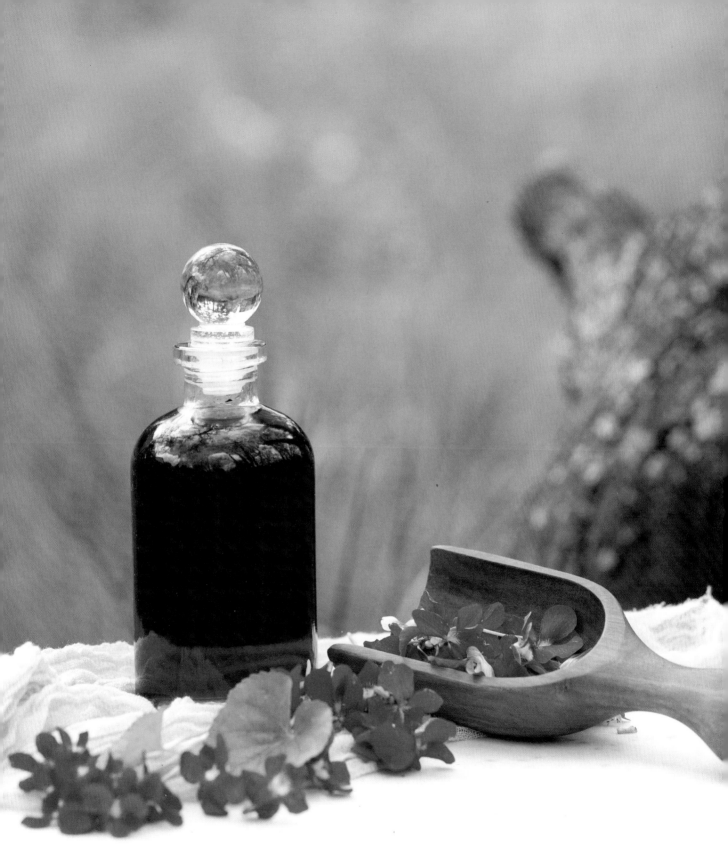

# Orange Viola Mocktail

YIELD: 2 drinks

2 cups sparkling water

½ cup pink grapefruit juice

¼ cup blood orange juice, or substitute orange juice

¼ cup Regal Violet Simple Syrup (page 406)

1½ teaspoons Dandy-Orange Bitters (page 264)

2 cups ice, to serve

My grandpa Joe was a storyteller of epic proportions. In his youth, he lived on a kibbutz that grew blood oranges, mythical citrus that figured prominently into his stories. I could only imagine the fruit, as they weren't in stores at that time. Decades later, when I first cut open a blood orange, I was overjoyed to finally meet this fabled fruit. Now that they are readily available, I honor my grandpa Joe every winter by inventing new drinks that feature the fruit's glorious crimson color. In this drink, the violet syrup and citrus combine into a glorious coral hue. If you can't find blood orange, it's fine to substitute orange juice—it will still be a pretty peach color.

Mix the sparkling water, grapefruit juice, orange juice, simple syrup, and bitters in a large jar and stir until evenly combined. Pour over 2 large glasses filled with ice.

# Grapefruit Violas

YIELD: 2 drinks

½ cup pink grapefruit juice

2 ounces vodka

2 tablespoons Regal Violet Simple Syrup (page 406)

2 cups ice, to serve

Ever need reassurance that things are peachy? I'm not quite sure that a drink alone can set your mind at ease, but combine it with deep breathing, flower-gazing, and a gratitude list, and you're well on your way to equanimity. For a mocktail version of this libation, leave out the vodka and add a dash of bitters.

Combine the grapefruit juice, vodka, and violet syrup in a jar and shake until combined. Pour over 2 cocktail glasses filled with ice and serve.

# Viola-ritas

YIELD: 2 drinks

2 cups crushed ice

¼ cup Regal Violet Simple Syrup (page 406)

2 ounces tequila

3 tablespoons lime juice (from 1 to 2 limes)

Lime wedge, to serve

Coarse salt or sugar, for the glasses (optional)

Here, we have a margarita steeped in the love-language of springtime: violet flowers. Omit the tequila and add a teaspoon of bitters for a nonalcoholic version.

In a jar, combine the ice, violet syrup, tequila, and lime juice; stir. To sugar or salt the rims, run a lime wedge around the rim of the empty glasses. Pour a small amount of sugar or salt onto a small plate, and invert each glass over the sugar or salt, twisting to evenly coat the rim. Carefully pour the iced margarita into the glasses, taking care not to disturb the rim.

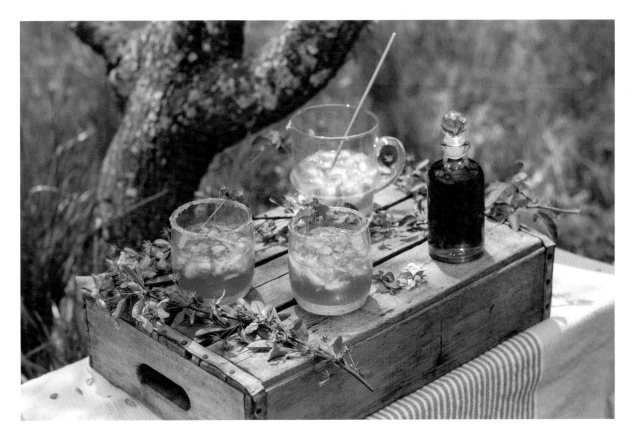

# Violet Hummus

YIELD: 2 cups

1 (15.5-ounce) can unsalted garbanzo beans or 1½ cups cooked garbanzo beans, drained

1 cup (48 grams) firmly packed violet leaves

¼ cup tahini

¼ cup extra-virgin olive oil, plus more for serving

2 tablespoons lime juice

2 garlic cloves

½ heaping teaspoon sea salt

Freshly ground black pepper, to taste

A pinch of the tiniest, fairy-sized violet leaves, for serving

This is one of the most kid-friendly recipes in this book and one of the easiest to prepare as well. I prefer the fresh flavor of home-cooked garbanzo beans, but I also keep cans on hand for those meal-in-a-pinch moments. Serve this emerald hummus with crudités, crackers, or chips or slather it on sandwiches and wraps.

Violet hummus is as heart-friendly as you can get, thanks to the garlic and the antioxidant vitamins found in the violet leaf. Then we have the healthy fats in the tahini and the soluble fiber in the violet (which whisks away LDL-cholesterol in a similar fashion to oatmeal). Tahini is rich in minerals, including calcium and phosphorus, and also contains B vitamins and omega-3 fatty acids. Garbanzo beans are a source of high-quality plant protein with a formidable fiber content that has also demonstrated LDL-cholesterol-lowering effects.

Combine the garbanzo beans, violet leaves, tahini, olive oil, lime juice, garlic, salt, and pepper in a food processor and process until smooth and silken. Serve in a wide bowl, drizzle with additional olive oil if you like, and garnish with miniature violet leaves. Store any excess in the refrigerator for up to a week.

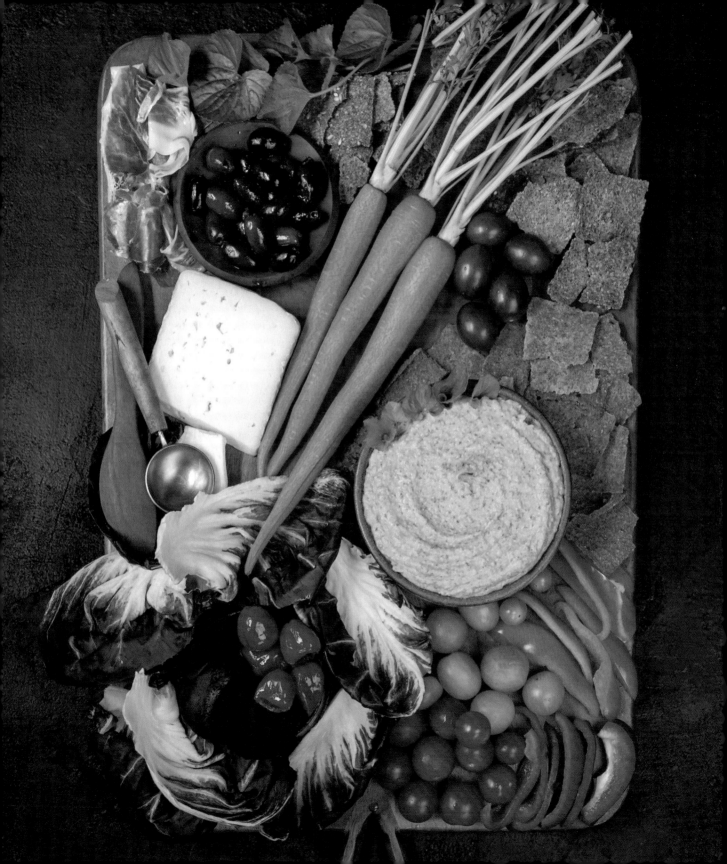

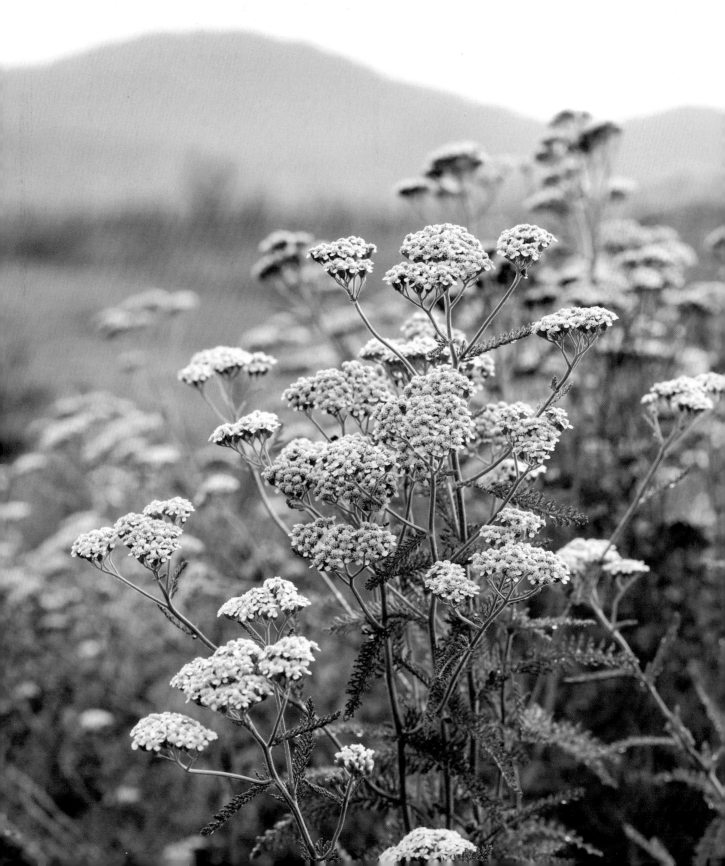

# YARROW

SCIENTIFIC NAME: *Achillea millefolium*
ASTERACEAE, aster family
AKA: milfoil, soldier's woundwort, bloodwort, staunchgrass, nosebleed plant, *plumajillo* ("little feather"), field hops

You can tell a lot about an herb by the number of legends, names, and mystical uses associated with the plant. Yarrow's scientific name *Achillea* is an homage to the Greek mythological character Achilles, who healed soldiers' wounds with the herb during the siege of Troy. Another tale ascribes his longevity in battle—including his ability to withstand arrow wounds—to his mother dipping him in a bath of yarrow. This legend is likely based on the fact that yarrow protects the skin with its qualities of vasoconstriction. The late Anishinaabe herbalist Keewaydinoquay Peschel tells a few stories from her youth about yarrow protecting the skin in the book *Plants Have So Much to Give Us, All We Have to Do Is Ask* by Mary Siisip Geniusz. Keewaydinoquay witnessed the fire-walking ceremonies of the Waabanoo, who soaked their skin in strong yarrow tea in anticipation of the rites. And her mother would soak her hands in an infusion of the herb to protect them when weaving baskets.

With a rich tradition as a divinatory and magical herb, yarrow plays an integral part in Chinese oracular ceremonies and Druidic weather prediction rites. Yarrow smoke features in Ojibwa medicine lodge ceremonies. The use of yarrow reaches far back in time and across species: remnants of the leaves were scraped from the teeth of a 50,000-year-old Neanderthal man in northern Spain. The herb has more than earned its legendary status with its ability to curb excessive bleeding, disinfect wounds, break fevers, and reduce sinus congestion.

Native to Europe, Asia, and North America, yarrow can be found in wildflower meadows and pastures, along roadsides, and throughout disturbed areas. The plant's scent evokes freshness, similar to the aroma of pine needles, chamomile, or lavender. Named "millefolium," the herb of 1,000 leaves, yarrow's foliage is so divided that it is feathery-fine. As a garden medicinal, its ability to attract beneficial insects and deter pests is unparalleled.

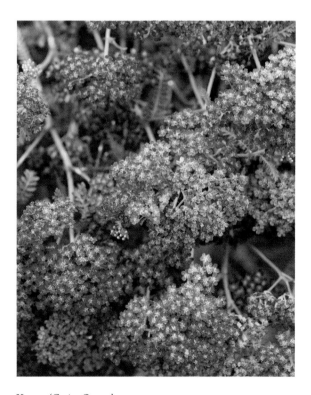

Yarrow 'Cerise Queen'

## Cultivation

ZONES: 2–9; full sun to light shade

SOIL: pH 5.5–7; fertile to poor soils with good drainage

SIZE: 1–3 feet tall; indefinitely wide

LIFESTYLE: Herbaceous perennial

PROPAGATION: Yarrow is most easily propagated through root division, which is the only way to maintain the desired characteristics of named varieties. Easy to grow from seed, yarrow can be sown on the surface of the soil (do not bury the seed) directly into the garden or in trays several weeks before the last frost, with germination in 10 to 14 days. Space the plants 1 foot apart, and they will expand in girth annually, forming a feathery verdant mound in no time.

SITING AND GARDEN CARE: Yarrow is a spreading groundcover that can take over if not curtailed by a semi-buried root barrier or the yearly removal of runners. It's one of the most carefree herbs you can grow and isn't especially fussy about the soil. The plant's one requirement is well-drained soil, so add pine bark fines, compost, and coarse sand if your soil is clayey. Yarrow's blooms and rich essential oil content make for a powerful companion plant in the garden. It attracts beneficial insects such as ladybugs, lacewings, parasitic wasps, and hoverflies and repels peskier insect visitors. It is known as an "aromatic pest confuser"—a permaculture term for plants that protect the garden at large by distracting and dissuading harmful pests with aromatic compounds. In addition, yarrow is a dynamic accumulator. When its leaves decompose, it concentrates valuable nutrients in the soil, especially phosphorus, potassium, and copper.

Many cultivars of yarrow are grown as ornamentals for their beautiful colors and soft foliage. These varieties may be medicinal, but they aren't necessarily used interchangeably. Some brightly colored varieties of *A. millefolium* include 'Cerise Queen', with hot-pink flowers, and 'Paprika', which has beautiful red-orange blooms. I grow these ornamental yarrows for beauty and their beneficial garden attributes, but I don't use them medicinally. Instead, I use the white wild strain of yarrow, which won't have a variety name and will simply be sold under the name of yarrow (*Achillea millefolium*).

PROBLEM INSECTS AND DISEASES: Yarrow is generally carefree but can be affected by powdery mildew and botrytis mold.

HARVESTING: The flowering clusters can be harvested directly into baskets and dried on screens or in loose-weaved baskets. Harvest the basal leaves with scissors early in the summer when they are perky and vital. Dry the same as the flowers. Alternatively, harvest the long flowering stalks when the plants are in full bloom and bundle to dry. Strip the leaves and flowers from the stems after drying. Be sure of your identification, as there are look-alikes, one of which is deadly poisonous (see the Precautions section on page 417).

## Medicinal Properties

PART USED: Leaves, flowers, and roots

MEDICINAL PREPARATIONS: Infusion, tincture, poultice, powder, wash, compress, infused oil, and salve

TINCTURE RATIOS AND DOSAGE: Leaf or flower: Fresh (1:2 95%) or dry (1:5 50%); either preparation 1–3 ml up to three times a day

TEA RATIOS AND DOSAGE: Infusion of 1 to 2 teaspoons dried leaves or flowers per 1 cup water up to three times a day. (Higher doses can cause nausea.)

ACTIONS: Styptic, antihemorrhagic, anti-inflammatory, decongestant, astringent, alterative, antimicrobial, vulnerary, diaphoretic, circulatory stimulant, hypotensive, emmenagogue, antispasmodic, bitter, and emetic in higher doses

ENERGETICS: Cooling or heating depending on the state of the body; drying

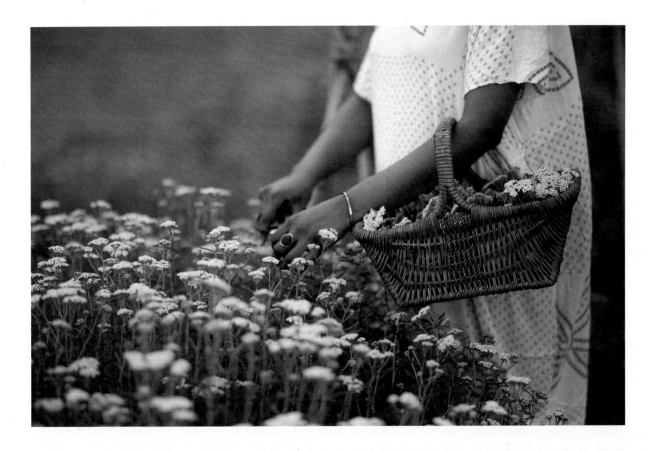

## Medicinal Uses

Yarrow is one of the most widely used herbs worldwide, with overlapping traditions in China, India, Europe, and North America. Both the leaves and flowers are medicinal, and many herbalists use them interchangeably. I prefer the leaves to the flowers when addressing excessive bleeding, but for all other uses, I prefer the flowers to the leaves.

### REPRODUCTIVE SYSTEM

Yarrow helps stem excessive uterine bleeding; its use is described on page 416 in the Circulatory System section. Combine with calendula, witch hazel, and garden sage to prepare a postpartum sitz bath to heal vaginal and perineal tears.

### IMMUNE SYSTEM

The flowers are a treasured remedy for colds and flu with their diaphoretic, decongestant, and antimicrobial qualities. Yarrow's antimicrobial and anti-inflammatory actions make it indispensable for clearing sinus congestion from respiratory infections. The herb offers similar relief from seasonal allergies. The flowers, along with blue vervain and elderflower, are helpful as a tea for breaking fevers in cold and flu. (See the recipe on page 417.) Diaphoretic herbs like yarrow help stimulate perspiration in low-grade fevers, which can help bring fever to a head and ultimately lower the fever, especially when combined with a hot bath, followed by burrowing under heavy blankets. Because diaphoretic herbs temporarily raise a fever, don't use them with fevers that are already high.

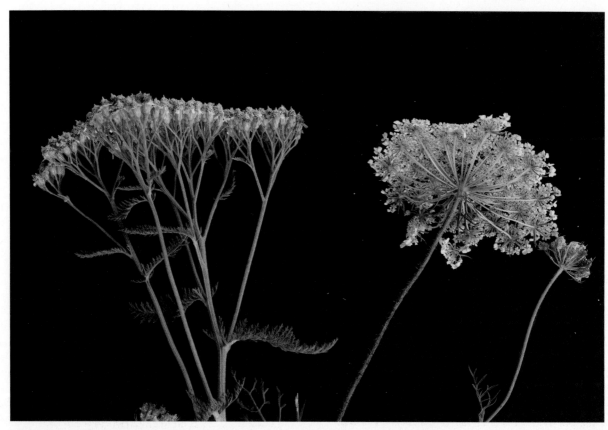

Yarrow (*Achillea millefolium*) on the left and Queen Anne's lace (*Daucus carota*) on the right

When I was sick as a child, my grandfather would make me drink a piping hot cup of tea and then wrap me up like a burrito in a bunch of wool blankets. At the time, I thought it old-fashioned and stifling, but it never failed to help: after a sick day with Grandpa Joe, my fever would always be gone, and I would be on the mend.

## TOPICAL USES

Yarrow is a powerful first aid medicine due to its antimicrobial and styptic qualities. The leaves or flowers can be prepared into a concentrated tea and applied to wounds, cuts, acne, and abrasions as a wash or compress. Alternatively, yarrow can be prepared into a poultice. I keep the dried powdered leaves in the first aid kit that I carry in my backpack. I've had more than one occasion taking groups into the wilderness where I was glad that I had yarrow at the ready. Yarrow tones the blood vessels and can be applied as a salve, compress, poultice, or wash to varicose veins, bruises, and hemorrhoids.

## CIRCULATORY SYSTEM

Yarrow is a classic remedy for stanching the blood, and is the first herb I turn to for deep cuts and excessive bleeding. Externally, the leaves slow the flow of blood from wounds and cuts. It is used internally, along with cinnamon and shepherd's purse, to slow bleeding from heavy menstruation, postpartum hemorrhage, and miscarriage.

## URINARY SYSTEM

Yarrow is a helpful remedy for urinary tract infections and can be combined with corn silk, marshmallow root, and uva-ursi. Ideally, the herbs should be prepared as an infusion that is allowed to cool to room temperature before drinking, which augments the tea's diuretic effect.

## "Influ-endsa" Tea

This tea blend is helpful for the aches and pains of flu and helps to increase sweating. It contains traditional antimicrobial, immunostimulating, and diaphoretic herbs. I will warn you that it's quite bitter! You can mask the bitterness a little with elderberry honey or maple syrup, but most children still will not appreciate the flavor. Alternatively, you can make this same blend as a tincture formula of equal parts; the dosage is 3 ml in 1 cup of very hot water or tea. Substitute 1 teaspoon of echinacea for the spilanthes if needed.

4 cups water

2 tablespoons dried elderflower (*Sambucus nigra*)

2 teaspoons dried yarrow flower (*Achillea millefolium*)

2 teaspoons dried blue vervain or European vervain leaf and flower (*Verbena hastata* or *V. officinalis*)

2 teaspoons dried spilanthes leaf and flower (*Acmella oleracea*)

2 teaspoons dried ginger root (*Zingiber officinale*)

In a small pot, bring the water to boil. Turn off the heat, and add all the herbs. Let sit, covered, for 20 minutes and then strain. Adults, drink up to three cups a day. Drink the tea warm to bring a fever higher by increasing sweating. Taking a warm bath and covering with blankets will increase the tea's diaphoretic qualities. If the fever is already dangerously high, do not drink the tea, as it may bring the fever up even higher. Use carefully with children as the tea can be nauseating and is potent. Calculate dosage for children following the directions on page 133.

**PRECAUTIONS:** Because of its emmenagogue effects, don't use yarrow internally during pregnancy. Internally and externally, yarrow may cause side effects (contact dermatitis, photosensitivity, and allergic reactions) for those with Asteraceae sensitivity, although reactions are very rare. Large doses can cause nausea, dizziness, and vomiting. Be sure of your yarrow identification, as there are poisonous look-alikes, two of which are described here.

Queen Anne's lace (*Daucus carota*), also known as wild carrot, is sometimes confused with yarrow, especially when they aren't in flower. It grows wild in pastures and meadows and has deeply divided leaves, hairy stems, and white clusters of flowers. Queen Anne's lace is in the carrot family and has a characteristic carroty odor. Its flowers appear in compound umbels (a larger umbel that bears secondary umbels). See the photo of yarrow and Queen Anne's lace side by side.

Poison hemlock (*Conium maculatum*) is yarrow's most dangerous look-alike—it is deadly poisonous and grows in similar habitats as yarrow. Poison hemlock has a smooth purple or darkly spotted hollow stem that is often coated with a prominent white bloom (as opposed to yarrow's hairy, fibrous stem). Its petiole (leaf stalk) clasps the stem, whereas yarrow's petiole does not. Poison hemlock's flowers—like those of Queen Anne's lace—are arranged in the classic double umbel of the carrot family. As with all plants, don't harvest if in doubt!

# Acknowledgments

Completing any book is a feat of determination. Add parenting and running a business into the mix, and you now need a troupe to usher the book into existence. When I set out to write and photograph this book, little did I know I would be facing two surgeries, a month without the ability to speak, and the beginning of the COVID-19 pandemic. (Surely, I would have turned heel.) To my family, friends, and team members: you sang this book into creation right alongside me. For starters, I couldn't have finished this project without the support of my partner, Tom, who put food on the table every night, nurtured our gardens and our daughter, and brought me lattes every morning. Thanks to my agent, Coleen O'Shea, for championing this book from its inception onward. A bow to my editor, Stephanie Fletcher, at Mariner Books for believing in the book and refining its pages. To Naomi Kim Eagleson and the team at the Artful Editors: thank you for your expert word wrangling.

To my culinary and horticultural partners in crime, Amber Brown and Eden May, I raise a glass of elderberry mead. Our recipe-testing days were my favorite part of creating this book. Eden, you are a formidable tower of skills. I couldn't imagine a better gardener to care for my plants when I'm away. Or a superior light-bouncer or research assistant. Amber, your silliness lightens our workdays and softens my heart. Everything is better with you around. Especially our food.

I'm blessed to work with an amazingly creative team of women, who lovingly tended my herbal school and taught our students while I worked on the book. Endless and heartfelt gratitude to Kathryn, Carrie Faye, Amber, Meghan, Christine, Sara, Sarah, and Melita. Meghan Gemma, thank you for always being ready to roll up your sleeves. Your research, editing, and assistance with the book were essential to my sanity and sleep. Kathryn Blau, your crystalline leadership has brought me to tears of gratitude more times than I can count. You keep it tight and right, mama. And you do it all with kindness, compassion, and clear communication.

To my soul sisters, for having my back and celebrating the milestones: Kathleen, Amber, McCayne, Asia, Maureen, Chelsea, Claudia, Mary Morgaine, and my dear Sarah S's, you make life that much sweeter and deeper. The heavens showered me with light when they gave me you as friends. Marc Williams, you are my role model of decency and integrity. I see your tireless dedication to sharing plant wisdom and earth knowledge. You are forever my brother.

A big thanks to our intrepid recipe testers, who helped us polish each recipe until it gleamed: Becky Starling, Brette Barclay Barron, Briana Cushman, Christine Borosh, Donna Ramos, Greta Dietrich, Heather Zloty, Karen Cooke, Karen B. Tyndall, Katie Kovach, Laura Denyes, Lori Valentine Rose, and Rhiannon Sundquist.

To my grandpa Joe (Joachim Naphtali Simon), who planted the seed of this book by sharing his love of nature, gardening, and the written word with me throughout my childhood. Above all, you taught me how to live a creative and authentic life and cultivate wonder. You also modeled how to listen and notice deeply and how to be a decent and generous person. I wouldn't be half the woman I am today without your patient tutelage and attention.

To my parents, Gil, Joanna, and Liz, thank you

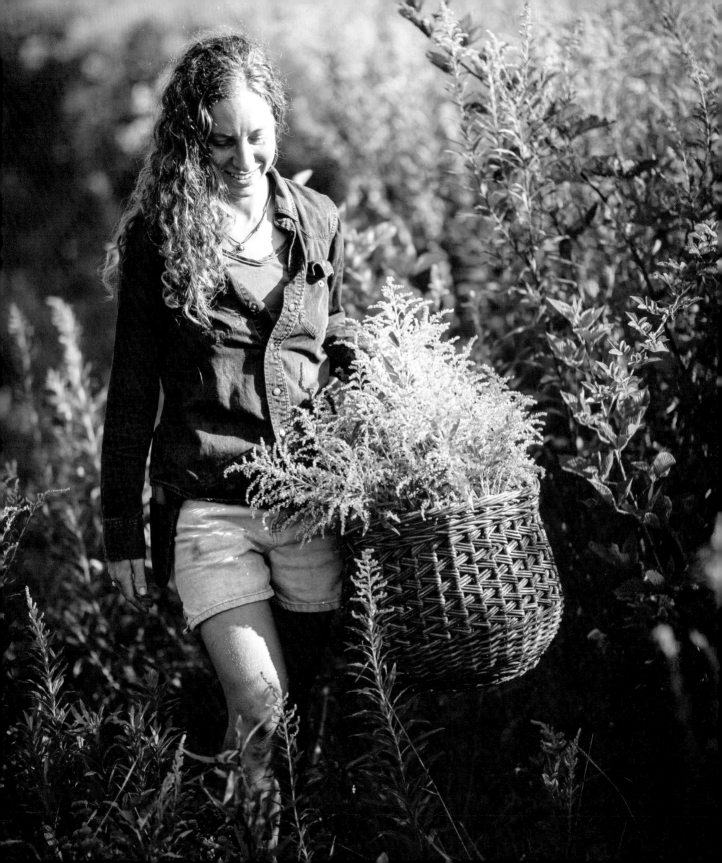

for supporting my path as a budding herbalist even when you didn't quite understand what in the heck I was up to. Mom, you taught me to think for myself, stand up to injustice, say what I mean, and be an independent woman. Dad, you showed me how hard work and genuine civic thinking can build successful small businesses *and* strengthen local communities. You are my greatest inspiration in the art of paying it forward. Liz, you have a wicked sense of humor, and you're one of the smartest and kindest people I know. We hit the jackpot when you joined our tribe.

My teachers have meant a great deal to me over the years, starting with my high school science teachers who nurtured my budding inner scientist. I'm forever indebted to my herbal teachers, Gloria Starita, 7Song, James Snow, and the late Michael Moore. 7Song, I couldn't imagine a funnier and more passionate mentor than you. I do so appreciate the meanderings of your mind and conscience. I thank my lucky stars that you are my dear friend and confidant. Your dedication to elevating our craft and offering free herbal care is inspirational. I have also learned a great deal from these herbalists (both living and ancestors), primarily from their writing: Rosemary Gladstar, Tieraona Low Dog, Amanda McQuade Crawford, Mary Siisip Genuisz, Keewaydinoquay Peschel, Juliette de Bairacli Levy, Tommie Bass, Dr. Jill Stansbury, Robin Rose Bennett, Steven Foster, Richo Cech, Kathi Keville, David Hoffmann, Kiva Rose Hardin, and Rosalee de la Foret. And an earnest thank-you to my precious students from over the years—you've made me a better herbalist and teacher.

To my dear plant brother, Frank Cook, who has traveled to the sky-fields of wild strawberries: you turned it *all* into a grand adventure of the heart. I was blessed to walk, learn, and teach alongside you. You fanned my wings when I was a young herbalist and helped me soar as a teacher and leader. I give you my word: after this book, I *will* slow down. I look forward to the day when we sit together in the sky-fields and eat homemade biscuits topped with chickweed and miner's lettuce. Until then, I'll toast to you with a bubbling mug of field-herbs mead.

Ruby Rose, it is my prayer that you someday know a passion that feeds your soul and drives your days. Thank you for sharing me with the plants all your years. You are loved and treasured beyond measure.

I'm grateful for all the gardeners and public gardens that allowed me to come and photograph their herbs. Thank you, Robison Herb Garden at Cornell Botanic Gardens in Ithaca, NY; Garden in the Woods at the headquarters of the Native Plant Trust in Framingham, MA; the Green Farmacy Garden (Jim and Peggy Duke) in Fulton, MD; Herb Mountain Farm (Mary Morgaine and Hart Squire) in Weaverville, NC; the permaculture gardens of Janell V. Kapoor in Asheville, NC; Longwood Gardens in Kennett Square, PA; Mountain Gardens (Joe Hollis) in Burnsville, NC; Rebecca Vann of Sacred Mountain Sanctuary; Chama Woydak's land of Homegrown Families in Asheville, NC; and Wild Abundance: School of Permaculture, Carpentry, Homesteading, Organic Gardening, and Primitive Skills (Natalie Bogwalker) in Weaverville, NC.

A deep bow to the lovely souls who poured potions, cooed over plants, and cradled harvests as I photographed them for this book. Here's a bit about how they live and how they love plants:

# Plant-Lovers & Herb Gardeners Featured in the Book

AMBER BROWN is a Native Alaskan from the Tlingit and Haida tribe of southeast Alaska. Amber is passionate about wild foods and medicine, as well as native trees and forest medicinals. She is a concoctress of small-batch, seasonal tinctures and essences and tends the Chestnut School's inner gardens. Find Amber at www.gloriousforestfarm.com.

CHIWA CLARK is a clay artist and has also worked with herbs since the early '80s when she was with Gaia Herbs in Massachusetts. It instilled a love of the plant and plant medicine world into her being. Learn more about Chiwa's pottery at www.riverartsdistrict.com/artist/chiwa-clark.

COCO VILLA is an interdisciplinary artist, botanical dyer, and the founder of Casa De Coco. She works with artists, designers, and other businesses to realize their creative branding and visual content needs through photography, movement, sustainable fashion design, and art direction. Find Coco Villa online at www.casadecoco.space and @_casadecoco_ on Instagram.

EDEN MAY is a community herbalist, homesteader, and wildcrafter working in the Southern Appalachian Mountains. She tends the gardens at the Chestnut School, processes the harvests, and makes medicine. Follow her on Instagram @eden.mayapple.

FLORA VENA RUBY's name was chosen out of her mother's great love of flowers, plants, and children. You can learn more about their gardening adventures at YummyYards.com and www.facebook.com/YummyYards.

INDY SRINATH is a Los Angeles–based urban gardener, mushroom cultivator, and food justice advocate. She's committed to increasing organic food access and health literacy in underserved populations. Find her work on Instagram @indyofficinalis.

MUNA HUSSEIN is currently a student of Acupuncture and Chinese Medical Arts. She has a passion for this medicine and the magical healing powers of herbal medicine. You can follow her on Instagram @herbsandpotsbymoon.

MEGHAN GEMMA is one of the Chestnut School's primary instructors and is the principal pollinator of the school's social media community. She has been in a steady relationship with the Chestnut School since 2010—as an intern and manager at the Chestnut Herb Nursery; as a plant-smitten student; and later as a part of the school's woman-powered professional team.

# References

Please see the HealingGardenGateway.com for the Recommended Reading and Bibliography.

## Chapter Eight References

Bombay A, Matheson K, Anisman H. Intergenerational trauma: convergence of multiple processes among First Nations Peoples in Canada. *J Aborig Heal*. 2009.

Cohen S, Janicki-Deverts D, Miller G. Psychological stress and disease. *J Am Med Assoc*. 2007.

Colton H, Altevogt B. *Sleep Disorders and Sleep Deprivation: An Unmet Public Health Problem*. National Academics Press; 2006.

Czeisler C. Perspective: casting light on sleep deficiency. *Nature*. 2013.

Duke University. Exercise may be just as effective as medication for treating major depression. https://www.sciencedaily.com/releases/1999/10/991027071931.htm.

Finan P, Goodin B, Smith M. The association of sleep and pain: an update and a path forward. *J Pain*. 2013.

Gardner Z, McGuffin M, eds. *American Herbal Products Association's Botanical Safety Handbook*, 2nd ed. CRC Press; 2013.

Huxtable R. Human health implications of pyrrolizidine alkaloids and herbs containing them. In: PR Cheeke, ed. *Toxicants of Plant Origin*. CRC Press; 1989.

Kroenke CH, Kubzansky LD, Schernhammer ES, Holmes MD, Kawachi I. Social networks, social support, and survival after breast cancer diagnosis. *J Clin Oncol*. 2006.

Menefee L, Cohen M, Anderson WR, Doghramji K, Frank ED, Lee H. Sleep disturbance and nonmalignant chronic pain: a comprehensive review of the literature. *Pain Med*. 2000.

Miller G, Blackwell E. Turning up the heat: inflammation as a mechanism linking chronic stress, depression, and heart disease. *Curr Dir Psychol Sci*. 2006.

National Sleep Foundation. The complex relationship between sleep, depression, and anxiety. https://sleepfoundation.org/excessivesleepiness/content/the-complex-relationship-between-sleep-depression-anxiety.

Neuman M, Cohen L, Opris M, Nanau RM, Hyunjin J. Hepatotoxicity of pyrrolizidine alkaloids. *J Pharm Pharm Sci*. 2015.

Passos G, Poyares D, et al. Effect of acute physical exercise on patients with chronic primary insomnia. *J Clin Sleep Med*. 2010.

Pham-Huy LA, He H, Pham-Huy C. Free radicals, antioxidants in disease and health. *Int J Biomed Sci*. 2008.

Uchino BN, Cacioppo JT, Kiecolt-Glaser JK. The relationship between social support and physiological processes: a review with emphasis on underlying mechanisms and implications for health. *Psychol Bull*. 1996.

Wulff K, Gatti S, et al. Sleep and circadian rhythm disruption in psychiatric and neurodegenerative disease. *Nat Rev Neurosci*. 2010.

## Basil

Satoh T, Sugawara Y. Effects on humans elicited by inhaling the fragrance of essential oils: sensory test, multi-channel thermometric study and forehead surface potential wave measurement on basil and peppermint. *Anal Sci*. 2003.

Srivastava U, Ojha S, Tripathi N, Singh P. In vitro antibacterial, antioxidant activity and total phenolic content of some essential oils. *J Environ Biol*. 2015.

Vlase L, Benedec D, Hanganu D, et al. Evaluation of antioxidant and antimicrobial activities and phenolic profile for *Hyssopus officinalis*, *Ocimum basilicum* and *Teucrium chamaedrys*. *Molecules*. 2014.

## Bee Balm

Armitage AM. *Armitage's Native Plants for North American Gardens*. Timber Press; 2006.

BONAP's North American Plant Atlas. TaxonMaps website. http://bonap.net/NAPA/TaxonMaps/Genus/County/Monarda.

Li H, Yang T, Li FY, Yao Y, Sun ZM. Antibacterial activity and mechanism of action of *Monarda punctata* essential oil and its main components against common bacterial pathogens in respiratory tract. *Int J Clin Exp Pathol*. 2014.

Monarda RK. The Medicine Women's Roots website. http://bearmedicineherbals.com/monards.html

Savickiene N, Dagilyte A, Barsteigiene Z, Kazlauskas S, Vaiciūniene J. Analysis of flavonoids in the flowers and leaves of *Monarda didyma* L. *Medicina*. 2002.

## Black Cohosh

Chung D, Kim H, Park K, Jeong K. Black cohosh and St. John's wort (GYNO-Plus®) for climacteric symptoms. *Yonsei Med J*. 2007.

Einbond LS, Mighty J, Redenti S, Wu H. Actein induces calcium release in human breast cancer cells. *Fitoterapia*. 2013.

Henneicke-von Zepelin H. 60 years of *Cimicifuga racemosa* medicinal products. *Wiener Medizinische Wochenschrift*. 2017.

Nappi R, Malavasi B, Brundu B. Efficacy of *Cimicifuga racemosa* on climacteric complaints: a randomized study versus low-dose transdermal estradiol. *Gynecol Endocrinol*. 2005.

Rostock M, Fischer J, Mumm A. Black cohosh (*Cimicifuga racemosa*) in tamoxifen-treated breast cancer patients with climacteric complaints—a prospective observational study. *Gynecol Endocrinol*. 2011.

Seidlová-Wuttke D, Hesse O, Jarry H, Christoffel V. Evidence for selective estrogen receptor modulator activity in a black cohosh (*Cimicifuga racemosa*) extract: comparison with estradiol-17beta. *Eur J Endocrinol.* 2003.

Uebelhack R, Blohmer J, Graubaum H. Black cohosh and St. John's wort for climacteric complaints: a randomized trial. *Obstet Gynecol.* 2006.

## Dandelion

USDA, Agricultural Research Service, National Plant Germplasm System. https://npgsweb.ars-grin.gov/gringlobal/taxonomydetail.aspx?80051.

## Echinacea

Schoop R, Klein P, Suter A, Johnston S. Echinacea in the prevention of induced rhinovirus colds: a meta-analysis. *Clin Ther.* 2006

## Elderberry

Barak V, Halperin T, Kalickman I. The effect of Sambucol, a black elderberry-based, natural product, on the production of human cytokines: I. Inflammatory cytokines. *Eur Cytokine Netw.* April–June 2001.

Bisset N, Wichtl M. *Herbal Drugs and Phytopharmaceuticals: A Handbook for Practice on a Scientific Basis.* Medpharm Scientific Publishers; 1994.

Forsell M. *The Herbal Grove.* Villard Books; 1995.

Home lawn and garden: Insect pests. Penn State Extension website. http://extension.psu.edu/plants/gardening/fphg/elderberries/insect-pests.

Hopman EE. *A Druid's Herbal of Sacred Tree Medicine.* Inner Traditions/Bear and Co.; 2008.

Poisoning from Elderberry Juice—California. Centers for Disease Control and Prevention website. https://www.cdc.gov/mmwr/preview/mmwrhtml/00000311.html.

Rose K. The Elder Mother. The Medicine Woman's Roots website. http://bearmedicineherbals.com/the-elder-mother.html.

Serkedijieva J, Manolova N, Zgórniak-Nowosielska I, Grzybek J. Antiviral activity of the infusion from flowers of *Sambucus nigra* L., aerial parts of *Hypericum perforatum* L, and roots of *Saponaria officinalis* L. against influenza and herpes simplex viruses. *Phytother Res.* 1990.

Turner NJ. *Food Plants of British Columbia Indians. Part I: Coastal Peoples.* British Columbia Provincial Museum; 1975.

Veberic R, Jakopic J, Stampar F, Schmitzer V. European elderberry (*Sambucus nigra*) rich in sugars, organic acids, anthocyanins, and selected polyphenols. *Food Chem.* 2009.

Zakay-Rones Z, Varsano N, Zlotnik M, et al. Inhibition of several strains of influenza virus in vitro and reduction of symptoms by an elderberry extract (*Sambucus nigra* L.) during an outbreak of influenza B Panama. *Journal Altern Complement Med.* 2007.

## Goldenrod

Goldenrod. Chicago Botanic Garden website. http://www.chicagobotanic.org/plantinfo/goldenrod.

## Goldenseal

Bergner, P. *The Healing Power of Echinacea and Goldenseal and Other Immune System Herbs.* Prima Lifestyles; 1997.

Bergner, P. *The Healing Power of Ginseng and the Tonic Herbs: The Enlightened Person's Guide.* Prima Publishing; 1996.

Elliott DD. *Wild Roots: A Forager's Guide to the Edible and Medicinal Roots, Tubers, Corms, and Rhizomes of North America.* Healing Arts Press; 1995.

Foster S. Goldenseal: masking of drug tests; from fiction to fallacy; an historical anomaly. *HerbalGram.* 1989.

French J. The indications for *Hydrastis canadensis. Am J Clin Med.* 1922.

Scazzocchio F, Cometa MF, Tomassini L, Palmery M. Antibacterial activity of *Hydrastis canadensis* extract and its major isolated alkaloids. *Planta Medica.* 2001.

Villinksi J, Dumas E, Chai HB, Pezzuto J, Angerhofer C, Gafner S. Antibacterial activity and alkaloid content of *Berberis thunbergii, Berberis vulgaris* and *Hydrastis canadensis. Pharm Biol.* 2003.

## Gotu Kola

Caldecott T, Tierra M. *Ayurveda: The Divine Science of Life.* Mosby Elsevier; 2006.

Khalsa KPS, Tierra M. *The Way of Ayurvedic Herbs: The Most Complete Guide to Natural Healing and Health with Traditional Ayurvedic Herbalism.* Lotus Press; 2008.

Lu L, Ying K, Wei S, et al. Asiaticoside induction for cell-cycle progression, proliferation and collagen synthesis in human dermal fibroblasts. *Int J Dermatol.* 2004.

Morisset R, Côté NG, Panisset JC, Jemni L, Camirand P, Brodeur A. Evaluation of the healing activity of hydrocotyle tincture in the treatment of wounds. *Phytother Res.* 1987.

## Hibiscus

Babalola SO, Babalola AO, Aworh OC. Compositional attributes of the calyces of roselle (*Hibiscus sabdariffa* L.). *J Food Technol Africa*. 2001.

Bamishaiye E, Olayemi F, Bamishaiye O. Effects of boiling time on mineral and vitamin C content of three varieties of *Hibiscus sabdariffa* drink in Nigeria. *World J Agric*. 2011.

Hopkins AL, Lamm MG, Funk JL, Ritenbaugh C. *Hibiscus sabdariffa* L. in the treatment of hypertension and hyperlipidemia: a comprehensive review of animal and human studies. *Fitoterapia*. 2013; 85:84–94.

Jung E, Kim Y, Joo N. Physicochemical properties and antimicrobial activity of Roselle (*Hibiscus sabdariffa* L.). *J Sci Food Agric*. 2013; 93(15):3769–3776.

Konczak I, Zhang W. Anthocyanins—more than nature's colours. *J Biomed Biotechnol*. 2004.

Lin TL, Lin HH, Chen CC, Lin MC, Chou MC, Wang CJ. *Hibiscus sabdariffa* extract reduces serum cholesterol in men and women. *Nut Res*. 2007; 27(3):140–145.

Mahmoud BM, Ali HM, Homeida MM, Bennett JL. Significant reduction in chloroquine bioavailability following coadministration with the Sudanese beverages aradaib, karkadi and lemon. *J Antimicrob Chemother*. 1994; 33(5):1005–1009.

McKay D, Chen C, Saltzman E. *Hibiscus sabdariffa* L. tea (tisane) lowers blood pressure in prehypertensive and mildly hypertensive adults. *J Nut*. 2010.

Stansbury J. High flavonoid herbs and vascular health. In: *Medicines from the Earth*. 2011.

Wilson FD, Menzel MY. Kenaf (*Hibiscus cannabinus*), roselle (*Hibiscus sabdariffa*). *Econ Bot*. 1964; 18(1):80–91.

## Lemon Balm

Auf'mkolk M, Ingbar JC, Kubota K, Amir SM, Ingbar SH. Extracts and auto-oxidized constituents of certain plants inhibit the receptor-binding and the biological activity of Graves' immunoglobulins. *Endocrinology*. 1985.

Auf'mkolk M, Ingbar JC, Kubota K, Amir SM, Ingbar SH. Inhibition by certain plant extracts of the binding and adenylate cyclase stimulatory effect of bovine thyrotropin in human thyroid membranes. *Endocrinology*. 1984.

Geuenich S, Goffinet C, Venzke S, et al. Aqueous extracts from peppermint, sage and lemon balm leaves display potent anti-HIV-1 activity by increasing the virion density. *Retrovirology*. 2008; 5(27).

Bown D. *New Encyclopedia of Herbs and Their Uses*. DK Publishing; 2001.

Koytchev R, Alken R, Dundarov S. Balm mint extract (Lo-701) for topical treatment of recurring herpes labialis. *Phytomedicine*. 1999; 6(4):225–230.

Petenatti M, Petenatti E, Del Vitto L, et al. Evaluation of macro and microminerals in crude drugs and infusions of five herbs widely used as sedatives. *Revista Brasileira de Farmacognosia*. 2011.

Pourghanbari G, Nili H, Moattari A, Mohammadi A, Iraji A. Antiviral activity of the oseltamivir and *Melissa officinalis* L. essential oil against avian influenza A virus (H9N2). *Virusdisease*. 2016

Schnitzler P, Schumacher A, Astani A, Reichling J. *Melissa officinalis* oil affects infectivity of enveloped herpes viruses. *Phytomedicine*. 2008; 15(9):734–740.

Yarnell E, Abascal K. Botanical medicine for thyroid regulation. *Altern Complement Ther*. 2006.

## Meadowsweet

Cwikla C, Schmidt K, Matthias A, Bone KM, Lehmann R, Tiralongo E. Investigations into the antibacterial activities of phytotherapeutics against *Helicobacter pylori* and *Campylobacter jejuni*. *Phytother Res* 2010; 24(5):649–656.

Lee JC. Effect of methyl salicylate-based lures on beneficial and pest arthropods in strawberry. *Environ Entomol* 2010; 39(2):653–660.

## Motherwort

Xia YX. The inhibitory effect of motherwort extract on pulsating myocardial cells in vitro. *J Tradit Chinese Med*. 1983; 3(3):185–188.

## Passionflower

Strachey W, Major RH. *The Historie of Travaile into Virginia Britannia*. Ebook. https://archive.org/details/historietravail00majogoog/page/n9/mode/2up

## Prickly Pear

Abascal K, Yarnell E. A review of prickly pear: the upscale medicinal food. *Altern Complement Ther*. 2000.

Baudar P. *The New Wildcrafted Cuisine: Exploring the Exotic Gastronomy of Local Terroir*. Chelsea Green Publishing; 2016.

Bown D. *New Encyclopedia of Herbs and Their Uses*. DK Publishing; 2001.

Cota-Sánchez J. Nutritional Composition of the Prickly Pear (*Opuntia ficus-indica*) Fruit. In: *Nutritional Composition of Fruit Cultivars*. Academic Press; 2016.

Gouws C, Georgousopoulou E, Mellor D, McKune A, Naumovski N. Effects of the consumption of prickly pear cacti (*Opuntia* spp.) and its products on blood glucose levels and insulin: A systematic review. *Medicina*. 2019.

Harvesters D. *Eat Mesquite and More: A Cookbook for Sonoran Desert Foods and Living*. Rainsource Press; 2018.

Hodgson WC. *Food Plants of the Sonoran Desert*. University of Arizona Press; 2001.

Linarès E, Thimonier C, Degre M. The effect of NeOpuntia on blood lipid parameters—risk factors for the metabolic syndrome (Syndrome X). *Adv Ther*. 2010.

Niethammer CJ. *Cooking the Wild Southwest: Delicious Recipes for Desert Plants*. University of Arizona Press; 2011.

Ota A, Ulrih N. An overview of herbal products and secondary metabolites used for management of type two diabetes. *Front Pharmacol*. 2017.

Schor J. Betalain-rich concentrate improves exercise performance. *Nat Med J*. 2017.

### Rose

Bender D. The Mythological Rose. Charenton Macerations website. http://www.charentonmacerations.com/2014/10/29/mythological-rose/.

Bennett RR. *The Gift of Healing Herbs: Plant Medicines and Home Remedies for a Vibrantly Healthy Life*. North Atlantic Books; 2014.

Bergner, P. Herbs for the spiritual heart. *Med Herbal: A J Clin Pract*. 2012; 27(2):13.

Erenturk S, Gulaboglu M. The effects of cutting and drying medium on the vitamin C content of rosehip during drying. *J Food Eng*. 2005; 68(4):513–518.

Giesecke A. *The Mythology of Plants: Botanical Lore from Ancient Greece and Rome*. J. Paul Getty Museum; 2014.

Haynes, J. History of Roses, Part 1. American Rose Society website. http://www.rose.org/wp-content/uploads/2012/01/History-of-Roses-Species-Part-A.pdf.

Pyke M, Melville R. Vitamin C in rosehips. *Biochem J*. 1942.

Rose K. Sweet Medicine: Healing with the Wild Heart of Rose. The Medicine Woman's Roots website. http://medicinewomansroots.blogspot.com/2007/05/sweet-medicine-healing-with-wild-heart.html.

Suler A. Oh, Roses: Medicine, Magic and Honey. *Woolgathering and Wildcrafting* website. https://woolgatheringwildcrafting.wordpress.com/2013/06/13/oh-roses-medicine-magic-honey/.

Vinokur Y, Rodov V, et al. Rose petal tea as an antioxidant-rich beverage: cultivar effects. *J Food Sci*. 2006; 71:S42–S47.

Vitamin C Factsheet for Health Professionals. National Institutes of Health: Office of Dietary Supplements website. https://ods.od.nih.gov/factsheets/VitaminC-HealthProfessional/.

Yoruk H, Turker M, et al. Fatty acid, sugar and vitamin contents in rose hip species. *Asian J Chem*. 2008; 20(2):1357–1364.

### Skullcap

Foster S. Adulteration of skullcap with American germander. *HerbalGram*. 2002.

Rose, K. Blisswort in Bloom: Subtleties and Specifics. The Medicine Woman's Roots website. http://bearmedicineherbals.com/blisswort-in-bloom-subtleties-specifics.html.

Sevensong. The Skullcaps: A *Scutellaria* Monograph. Northeast School of Botanical Medicine website. http://7song.com/blog/2012/02/the-skullcaps-a-scutellaria-monograph/.

### Spilanthes

Duke J. *Duke's Handbook of Medicinal Plants of Latin America*. CRC Press; 2008.

Hind N, Biggs N. Plate 460. Acmella oleracea compositae. *Curtis's Bot Mag*. 2003; 20(1):31–39.

O'Neil L. Barcode: High-voltage cocktails at Haru. *Boston Globe*. http://archive.boston.com/ae/food/restaurants/articles/2010/03/19/barcode_high_voltage_cocktails_at_haru/.

Shimizu K. The electric paracress. *Saveur*. http://www.saveur.com/article/Kitchen/The-Electric-Paracress.

Tiwari K, Jadhav S, Joshi V. An updated review on medicinal herb genus *Spilanthes*. *J Chin Integr Med*. 2011; 9(11):1170–1178.

Van Wyk BE, Wink M. *Medicinal Plants of the World: An Illustrated Scientific Guide to Important Medicinal Plants and Their Uses*. Timber Press; 2004.

Prachayasittikul S, Suphapong S, Worachartcheewan A, Lawung R, Ruchirawat S, Prachayasittikul V. Bioactive metabolites from Spilanthes acmella Murr. *Molecules*. 2009; 14(2):850–867.

### Stinging Nettles

Mittman P. Randomized, double-blind study of freeze-dried *Urtica dioica* in the treatment of allergic rhinitis. *Planta Medica*. 1990.

### Tulsi

Cambie RC, Brewis A. *Anti-Fertility Plants of the Pacific*. CSIRO Publishing; 1997.

Cech R. Tulsi, Rama—Holy Basil. *Strictly Medicinal Seeds* website. https://www.strictlymedicinalseeds.com/product.asp?specific=883.

Cohen MM. Tulsi—*Ocimum sanctum*: A herb for all reasons. *J Ayurveda Integr Med*. 2014; 5(4):251–259.

Dass V. *Ayurvedic Herbology East and West: An Ayurvedic Approach to Medicinal Herbs*. Lotus Press; 2013.

Jürges G, Sahi V, Rodriguez D, et al. Product authenticity versus globalisation—the tulsi case. *PLOS ONE*. 2018.

Narasimhulu CA, Vardhan S. Therapeutic potential of *Ocimum tenuiflorum* as MPO inhibitor with implications for atherosclerosis prevention. *J Med Food*. 2015; 18(5):507–515.

Rai V, Mani UV, Iyer UM. Effect of *Ocimum sanctum* leaf powder on blood lipoproteins, glycated proteins and total amino acids in patients with non-insulin-dependent diabetes mellitus. *J Nutr Environ Med*. 1997; 7(2):113–118.

Sethi J, Yadav M, Sood S, Dahiya K, Singh V. Effect of tulsi (*Ocimum sanctum* Linn.) on sperm count and reproductive hormones in male albino rabbits. *Intern J Ayurveda Res*. 2010; 1(4):208–210.

Effect of *Ocimum sanctum* fixed oil on blood pressure, blood clotting time and pentobarbitone-induced sleeping time. *J Ethnopharmacol*. 2001; 78(2):139–143.

### Yarrow

Aikman J. Yarrow: On love and marriage and ale. Gather website. https://gathervictoria.com/2016/05/27/on-yarrow-love-marriage-ale/.

Buhner SH. *Sacred and Herbal Healing Beers: The Secrets of Ancient Fermentation*. Brewers Publications; 1998.

Hardy K, Buckley S, Collins M, et al. Neanderthal medics? Evidence for food, cooking, and medicinal plants entrapped in dental calculus. *Naturwissenschaften* 2012; 99(8):617–626.

# Herbal Resources

## Chestnut School of Herbal Medicine

THE HEALING GARDEN GATEWAY An online portal to exclusive bonuses and resources *just* for folks who have purchased *The Healing Garden*. Bonuses include The Healing Garden herb cultivation mini-course, printable seed and propagation charts, regional herb gardening profiles, and brand new recipes. You'll find extensive lists of herbal and gardening resources in the gateway. HealingGardenGateway.com

BLOG CASTANEA This is my personal blog! Come join me (and some special guest bloggers) for a hearty dose of bioregional herbalism. You'll also find destination hubs on Medicinal Herb Gardening, Container Herb Gardening, Sustainable Herbalism, Foraging, and more. chestnutherbs.com/blog

MEDICINAL HERB GARDENING HUB From seeds to sprouts, this hub is an online collection of our articles and expertise on cultivating medicinal plants. chestnutherbs.com/medicinal-herb-gardening

OUR FAVORITE HERBAL BLOGS, PODCASTS, AND YOUTUBE CHANNELS A roundup of our most-trusted online herbal resources for you to peruse. chestnutherbs.com/our-favorite-herbal-blogs-podcasts-and-youtube-channels

THE BUDDING HERBALIST GUIDE A free 95-page guide filled with herbal tips and trade secrets for up-and-coming herbalists. This free digital guide includes herbal resources, organizations, conferences, and associations. chestnutherbs.com/budding-herbalist-guide

ONLINE HERBAL COURSES We offer outstanding online herbal programs with a sustainable, plant-centered focus. Topics include medicine making, herb cultivation, and sustainable foraging. chestnutherbs.com

## Medicinal Seed Companies & Herbal Nurseries

HERBAL SEED SUPPLIERS AND NURSERIES: ETHICAL SOURCES FOR MEDICINAL PLANTS AND SEEDS This is our roll call of medicinal seed suppliers and nurseries, including small-scale and regional suppliers, in the U.S.A. and Canada—*many of whom ship internationally!* chestnutherbs.com/herbal-seed-suppliers-and-nurseries

STRICTLY MEDICINAL SEEDS Formerly known as Horizon Herbs, this Oregon-based business has the largest collection of organically grown medicinal herb seeds and plants. One of my go-to's for over two decades. strictlymedicinalseeds.com

FEDCO SEEDS A cooperatively owned seed and garden supply company based in Maine. Offers a wide variety of medicinal and culinary herbs, native plants, and edible shrubs and trees. Specializes in cold-hardy varieties. fedcoseeds.com

JOHNNY'S SELECTED SEEDS Large selection of seeds and plants, with organic options. A great go-to site for general farm supply needs, including garden tools, seed trays, and soil amendments. johnnyseeds.com

RICHTERS HERBS Canadian nursery offering a vast selection of herb seeds and plants, including rare and hard-to-find herbs. Based in Toronto. richters.com

## Bulk Medicinal Herbs & Supplies

ROSALEE DE LA FORÊT'S LIST OF SUSTAINABLE HERB FARMS AND ETHICAL WILDCRAFTERS A handy list of sustainable herb farms and ethically wildcrafted herbal suppliers in the United States and Canada. herbalremediesadvice.org/Herb-Farms-Wildcrafters.html

MOUNTAIN ROSE HERBS A quality source for bulk ingredients, including organic and wildcrafted dried herbs, as well as carrier oils and essential oils for natural body care. They also sell medicine-making supplies. Mountainroseherbs.com

PACIFIC BOTANICALS One of the largest medicinal herb farms and suppliers in North America. Supplies fresh and dried herbs. pacificbotanicals.com

ZACH WOODS HERB FARM An excellent source of organically grown and ethically wildcrafted fresh and dried herbs. Based in Vermont. zackwoodsherbs.com

HERBIARY A well-stocked online apothecary of bulk herbs and teas, as well as essential oils, medicine-making supplies, and fun herbal miscellany. herbiary.com

## Herbal Organizations

UNITED PLANT SAVERS The mission of this non-profit organization is to protect the native medicinal plants of the United States and Canada (and their native habitat) while ensuring an abundant renewable supply of medicinal plants for generations to come. unitedplantsavers.org

AMERICAN BOTANICAL COUNCIL The ABC publishes *HerbalGram* quarterly, which focuses on the herbal industry and medical herbalism. Their website has many searchable databases related to scientific research on medicinal herbs. abc.herbalgram.org

AMERICAN HERBALISTS GUILD An association of registered herbal practitioners. Membership includes many educational benefits. americanherbalistsguild.com

SUSTAINABLE HERBS PROJECT Created by writer, plant-lover, and anthropologist Ann Armbrecht. Their goal is to create a movement supporting high-quality herbal remedies, sustainable and ethical sourcing, and greater transparency in the herbal supply chain. sustainableherbsproject.com

## Bibliography and Recommended Reading

Our list of treasured resources, organized by topic. HealingGardenGateway.com.

# Common to Scientific Name Index

| COMMON NAME | SCIENTIFIC NAME |
|---|---|
| Alder | *Alnus* spp. |
| Alfalfa | *Medicago sativa* |
| Aloe | *Aloe vera* |
| Amaranth | *Amaranthus* spp. |
| Angel trumpet | *Brugmansia* spp. |
| Angelica | *Angelica archangelica*, and other species |
| Anise | *Pimpinella anisum* |
| Anise hyssop | *Agastache foeniculum* |
| Arizona cypress | *Cupressus arizonica* |
| Arnica | *Arnica chamissonis*, and other species |
| Artichoke | *Cynara cardunculus* var. *scolymus* |
| Ash | *Fraxinus* spp. |
| Ashwagandha | *Withania somnifera* |
| Astragalus | *Astragalus propinquus*, formerly *A. membranaceus* |
| Autumn olive | *Elaeagnus umbellata* |
| Balm of Gilead | *Populus balsamifera, P. trichocarpa*, and others |
| Barbary fig | *Opuntia ficus-indica* |
| Basil | *Ocimum basilicum* |
| Basswood | *Tilia* spp. |
| Bay laurel | *Laurus nobilis* |
| Bayberry | *Morella cerifera*, formerly *Myrica cerifera* |
| Bee balm | *Monarda didyma* and other species |
| Bee balm, lemon | *Monarda citriodora* |
| Beech | *Fagus* spp. |
| Birch | *Betula* spp. |
| Birch, black | *Betula lenta* |
| Black cohosh | *Actaea racemosa* |
| Black haw | *Viburnum prunifolium* |
| Blackberry | *Rubus* (various species) |
| Bloodroot | *Sanguinaria canadensis* |
| Blue cohosh | *Caulophyllum thalictroides* |
| Blueberry | *Vaccinium* spp. |
| Boneset | *Eupatorium perfoliatum* |

| COMMON NAME | SCIENTIFIC NAME |
|---|---|
| Borage | *Borago officinalis* |
| Brahmi | *Bacopa monnieri* |
| Bugleweed | *Lycopus virginicus* |
| Burdock | *Arctium lappa, A. minus* |
| Butterbur | *Petasites* spp. |
| Butterfly weed | *Asclepias tuberosa* |
| Calamus/Sweet flag | *Acorus calamus, A. americanus* |
| Calendula | *Calendula officinalis* |
| California poppy | *Eschscholzia californica* |
| Cannabis/Marijuana | *Cannabis sativa, C. indica* |
| Cardamom | *Elettaria cardamomum* |
| Cat's ear | *Hypochaeris radicata* |
| Catmint | *Nepeta x faassenii* |
| Catnip | *Nepeta cataria* |
| Cayenne | *Capsicum annuum* |
| Chamomile, German | *Matricaria recutita* |
| Chamomile, Roman | *Chamaemelum nobile* |
| Cherry | *Prunus*, various species |
| Chia | *Salvia hispanica* |
| Chickweed | *Stellaria media* |
| Chickweed, mouse ear | *Cerastium* spp. |
| Chicory | *Cichorium intybus* |
| Chives | *Allium schoenoprasum* |
| Cilantro | *Coriandrum sativum* |
| Cinnamon | *Cinnamomum verum, C. cassia, C. burmannii* |
| Citrus | *Citrus* spp. |
| Cleavers | *Galium aparine* |
| Clove | *Syzygium aromaticum* |
| Clover, red | *Trifolium pratense* |
| Clover, sweet | *Melilotus officinalis* |
| Clover, white | *Trifolium repens* |
| Coltsfoot | *Tussilago farfara* |
| Comfrey | *Symphytum officinale* |
| Coriander | *Coriandrum sativum* |

| COMMON NAME | SCIENTIFIC NAME |
|---|---|
| Corn silk | *Zea mays* |
| Cowpea | *Vigna unguiculata* |
| Cramp bark | *Viburnum opulus* |
| Cranberry | *Vaccinium oxycoccos, V. macrocarpon* |
| Culver's root | *Veronicastrum virginicum* |
| Curry plant | *Helichrysum italicum* |
| Damiana | *Turnera diffusa* |
| Dandelion | *Taraxacum officinale* |
| Dill | *Anethum graveolens* |
| Doll's eye | *Actaea pachypoda* |
| Douglas fir | *Pseudotsuga menziesii* |
| Echinacea, narrow-leafed | *Echinacea angustifolia* |
| Echinacea, or purple coneflower | *Echinacea purpurea* |
| Elderberry | *Sambucus nigra, S. nigra* var. *canadensis* |
| Elderberry, blue | *Sambucus cerulea, S. nigra* ssp. *cerulea* |
| Elderberry, red | *Sambucus racemosa* |
| Elecampane | *Inula helenium* |
| Eleuthero/Siberian ginsing | *Eleutherococcus senticosus* |
| Ephedra/*Ma huang* | *Ephedra sinica* |
| Eucalyptus | *Eucalyptus* spp. |
| False unicorn root | *Chamaelirium luteum* |
| Fennel | *Foeniculum vulgare* |
| Fenugreek | *Trigonella foenum-graecum* |
| Feverfew | *Tanacetum parthenium* |
| Foxglove | *Digitalis purpurea* |
| Fraser magnolia | *Magnolia fraseri* |
| Fringe tree | *Chionanthus virginicus* |
| Garlic | *Allium sativum* |
| Gentian | *Gentiana* spp. |
| Germander | *Teucrium* spp. |
| Ginger | *Zingiber officinale* |
| Ginkgo | *Ginkgo biloba* |
| Ginseng | *Panax quinquefolius, P. ginseng* |
| Goldenrod | *Solidago* spp. |

| COMMON NAME | SCIENTIFIC NAME |
|---|---|
| Goldenrod, Canadian | *Solidago canadensis* |
| Goldenrod, European | *Solidago virgaurea* |
| Goldenrod, sweet | *Solidago odora* |
| Goldenseal | *Hydrastis canadensis* |
| Gotu kola | *Centella asiatica* |
| Grindelia/Rosinweed | *Grindelia squarrosa* |
| Gumi/Goumi | *Elaeagnus multiflora* |
| Hawthorn | *Crataegus* spp. |
| Heart's-ease/Johnny jump-up | *Viola tricolor* |
| Hemlock | *Tsuga* spp. |
| Henbane | *Hyoscyamus niger* |
| Hibiscus, Chinese | *Hibiscus rosa-sinensis* |
| Hibiscus, cranberry | *Hibiscus acetosella* |
| Hibiscus, roselle | *Hibiscus sabdariffa* |
| Hickory | *Carya* spp. |
| Honeysuckle | *Lonicera japonica* |
| Hops | *Humulus lupulus* |
| Horehound | *Marrubium vulgare* |
| Horsemint | *Monarda punctata* |
| Horseradish | *Armoracia rusticana* |
| Horsetail | *Equisetum* spp. |
| Hyssop | *Hyssopus officinalis* |
| Ironweed | *Vernonia* spp. |
| Jack-in-the-pulpit | *Arisaema triphyllum* |
| Jiaogulan | *Gynostemma pentaphyllum* |
| Jojoba | *Simmondsia chinensis* |
| Juniper | *Juniperus communis* (and other species) |
| Kava kava | *Piper methysticum* |
| Korean licorice mint | *Agastache rugosa* |
| Lady's mantle | *Alchemilla vulgaris* |
| Lamb's-quarters | *Chenopodium album* |
| Lavender | *Lavandula angustifolia,* and other species |
| Lavender, spike | *Lavandula latifolia* |
| Lemon balm | *Melissa officinalis* |
| Lemon verbena | *Aloysia citriodora* |

| Common Name | Scientific Name |
|---|---|
| Lemongrass | *Cymbopogon citratus* |
| Licorice | *Glycyrrhiza glabra, G. uralensis* |
| Life root | *Packera aurea* |
| Linden/Lime tree | *Tilia* spp. |
| Lion's mane | *Hericium erinaceus* |
| Lobelia | *Lobelia inflata* |
| Loquat | *Eriobotrya japonica* |
| Lovage | *Levisticum officinale* |
| Maitake | *Grifola frondosa* |
| Maple | *Acer* spp. |
| Maple, red | *Acer rubrum* |
| Maple, sugar | *Acer saccharum* |
| Marigold | *Tagetes* spp. |
| Marjoram | *Origanum majorana* |
| Marshmallow | *Althaea officinalis* |
| Meadowsweet | *Filipendula ulmaria* |
| Milk thistle | *Silybum marianum* |
| Milkvetch | *Astragalus canadensis*, and other species |
| Milkweed, common | *Asclepias syriaca* |
| Milky oats | *Avena sativa* |
| Mimosa | *Albizia julibrissin* |
| Mint, most varieties | *Mentha* spp. |
| Mint, water | *Mentha aquatica* |
| Motherwort | *Leonurus cardiaca* |
| Motherwort, Asian | *Leonurus japonicus* |
| Mountain laurel | *Kalmia latifolia* |
| Mugwort | *Artemisia vulgaris* |
| Mugwort, western | *Artemisia douglasiana* |
| Mulberry, white | *Morus alba* |
| Mullein | *Verbascum thapsus, V. olympicum* |
| Mustard | *Brassica* spp. |
| Nasturtium | *Tropaeolum majus* |
| Oak | *Quercus* spp. |
| Oatstraw | *Avena sativa* |
| Olive | *Olea europaea* |
| Opium poppy | *Papaver somniferum* |
| Orange | *Citrus x sinensis* |
| Oregano | *Origanum vulgare* |
| Oregon grape | *Mahonia aquifolium* |
| Pansy | *Viola*, various species |
| Parsley | *Petroselinum crispum* |
| Partridgeberry | *Mitchella repens* |
| Passionflower | *Passiflora incarnata* |
| Pedicularis, eastern | *Pedicularis canadensis* |
| Pedicularis, elephanthead | *Pedicularis groenlandica* |
| Pennyroyal | *Mentha pulegium* |
| Pepper, black | *Piper nigrum* |
| Peppermint | *Mentha x piperita* |
| Pine | *Pinus* spp. |
| Pink lady's slipper | *Cypripedium acaule* |
| Pipsissewa | *Chimaphila umbellata, C. maculata* |
| Plantain | *Plantago* spp. |
| Poison hemlock | *Conium maculatum* |
| Prickly ash | *Zanthoxylum clava-herculis, Z. americanum* |
| Prickly pear | *Opuntia* spp. |
| Purple coneflower | *Echinacea purpurea* |
| Purple dead nettle | *Lamium purpureum* |
| Queen Anne's lace | *Daucus carota* |
| Ragweed | *Ambrosia* spp. |
| Ragworts | *Jacobaea* spp., *Senecio* spp. |
| Raspberry | *Rubus* (various species) |
| Red root/New Jersey tea | *Ceanothus* spp. |
| Reishi | *Ganoderma tsugae, G. lucidum* |
| Rhodiola | *Rhodiola rosea* |
| Rhododendron | *Rhododendron* spp. |
| Rocky Mountain bee plant | *Cleome serrulata* |
| Rose | *Rosa* spp. |
| Rose of Sharon | *Hibiscus syriacus* |
| Rose, cabbage | *Rosa centifolia* |
| Rose, damask | *Rosa x damascena* |
| Rose, multiflora | *Rosa multiflora* |
| Rose, musk | *Rosa moschata* |
| Rose, ramanas | *Rosa rugosa* |
| Rosemary | *Salvia rosmarinus* |
| Rue | *Ruta graveolens* |

| COMMON NAME | SCIENTIFIC NAME |
|---|---|
| Sage, black | *Salvia mellifera* |
| Sage, garden | *Salvia officinalis* |
| Sage, Mexican | *Salvia leucantha* |
| Sage, pineapple | *Salvia elegans* |
| Sage, purple | *Salvia officinalis* 'Purpurascens' |
| Sage, white | *Salvia apiana* |
| Sassafras | *Sassafras albidum* |
| Saw palmetto | *Serenoa repens* |
| Scarlet pimpernel | *Anagallis arvensis* |
| Schisandra | *Schisandra chinensis* |
| Sea buckthorn | *Hippophae rhamnoides* |
| Sesame | *Sesamum indicum* |
| Shepherd's purse | *Capsella bursa-pastoris* |
| Shiitake | *Lentinula edodes* |
| Shiso | *Perilla frutescens* |
| Sichuan pepper | *Zanthoxylum piperitum* |
| Skullcap | *Scutellaria lateriflora* |
| Slippery elm | *Ulmus rubra* |
| Solomon's seal | *Polygonatum biflorum* |
| Sorrel, French | *Rumex acetosa* |
| Sow thistle | *Sonchus* spp. |
| Spearmint | *Mentha x spicata* |
| Speedwell | *Veronica* spp. |
| Spikenard | *Aralia racemosa* |
| Spilanthes | *Acmella oleracea* |
| Spruce | *Picea* spp. |
| St. John's wort | *Hypericum perforatum* |
| Stevia | *Stevia rebaudiana* |
| Stinging nettles | *Urtica dioica* |
| Sweetfern | *Comptonia peregrina* |
| Sweet gale | *Myrica gale* |
| Sweet woodruff | *Galium odoratum* |
| Tarragon, French | *Artemisia dracunculus* |
| Tarragon, Mexican | *Tagetes lucida* |
| Tea | *Camellia sinensis* |
| Thyme | *Thymus* spp. |
| Tobacco | *Nicotiana* spp. |
| Trillium | *Trillium* spp. |
| Tulip poplar | *Liriodendron tulipifera* |
| Tulsi | *Ocimum tenuiflorum* |
| Turkey tail | *Trametes versicolor* |
| Turmeric | *Curcuma longa* |
| Usnea | *Usnea* spp. |
| Uva-ursi | *Arctostaphylos uva-ursi* |
| Valerian | *Valeriana officinalis* |
| Vervain, blue | *Verbena hastata* |
| Vervain, European | *Verbena officinalis* |
| Violets | *Viola* spp. |
| Violet, common blue | *Viola sororia* |
| Violet, sweet | *Viola odorata* |
| Vitex/Chaste tree | *Vitex agnus-castus* |
| Water hemlock | *Cicuta* spp. |
| Wax myrtle | *Morella cerifera*, formerly *Myrica cerifera* |
| White ash | *Fraxinus americana* |
| Wild bergamot | *Monarda fistulosa* |
| Wild cherry | *Prunus serotina* |
| Wild geranium | *Geranium maculatum* |
| Wild ginger | *Asarum canadense* |
| Wild indigo | *Baptisia tinctoria* |
| Wild lettuce | *Lactuca* spp. |
| Wild yam | *Dioscorea villosa* |
| Willow | *Salix* spp. |
| Wintergreen | *Gaultheria procumbens* |
| Witch hazel | *Hamamelis virginiana* |
| Wood nettle | *Laportea canadensis* |
| Wormwood | *Artemisia absinthium* |
| Yarrow | *Achillea millefolium* |
| Yaupon holly | *Ilex vomitoria* |
| Yellow buckeye | *Aesculus flava* |
| Yellow dock | *Rumex crispus, R. obtusifolius* |
| Yellowroot | *Xanthorhiza simplicissima* |
| Yerba mansa | *Anemopsis californica* |
| Yucca | *Yucca* spp. |

# Index

*Note:* **Bold** page numbers indicate herbal profiles.

## A

Actinorhizal medicinal herbs, 60
Actinorhizal plants, 59
Actions of herbs, terminology for, 194, 196
Adaptogen (term), 196
Alaska mix nasturtium, 79
Alcohol, 139–40
Alfalfa (*Medicago sativa*), 58, 60, 70
Aloe (*Aloe vera*), 40, 41, 81–83
Alterative (term), 196
Amethyst improved basil, 216
Amethyst purple basil, 79
Analgesic/anodyne (term), 196
Angelica (*Angelica archangelica*), 71, 108
Angelica (*Angelica* spp.), 40, 69, 70
Anise (*Pimpinella anisum*), 209
Anise hyssop (*Agastache foeniculum*), 40, 67, 69–71, 79, 108, 178, **208–11**
Antianxiety (term), 196
Antidepressant (term), 196
Anti-inflammatory (term), 196
Antimicrobial (term), 196
Antirheumatic (term), 196
Antispasmodic (term), 196
Antiviral (term), 196
Aphids, 72–74
Aphrodisiac (term), 196
Apothecary, 138
Apple blossoms, 178
Applying fertilizers, 49–52
Arid-climate herbs, 41, 81
Arizona cypress (*Cupressus arizonica*), 41
Arnica (*Arnica chamissonis, A. montana*), 89, 108
Artemisia species (*Artemisia* spp.), 70
Ashwagandha (*Withania somnifera*), 41, 42, 72, 91, 108, **212–15**
Aster yellows, 72, 73
Astragalus (*Astragalus propinquus*), 58, 108
Astringent, 194, 196
Austin, Alfred, 13

## B

Barbary fig (*Opuntia ficus-indica*), 351
Basil (*Ocimum basilicum*), 42, 79, 108, **216–19**
Baskets, 29, 124
Basswood tree (*Tilia* spp.), 39
Baths, 160–61
Bay (*Laurus nobilis*), 108
Bayberry (*Morella cerifera*), 38, 59, 60
Bayberry (*Morella* spp.), 6, 70, 108
Bay laurel (*Laurus nobilis*), 41
Bee balm (*Monarda didyma*), 71, 178, 222, 223, 227
Bee balm (*Monarda fistulosa*), 224
Bee balm (*Monarda* spp.), 40, 69, 70, 108, 178, **222–27**
Beneficial insects, 69–71
Bergamots, 223, 224
Berry, Wendell, 45
Biodegradable seed pots, 94
Bitter (term), 196
Blackberry (*Rubus* spp.), 70, 105, 113, 197
Black cohosh (*Actaea racemosa*), 31, 39, 81, 108, **228–33**
Black haw (*Viburnum prunifolium*), 109
Black locust (*Robinia pseudoacacia*), 178
Bloodroot (*Sanguinaria canadensis*), 32, 39, 109
Blueberry (*Vaccinium* spp.), 105
Blue cohosh (*Caulophyllum thalictroides*), 33, 39, 81, 90, 109
Blue flag (*Iris versicolor*), 38
Boneset (*Eupatorium perfoliatum*), 38, 40, 69, 70, 82, 109
Borage (*Borago officinalis*), 109
Botanical medicine. *See* Herbal medicine (herbalism)
Brahmi (*Bacopa monnieri*), 38, 42
Breastfeeding, 198–99, 201
Buckets, 29
Bundling and hanging herbs, 124–26
Burdock (*Arctium lappa, A. minus*), 109
Butterfly weed (*Asclepias tuberosa*), 70, 105, 109

## C

Calamus (*Acorus calamus*), 38, 40, 82, 109
Calendula (*Calendula officinalis*), 8, 42, 67, 70, 79, 109, 178, **234–38**
California lilac (*Ceanothus* spp.), 41
California poppy (*Eschscholzia californica*), 41, 110
Car-as-greenhouse drying method, 126
Cardamom (*Elettaria cardamomum*), 42
Cardiotonic (term), 196
Carminative (term), 196
Carnation (*Dianthus caryophyllus*), 178
*Castanea* blog, 8
Catmint (*Nepeta* x *faassenii*), 41
Catnip (*Nepeta cataria*), 105, 110
Cayenne (*Capsicum annuum*), 41, 42
Chamomile (*Matricaria chamomilla*, syn. *M. recutita*), 60, 70, 110
Chamomile, Roman (*Chamaemelum nobile*), 110
Cherry, flowering (*Prunus* spp.), 178
Chestnut Herb Nursery, 8
Chestnut School of Herbal Medicine, 8
Chickweed (*Stellaria media*), 42, 60, 110, **246–50**
Children
   giving medicine to, 133
   and PA-containing plants, 201
Chinese chives (*Allium tuberosum*), 178

Chinese licorice (*Glycyrrhiza uralensis*), 58, 112
Chives (*Allium schoenoprasum*), 70, 79, 110, 178
Cholagogue (term), 196
Cilantro/coriander (*Coriandrum sativum*), 70, 110
Cinnamon (*Cinnamomum verum*), 42, 105
Citrus (*Citrus* spp.), 41, 81, 105
Cleaning seeds, 106–7
Cleavers (*Galium aparine*), 40, 110
Climate, 14, 41, 42, 81
Cold conditioning, 87–89
Cold-sensitive herbs, 81
Comfrey (*Symphytum officinale*), 40, 60, 70, 110, 200
Common milkweed (*Asclepias syriaca*), 70, 112
Companion plants, 68–71
Composting, 22, 51, 61–63
Compound butters, 164–67
Compresses, 160–61
Connection, 1, 17
Containers, 25, 76–83, 92–94
Cottage gardens, 20–21
Cough syrups, quick, 154
Cover crops, 54
Crabapple flowers, 178
Cramp bark (*Viburnum opulus*), 110
Cranberry (*Vaccinium oxycoccos, V. macrocarpon*), 38
Crop rotation, 68
Culinary herbs, 16, 87, 127. *See also* Healing foods; Herbal profiles
Cultivars, 86
Cultivation, 206. *See also* Herbal profiles
Culver's root (*Veronicastrum virginicum*), 38, 110, 222
Curry leaf (*Murraya koenigii*), 42
Curry plant (*Helichrysum italicum*), 41

D
Dandelion (*Taraxacum officinale*), 60, 70, 110, 178, **256–61**
Daylily (*Hemerocallis fulva*), 178
Decoctions, 145–48
Decongestant (term), 196
Dehydrators, 124
Demulcent (term), 196
Desert willow (*Chilopsis linearis*), 41
Designing herbal landscapes, 15–23
    garden materials and hardscaping, 21–23
    how many of each herb, 18
    plant communities: interplanting, 20–22
    theme gardens, 19
    where to plant and garden beds, 18–19
    which herbs to plant, 17–18
Diaphoretic (term), 196
Diatomaceous earth (DE), 75
Digging fork, 28
Dill (*Anethum graveolens*), 70, 110
Direct seeding, 92
Disease and pest management, 14, 64–75. *See also* Herbal profiles
    attracting and nourishing beneficials, 69–72
    damage control, 74–75
    identifying causes of, 73
    preventive practices for, 66, 68
    strategies for, 73–75
Diuretic, 194, 196
Diversity, planting for, 68
Double boilers, 136
Double tilling, 34–37
Drying herbs, 124–26
Duke, Jim, 14
Dynamic accumulators, 60

E
Eastern black swallowtail, 71

Eastern tiger swallowtail, 71
Echinacea (*Echinacea purpurea*, other *Echinacea* spp.), 4, 70, 110, **266–69**
Eclectics, 6
Edible flowers, 176–181
Elderberry (*Sambucus nigra, S. canadensis*), 38, 40, 70, 105, 110, **270–75**
Elderflower (*Sambucus nigra* var. *canadensis*), 9, 274, 275
Elecampane (*Inula helenium*), 40, 70, 110, **276–79**
Elephant garlic (*Allium ampeloprasum*), 42
Eleuthero/Siberian ginseng (*Eleutherococcus senticosus*), 40
Emetic (term), 196
Emmenagogue (term), 196
Energetics of herbs, 197
Epazote (*Dysphania ambrosioides*), 41, 42
Ephedra (*Ephedra sinica*), 41, 81
Eucalyptus (*Eucalyptus* spp.), 42
European angelica (*Angelica archangelica*), 71
European licorice (*Glycyrrhiza glabra*), 112
Expectorant (term), 196

F
False roselle (*Hibiscus acetosella*), 299, 303
False unicorn root (*Chamaelirium luteum*), 39, 111
Fennel (*Foeniculum vulgare*), 41, 69, 70, 111, 178
Fenugreek (*Trigonella foenum-graecum*), 56, 57
Fertility of soil, 14, 47–48
Fertilizers, 49–53, 56, 96
Feverfew (*Tanacetum parthenium*), 70
Feverfew (*Tanacetum vulgare*), 111
Finishing salts, 168–71
Flea beetles, 72, 73

Flower fly, 67
Flowers, 120, 176–181
Foliar feeding, 50, 52, 96
Forsythia (*Forsythia suspensa*), 105
Foxglove (*Digitalis purpurea*, and other *Digitalis* species, Plantaginaceae), 200
Fringe tree (*Chionanthus virginicus*), 33, 39, 42

### G

Gaia Herbs, 4, 5, 421
Galactagogue (term), 196
Garden beds, 18–19, 35–36
Garden cart, 29
Gardening, 1, 9
Gardening tools, 28, 29
Garden materials and hardscaping, 21–23
Garden shears, 28, 29
Garden tubs, 29
Garlic and hot pepper soap spray, 75
Garlic chives (*Allium tuberosum*), 42, 178
Genovese basil, 216, 217
Gentian (*Gentiana* spp.), 111
Germinating herbs, 87–91
Ginger (*Zingiber officinale*), 40, 42, 81
Ginkgo (*Ginkgo biloba*), 105, 111
Ginseng (*Panax* spp.), 39, 111
Gloves, 29
Goldenrod (*Solidago* spp.), 70, 71, 111, **280–84**
Golden sage, 83
Goldenseal (*Hydrastis canadensis*), 31, 32, 39, 81, 111, **286–91**
Gotu kola (*Centella asiatica*), 38, 40, 42, 79, 81, 111, **292–97**
Green Farmacy Gardens, 13–15
Greenhouses, 92
Green manures, 54, 63
Groundsels, 200
Grow lights, 92

### H

Hardening off, 98
Hardscaping. *See* Garden materials and hardscaping

Harvesting herbs, 118–23. *See also* Herbal profiles
Harvesting seeds, 106
Hawthorn (*Crataegus* spp.), 105, 111
Healing foods, 164–89
 compound butters, 164–67
 culinary oils, 182–83
 edible flowers, 176–81
 finishing salts, 168–71
 herbal-infused rich syrups, 188–89
 immunity broth concentrate, 174–75
 pestos, 172–73
 vinegars, 184–87
Healthy plants, 68
Heart's-ease (*Viola tricolor*), 111, 178, **401–5**
Hemostatic (term), 196
Hepatic (term), 196
Herbal dietary supplements, 5
Herbal fertilizers, 52–53
Herbal-infused rich syrups, 188–89
Herbal medicine (herbalism), 1, 5, 192–201. *See also* Medicinal preparations
 conditions helped by, 130
 energetics of herbs, 197
 locally grown herbs, 5
 safety in, 198–201
 teachers of, 6
 terminology for actions of herbs, 194, 196
Herbal profiles, 202–417
 anise hyssop, licorice mint, 208–11
 ashwagandha, 212–15
 basil, 216–19
 bee balm, wild bergamot, 222–27
 black cohosh, 228–33
 calendula, 234–38
 chickweed, 246–50
 dandelion, 256–61
 echinacea, purple coneflower, 266–69
 elderberry, 270–75
 elecampane, 276–79
 goldenrod, 280–84
 goldenseal, 286–91
 gotu kola, 292–97
 hibiscus, roselle, 298–303

 how to use, 204–6
 lavender, 310–14
 lemon balm, 318–21
 meadowsweet, 322–26
 medicinal properties, 207
 milky oats, 328–33
 mints, 334–37
 motherwort, 340–43
 passionflower, 344–49
 prickly pear, 350–55
 rose, 358–62
 skullcap, 366–69
 spilanthes, 370–75
 stinging nettles, 376–81
 tulsi, 386–90
 valerian, 392–95
 vervain, 396–99
 violet, common and sweet, 400–405
 yarrow, 412–17
Herb Mountain Farm, 26, 27
Herb propagation chart, 108–15
Herbs as medicine, 1. *See also* Medicinal herbs
Hibiscus, Chinese (*Hibiscus rosa-sinensis*), 178, 299
Hibiscus, cranberry (*Hibiscus acetosella*), 42, 299, 303
Hibiscus, roselle (*Hibiscus sabdariffa*), 42, 70, 81, 111, 178, **298–303**
Hidcote lavender "Super Blue," 79
Hi-ho silver thyme, 79
Hildegard of Bingen, 193
Hollyhock (*Alcea rosea*), 178
Honesty (*Lunaria annua*), 178
Honeybee, 71
Honeys, 149–54
Honeysuckle (*Lonicera japonica*), 105
Hops (*Humulus lupulus*), 41, 105, 111
Horehound (*Marrubium vulgare*), 41, 112
Hori-hori, 28, 29
Horsemint (*Monarda punctata*), 41, 108, 224–26
Horsetail (*Equisetum* spp.), 38, 60, 82
Hoverfly, 71
Humid climate herbs, 42
Hypnotic (term), 196

Hypoglycemic (term), 196
Hypotensive (term), 196
Hyssop, true (*Hyssopus officinalis*), 41, 112, 209

I

Immune tonic (term), 196
Immunity broth concentrate, 174–75
Immunomodulator (term), 196
Immunostimulant (term), 196
Infusions, 145–48
Inoculants, 55, 56
Insects, 69–71. See also Disease and pest management
Interplanting, 20–22
Invasive species, 26, 112, 114

J

Jamaican dogwood (*Piscidia piscipula*), 42
Jiaogulan (*Gynostemma pentaphyllum*), 40, 81, 83, 112
Johnny jump-ups (*Viola tricolor*), 178
Juniper (*Juniperus* spp.), 41, 105

K

Kapoor, V., 25, 26, 42
Kava kava (*Piper methysticum*), 42
Kimmerer, Robin Wall, 2
Korean licorice mint (*Agastache rugosa*), 209

L

Labeling, 94, 95, 137, 139
Lady's mantle (*Alchemilla mollis*), 81
Lady's mantle (*Alchemilla vulgaris*), 40, 112
Lavandin (*Lavandula x intermedia*), 311
Lavender (*Lavandula angustifolia*), 41, 81, 83, 112, 178, **310–14**
Lavender (*Lavandula* spp.), 70, 105, 178
Laxative (term), 196
Layering, 103
Leaf mold, 62, 63
Leaves, harvesting, 120, 121
Lemon (*Citrus x limon*), 41, 42

Lemon balm (*Melissa officinalis*), 40, 41, 70, 112, **318–21**
Lemon bee balm (*Monarda citriodora*), 178, 223, 224, 226
Lemon bergamot (*Monarda citriodora*), 223–26
Lemongrass (*Cymbopogon citratus*), 41, 42, 81, 83, 112
Lemon verbena (*Aloysia citriodora*), 41, 81, 105, 112, 121
Licorice (*Glycyrrhiza glabra*), 58, 60, 70, 112, 209
Licorice mint (*Agastache* sp.), 71. See also Anise hyssop (*Agastache foeniculum*)
Life root, 200
Light-dependent germination, 90
Lilac (*Syringa vulgaris*), 178
Lime basil, 79, 216
Lime tree (*Tilia* spp.), 39
Linden tree (*Tilia* spp.), 39, 60, 70
Linnaeus, Carl, 204
Lobelia (*Lobelia inflata*), 112
Locust borer, 71
Longwood Gardens, 16
Lovage (*Levisticum officinale*), 70, 112
Lucansky, Terry, 6
Lymphagogue (term), 196

M

*Ma huang*, 41, 81
Manygrowing, 21
Marshmallow (*Althaea officinalis*), 38, 40, 70, 82, 112, 123
Meadowsweet (*Filipendula ulmaria*), 38, 40, 52, 82, 112, 127, **322–26**
Measurements, weight vs. volume, 136
Medical care, seeking, 199
Medicinal herbs, 15, 16. See also individual herbs; specific topics
  actinorhizal, 60
  identifying, 205
  nitrogen-fixing, 56–59
  profiles of (*See* Herbal profiles)
  saving seeds of, 105–7
  siting chart for, 39

Medicinal preparations, 128–63
  choosing herbal teas vs. tinctures, 132–33
  giving medicine to children, 133
  herbal honeys and syrups, 149–54
  herbal poultices, 162–63
  herbal soaks, compresses, and baths, 160–61
  herbal tinctures, 139–44
  infused oils and salves, 155–59
  infusions and decoctions, 145–48
  labeling, 137, 139
  quick cough syrups, 154
  sterilizing jars and bottles, 136
  storing and organizing medicine, 138
  straining and pressing, 137
  supplies and tools for, 134–36
  uses of (*See* Herbal profiles)
  weight vs. volume measurements, 136
Medicinal properties. See Herbal profiles
Medicine, 1, 130
Mexican tarragon (*Tagetes lucida*), 41
Milk thistle (*Silybum marianum*), 112
Milky oats (*Avena sativa*), **328–33**
Mimosa (*Albizia julibrissin*), 41, 42, 46, 57, 58, 105, 112
Mint (*Mentha* spp.), 70, 112, **334–37**
Moist climate herbs, 42
Money plant (*Lunaria annua*), 178
Moore, Michael, 6, 8
Motherwort (*Leonurus cardiaca*), 112, **340–43**
Mountain Gardens, 107
Mrs. Burns' lemon basil, 216
Mugwort, Western (*Artemisia douglasiana*), 41
Mulberry, white (*Morus alba*), 41
Mulch, 22, 66
Mullein (*Verbascum thapsus*, *V. olympicum*), 41, 113
Multicycle germinators, 88, 90
Multiflora rose (*Rosa multiflora*), 360
Mustard (*Brassica* spp.), 178

## N

Names of herbs, scientific and common, 204–5, 428–31
Nasturtium (*Tropaeolum* spp.), 79, 178
Natural rooting preparations, 102
Nectary plants, 69–71
Nervine (term), 196
New Jersey tea (*Ceanothus* spp.), 41, 113
Nitrogen-fixing plants, 54–60
North Carolina Arboretum, 24, 25
Nutrients for plants, 48

## O

Oats (*Avena sativa*), 113, **329–33**
Ocotillo (*Fouquieria splendens*), 41
Oils, 155–59, 182–83
Olive (*Olea europaea*), 41, 81
Opportunistic plant allies, 21
Oregano (*Origanum vulgare*), 41, 70, 113
Oregano "Kent Beauty," 79
Oregon grape (*Mahonia* spp.), 39–41, 105, 113
Organic holistic herb gardening, 13–14
Organic matter, 47
Oswego tea (*Monarda didyma*), 224

## P

Pansy (*Viola* spp.), 79, 178, 402
Parsley (*Petroselinum crispum*), 113
Partial-shade herbs, 39, 81
Partridgeberry (*Mitchella repens*), 39
Parturient (term), 196
Partus preparator (term), 196
Passionflower (*Passiflora incarnata*), 41, 42, 70, 105, 113, **344–49**
Pathways, 21–23
Pedicularis, eastern (*Pedicularis canadensis*), 39
Pennyroyal (*Mentha pulegium*), 335
Peppermint (*Mentha* x *piperita*), 40, **335–37**
Perennial Gussy Blend, 50
Peschel, Keewaydinoquay, 129
Pestos, 172–73
Phytoestrogen (term), 196
Pineapple guava (*Acca sellowiana*), 178
Pine bark, 51
Pink lady's slipper (*Cypripedium acaule*), 33, 39
Pipsissewa (*Chimaphila umbellata*; *C. maculata*), 39
Planning herbal landscapes, 12–43
  controlling spreading, 26
  designing the landscape, 15–23
  essential gardening tools, 28–29
  organic holistic herb gardening, 13–14
  siting charts: herbal habitats, 38–42
  small gardens, 24–25
  tilling new garden beds, 34–37
  woodland herb cultivation, 30–33
Plant communities, 20–22
Plastic seed trays, 93
Poison hemlock (*Conium maculatum*, Apiaceae), 200, 417
Poisonous plants, 199–201, 205
Polycultures, 21
Poor man's ginseng (*Codonopsis pilosula*), 40
Poultices, 162–63
Praying mantises, 67
Predatory insects, 69–71
Pregnancy, 198, 201
Pressing preparations, 137
Prickly ash (*Zanthoxylum clava-herculis*, *Z. americanum*), 41, 42
Prickly pear (*Opuntia* spp.), 41, 42, 70, 81, 105, 113, **350–55**
Propagating plants, 84–115. *See also* Herbal profiles
  herb propagation chart, 108–15
  preparing seed trays and sowing seeds, 92–99
  root division, 100–102
  saving seeds of medicinal herbs, 105–7
  stem cuttings, 102–5
  strategies for germinating herbs, 87–91
Pruners, 28, 29
Purple coneflower. *See* Echinacea
Purple dead nettle (*Lamium purpureum*), 178
Purple sage, 83
Pyrrolizidine alkaloid-containing plants, 200–201

## Q

Queen Anne's lace (*Daucus carota*), 417
Quince (*Cydonia oblonga*), 178

## R

Ragworts, 200
Ramanas rose (*Rosa rugosa*), 359, 363
Raspberry (*Rubus* spp.), 70, 105, 113
Recipe measurements, 207
Recipes, 9
  Anise Hyssop Simple Syrup, 189
  Antibacterial & Immune-Stimulating Formula, 291
  Antiviral & Immune-Stimulating Formula, 275
  Basil-Cucumber-Lemon Water, 220
  Basilicious Benediction Pesto, 391
  Basil Invocation Oil, 183
  Bergamot, Pepper & Anise Hyssop Vinegar, 186
  Calendula Tulsi Chai Concentrate, 244
  Charred Rosemary Simple Syrup, 189
  Chickweed Crepes with Chickweed Pesto & Chickweed Garnish, 251–53
  Chickweed Pesto, 254
  Chive-Garlic Compound Butter, 166
  Cilantro-Lime-Serrano Compound Butter, 166
  Compound Butters, 166–67
  Cranberry-Orange Compound Butter, 166
  Creamy Nettles Potato Soup, 383
  Crimson Cajun Salt, 171
  Dandelion Galette, 263
  Dandy-Orange Bitters, 264
  Dusky Desert Finishing Salt, 170
  Fairy-Floral Springtime Spread, 181
  Finishing Salts, 170–71
  Floral Serum: Rose-Calendula-Elder Oil, 364
  Focus & Clarity Tea Blend, 296
  Free and Clear Sinuses Formula, 284
  Gastrointestinal Inflammation Tea, 326

Ginger-Lemongrass Sesame Oil, 183
Grapefruit Violas, 408
Herbal Culinary Oils, 183
Herbal Immunity Broth Concentrate, 174–75
Herbal-Infused Syrups, 189
Herbal Vinegars, 186–87
Hibiscus Limeade, 305
Hibiscus-Pomegranate Fire Cider, 187
Hibiscus-Raspberry-Orange Compound Butter, 167
Hibiscus-Raspberry-Rose Margarita, 306
Hibiscus-Strawberry Ice Pops, 309
Hope Tea Blend, 390
Hormone-Balancing Formula, 232
Immune-Stimulating Formula, 269
"Influ-endsa" Tea, 417
Juniper-Rosemary-Pepper Oil, 183
Juniper-Sage Compound Butter, 166
Lavender-Lemon Bundt Cake, 315–16
Lavender-Rose Simple Syrup, 189
Lemon Balm Pesto, 173
Lemon–White Sage Finishing Salt, 170
Lemony Tea Blend, 321
Menstrual Cramp Tincture Formula, 343
Midnight Nettles Gomasio, 171
Mineral-Rich Herbal Infusion, 333
Mint Chutney, 338
Minty Dreams of Kitties & Butterflies Tea, 211
Minty Meadow Tea, 326
Minty Sunrise Iced Tea, 339
Musculoskeletal Anti-Inflammatory Formula, 232
Nettles Pâté, 384
Nourishing Skin Tea, 261
Orange Viola Mocktail, 408
Pain-Relieving Formula, 369
The Pompeii, 264
Quick Cough Syrup for Dry, Spasmodic Coughs, 154
Quick Cough Syrup for Productive Coughs, 154
Quick Herbal Broth, 241

Rainbow Nopales Salsa, 356
Raspberry-Rose-Lime Bubbly, 365
Raspberry-Rose-Lime Simple Syrup, 189
Recovery Tea Blend, 296
Regal Violet Simple Syrup, 406
Rejuvenation & Equanimity Formula, 390
Relaxation and Clarity Tea, 333
Resilience Vinegar for Strong Bones & Teeth, 187
Rest Easy Tincture Formula, 349
Sensual Tea, 362
Smoky BBQ Salt Rub, 171
Soothing Respiratory Tea, 405
Spiced Rose Compound Butter, 167
Sunlight Breaking Through the Clouds Formula, 314
Sweet Potato Shiitake Filling, 253
Thai Calendula Chicken Soup, 239–41
Urinary Tract "Back on Track" Tea, 290–91
Viola-ritas, 409
Violet Hummus, 410
Warming Elderberry Syrup & Elderberry Honey, 152
Warming Respiratory Tea, 279
Weedy & Wonderful Soothing Salve, 158
Whipped Calendula Body Butter, 242–43
Red bay (*Persea borbonia*), 42
Redbud (*Cercis canadensis*), 178
Red clover (*Trifolium pratense*), 57–60, 113, 178
Red root (*Ceanothus americanus*), 59, 70, 105, 113
Red root (*Ceanothus* spp.), 41
Regenerative root harvesting, 122
Relationship with healing plants, 2–3
Repeat harvesting, 25
Rhizobia, 55
Rhodiola, roseroot (*Rhodiola rosea*), 113
Robison Herb Garden, 22, 23, 266
Root bark, 6
Root division, 100–102

Roots, 120–23
Rose (*Rosa* spp.), 105, 113, 178, **358–62**
Rosemary (*Rosmarinus officinalis*), 41, 70, 81, 105, 113, 178
Rose of Sharon (*Hibiscus syriacus*), 113, 178, 299
Rotating crops, 68
Row covers, 74
Rue (*Ruta graveolens*), 42, 113
Runners, 26

S

Safety with herbs, 8, 198–201
Sage, black (*Salvia mellifera*), 41
Sage, common (*Salvia officinalis*), 41, 113
Sage, garden (*Salvia officinalis*), 81, 178
Sage, Mexican (*Salvia leucantha*), 81
Sage, pineapple (*Salvia elegans*), 41, 178
Sage, white (*Salvia apiana*), 41, 70, 81, 83, 114, 121
Sage species (*Salvia* spp.), 105
Saint John's wort (*Hypericum perforatum*), 41, 105, 114
Salts, finishing, 168–71
Salves, 155, 157–58
Sams, Jamie, 65
Sassafras (*Sassafras albidum*), 39
Saw palmetto (*Serenoa repens*), 42
Scarification, 90–91
Schisandra (*Schisandra chinensis*), 40, 114
Screens, 107, 124
Seaweed, for rooting, 102
Seeds, saving, 105–7
Seed-starting soil mixes, 94
Seed trays and sowing, 92–99
  bottom heat to enhance germination, 93
  common problems with seedlings, 97
  containers for seedlings, 93–94
  direct seeding vs. sowing in containers, 92
  fertilizing seedlings, 96
  germination setups, 92–93
  hardening off, 98
  seeding and labeling, 94–95
  seed-starting soil mixes, 94

Seed trays and sowing (*cont.*)
   sterilization, 94
   transplanting, 98, 99
   watering, 96
Self-heal (*Prunella vulgaris*), 40
Self-sowing herbs, 26
7Song, 6
Shade-loving herbs, 39, 40, 81
Shade-tolerant herbs, 40
Shibayama, Zenkei, 119
Shiso (*Perilla frutescens*), 114
Shovels, 29
Shrubs. *See* Medicinal herbs
Sialogogue (term), 196
Simon, Joachim Naphtali, 5
Siting, 38–42. *See also* Herbal profiles
Skullcap (*Scutellaria lateriflora*), 38, 40, 82, 114, **366–69**
Slippery elm (*Ulmus rubra*), 39
Slugs, 72, 73
Small gardens, 24–25
Smushing insects, 74
Snails, 73
Snapdragon (*Antirrhinum majus*), 178
Snow, James, 6
Soaks, 160–61
Soap spray, 75
Soil, 44–63
   actinorhizal medicinal herbs, 60
   amendments and fertilizers, 49–53
   building fertility of, 14, 47–48
   composition of, 45, 46
   composting, 61–63
   for containers, 80
   cover crops and green manures, 54
   dynamic accumulators, 60
   healthy, for disease and pest management, 66
   nitrogen-fixing plants, 54–60
   and organic matter, 47
   seed-starting soil mixes, 94
   for specific types of herbs (*See individual herbs*)
Soil amendments, 22, 49
Soil blocks, 94
Soil pH, 48

Soldier beetles, 67
Solomon's seal (*Polygonatum biflorum*), 39, 114
Solvents, 131–32, 139–40
Soothing Herbal Poultice, 163
Sorrel, 60
Southern ginseng (*Gynostemma pentaphyllum*), 81
Sowing seeds. *See* Seed trays and sowing
Spearmint (*Mentha spicata*), 40, **334–37**
Spike lavender (*Lavandula latifolia*), 311
Spikenard (*Aralia racemosa*), 39, 40, 114
Spilanthes (*Acmella oleracea*), 42, 114, **370–75**
Spotted bee balm (*Monarda punctata*), 223, 224
Spraying pests, 74, 75
Spreading, controlling, 26
Squash (*Cucurbita pepo*), 178
Staggerweed, 200
Stem cuttings, 102–5
Sterilizing equipment, 94, 136
Stevia (*Stevia rebaudiana*), 42
Stinging nettles (*Urtica dioica*), 38, 40, 53, 60, 72, 114, **376–81**
Stock, hoary (*Matthiola incana*), 178
Storing herbs, 127
Storing medicines, 138
Storing seeds, 107
Straining preparations, 137
Stratification, 87–89
Styptic (term), 196
Subtropical herbs, 42
Sunflower (*Helianthus annuus*), 178
Sweetfern (*Comptonia peregrina*), 38, 59, 60, 114
Sweet flag (*Acorus calamus* var. *americanus*), 38, 40, 109
Sweet gale (*Myrica gale*), 60
Sweet leaf (*Monarda fistulosa*), 224
Sweet woodruff (*Galium odoratum*), 40, 114
Swiss chard, 79
Syrphid fly, 67, 71
Syrups, 149–54, 188–89

T
Tea, green and black (*Camellia sinensis*), 40, 81, 105, 114
Teas, herbal, 132–33, 145–48
Theme gardens, 19
Thyme (*Thymus vulgaris*, other *Thymus* spp.), 41, 70, 81, 105, 114, 178
Tilling, 34–37
Tilth, 46
Tinctures, 132–33, 139–44, 185
Toads, 67
Tools, 28, 29
Transplanting seedlings, 98, 99
Trees, 16. *See also* Medicinal herbs
Tricolor sage, 83
Trillium (*Trillium* spp.), 39
Tropical herbs, 42
Tulsi (*Ocimum tenuiflorum*), 42, 70, 82, 83, 115, **386–90**
Turmeric (*Curcuma longa*), 40, 42, 81

U
Uva-ursi/bearberry (*Arctostaphylos uva-ursi*), 40, 41

V
Valerian (*Valeriana officinalis*), 38, 40, 115, **392–95**
Vasodilator (term), 196
Vegetative propagation, 86
Vermifuge (term), 196
Vertical gardening, 24, 25
Vervain (*Verbena* spp.), 115, **396–99**
Vervain, blue (*Verbena hastata*), 38, 40, 82, 115, **396–99**
Vervain, European (*Verbena officinalis*), 79, 115, **397–99**
Vinegars, 184–87
Violet, common and sweet (*Viola* spp.), 38, 40, 115, 178, **400–405**
Vitex, chaste berry/chaste tree (*Vitex agnus-castus*), 41, 70, 105, 115
Vulnerary (term), 196

## W

Wasabi (*Wasabia japonica*), 38
Watercress (*Nasturtium officinale*), 38
Water hemlock (*Cicuta* spp., Apiaceae), 200
Watering seedlings, 96
Water lily (*Nymphaea odorata*), 38
Water-loving herbs, 38
Wax myrtle (*Morella cerifera*), 60, 108
Weeding knife, 29
Wellness, 130
Wetland herbs, 38, 82
Wheelbarrow, 29
Where to plant, 18–19
Wild bergamot (*Monarda fistulosa*), 40, 41, 67, 69, 70, 108, 178, **223–27**
Wild cherry (*Prunus* spp.), 70
Wild geranium (*Geranium maculatum*), 39, 40, 81, 115
Wild indigo (*Baptisia tinctoria*), 40, 41, 57, 59, 70, 115
Wild yam (*Dioscorea villosa*), 39, 115
Willow (*Salix* spp.), 38, 115
Willow twigs, for rooting, 102
Winter field peas (*Pisum sativum*), 55
Wintergreen (*Gaultheria procumbens*), 39, 40
Witch hazel (*Hamamelis virginiana*), 38, 39, 105, 115
Woad (*Isatis tinctoria*), 115
Woodland herbs, 30–33, 39
Wood nettle (*Laportea canadensis*), 379
Worm castings, 51
Wormwood (*Artemisia absinthium*), 41, 105, 115

## Y

Yarrow (*Achillea millefolium*), 41, 60, 67, 70, 71, 115, **412–17**
Yaupon holly (*Ilex vomitoria*), 41, 42
Yellow basil, 79
Yellow coneflower (*Echinacea paradoxa*), 267
Yellow dock (*Rumex* spp.), 60, 115
Yellowroot (*Xanthorhiza simplicissima*), 82
Yellow spilanthes, 83
Yellow trillium (*Trillium luteum*), 33
Yerba mansa (*Anemopsis californica*), 82

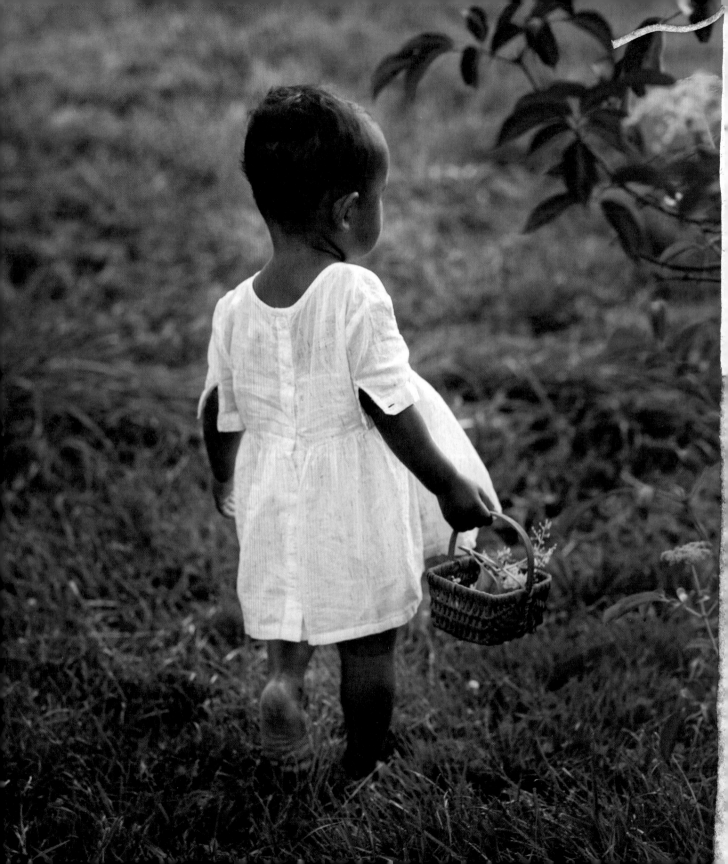

"Juliet Blankespoor has gifted us with a book of rare insight into the world of herbal plants! Her style of herbalism considers the 'whole person' and her gardening approach values 'the greater whole' as if it matters deeply, which of course, is the best way to grow and work with plants. This book is beautiful, extremely practical, and allows anyone, regardless of their level of expertise (from beginner to professional), to find a great many ways to turn the reading of words into the act of a holistic lifestyle. This book is sure to find a prominent place in the library of those interested in plants and herbal medicine."

—Tammi Hartung, co-owner of Desert Canyon Farm and author of *Homegrown Herbs* and *Cattail Moonshine & Milkweed Medicine*

"*The Healing Garden* is like an accomplished friend who leads you down the garden path into a sure relationship with whole plant medicine—as dependable as yarrow, as pretty as violet, as quenching to the question 'How do I go about this?' as cold spring water is to thirst."

—Richo Cech, author of *Making Plant Medicine* and founder of Strictly Medicinal Seeds

"*The Healing Garden* is a well-woven tapestry of education and inspiration that teaches and empowers the reader to grow medicinal plants—from garden planning and soil to fertilizers and propagation; from building sustaining relationships with a diverse group of plants to making herbal remedies and healthy herbal meals and snacks. Juliet Blankespoor imparts her wisdom of cultivating medicinal plants and herbal medicine making alongside breathtakingly beautiful photography. Her passionate writing along with well-selected and illuminating quotes will keep you enthralled with *The Healing Garden* and energized to manifest your own. *The Healing Garden* is truly a gift of knowledge for those who seek to further cultivate their relationship with medicinal plants and herbs as food and medicine. It will hold a sacred place in my library."

—Jade Shutes, founder of The School for Aromatic Studies

"*The Healing Garden* is one of the most imminently useful herbal books I know. It combines so many of the author's skills. It is beneficial for almost anyone interested in plants, with its detailed sections on cultivation, preparation, and processing herbs both as food and medicine. The photos are both beautiful and useful, treating the reader's eye and adding depth to the written information. This book is also superbly organized, making it easy to find and gain the information you seek. This is an elegant, practical book written by an insightful and thoughtful author."

—7Song, Director and main instructor at the Northeast School of Botanical Medicine and clinical herbalist and Director of Holistic Medicine at the Ithaca Free Clinic

"This book belongs on the shelf of every herb gardener and herbalist—beginner and advanced—and I think commercial herb growers would benefit from having it as a reference book, too. It is a feast for the eyes with beautiful, inspiring photographs of useful herbs, gardens, tools, food, and medicine. Part One is a very complete, permaculture-oriented guide to growing herbs. Part Two contains a delightful chapter filled with detailed recipes for making herbal remedies, foods, and beverages. And Part Three is composed of a thorough but easy-to-understand treatise on the basics of herbalism, herb safety, and thirty-two herb profiles."

—Dr. Jeanine Davis, horticulture professor and extension specialist with North Carolina State University and lead author of *Growing and Marketing Ginseng, Goldenseal, and Other Woodland Medicinals*

"If you want to learn about medicinal herbs, one of the best ways is to grow them, get to know them, and make medicine from them. That may sound daunting, but Juliet Blankespoor has created an absolutely gorgeous, easy-to-understand, and well-thought-out guide to making your herbal dreams and gardens come true."

—David Winston, RH(AHG) and co-author of *Adaptogens: Herbs for Strength, Stamina, and Stress Relief*